Endocrine and Metabolic Disorders

SOURCEBOOK

FOURTH EDITION

Health Reference Series

Endocrine and Metabolic Disorders
SOURCEBOOK

FOURTH EDITION

Basic Consumer Health Information about Hormonal and Metabolic Disorders That Affect the Body's Growth, Development, and Functioning, Including Disorders of the Pancreas, Ovaries and Testes, and Pituitary, Thyroid, Parathyroid, and Adrenal Glands, with Facts about Growth Disorders, Addison Disease, Cushing Syndrome, Pancreatic and Diabetic Disorders, Multiple Endocrine Neoplasia Type 1, Inborn Error of Metabolism, and More

Along with Information about Endocrine Functioning, Diagnostic and Screening Tests, a Glossary of Related Terms, and Directory of Additional Resources

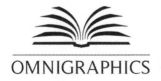

OMNIGRAPHICS

615 Griswold St., Ste. 520, Detroit, MI 48226

Bibliographic Note
Because this page cannot legibly accommodate all the copyright notices, the Bibliographic
Note portion of the Preface constitutes an extension of the copyright notice.

* * *

OMNIGRAPHICS
Angela L. Williams, *Managing Editor*
* * *

Copyright © 2020 Omnigraphics

ISBN 978-0-7808-1733-3
E-ISBN 978-0-7808-1734-0

Library of Congress Cataloging-in-Publication Data

Library of Congress Cataloging-in-Publication Data

Names: Williams, Angela L., editor.

Title: Endocrine and metabolic disorders sourcebook: basic consumer health
information about hormonal and metabolic disorders that affect the body's growth,
development, and functioning, including disorders of the pancreas, ovaries and testes,
and pituitary, parathyroid, and adrenal glands, with facts about growth disorders,
addison disease, cushing syndrome, conn syndrome, diabetic disorders, multiple
endocrine neoplasia, inborn error of metabolism, and more; along with Information
about endocrine functioning, diagnostic and screening tests, a glossary of related
terms, and directories of additional resources / [edited by] Angela L. Williams.

Description: Fourth edition. | Detroit: Omnigraphics, Inc., 2019. | Series: Health
reference series | Includes bibliographical references and index. | Summary:
"Provides basic consumer health information about diagnosis and treatment of
endocrine system and metabolic function disorders. Includes index, glossary of related
terms, and other resources"--Provided by publisher"-- Provided by publisher.

Identifiers: LCCN 2019031611 (print) | LCCN 2019031612 (ebook) | ISBN
9780780817333 (library binding) | ISBN 9780780817340 (ebook)

Subjects: LCSH: Endocrine glands--Diseases--Popular works. | Metabolism--
Disorders--Popular works.

Classification: LCC RC648.E418 2019 (print) | LCC RC648 (ebook) | DDC 616.4--dc23

LC record available at https://lccn.loc.gov/2019031611

LC ebook record available at https://lccn.loc.gov/2019031612

Table of Contents

Part II: The Pituitary Gland and Growth Disorders

Part III: Thyroid and Parathyroid Gland Disorders

Part IV: Adrenal Gland Disorders

Part V: Pancreatic and Diabetic Disorders

Part VI: Disorders of the Ovaries and Testes

Part VII: Other Disorders of Endocrine and Metabolic Functioning

Part VIII: Additional Help and Information

Preface

About This Book

In the United States, the most common endocrine disease is diabetes. The endocrine system includes the pituitary, adrenal, and thyroid glands, the pancreas, and the ovaries and testes. These glands secrete hormones that regulate metabolism, the process that supplies the body's cells with energy. Abnormal levels of hormones, whether too high or too low, disrupt normal functioning and compromise health. Sometimes the symptoms of dysfunctioning appear so gradually that they are hardly noticed. Hypothyroidism, for example, can remain undetected for years.

Endocrine and Metabolic Disorders Sourcebook, Fourth Edition provides updated information about the endocrine system and its role in the regulation of human growth, organ function, and metabolic control. Readers will learn about growth disorders, hypothyroidism, pancreatic and diabetic disorders, Addison disease, Cushing syndrome, pheochromocytoma, multiple endocrine neoplasia type 1, and inborn errors of metabolism. It gives information about disorders in the ovaries and testes. It includes facts about symptoms, diagnosis, and treatment. A glossary of terms and directory of resources provide additional help and information.

How to Use This Book

This book is divided into parts and chapters. Parts focus on broad areas of interest. Chapters are devoted to single topics within a part.

Part One: Endocrine Functioning and Metabolism describes the endocrine system, the various endocrine glands and their hormones, and the processes of metabolism, along with biological pathways and energy balance. It also describes chemicals that disrupt the endocrine process, along with diagnostic tests and procedures for endocrine and metabolic disorders. Individual chapters explain prenatal tests, newborn screening, genetic counseling, and chromosomal abnormalities.

Part Two: The Pituitary Gland and Growth Disorders discusses common growth disorders in children, the growth hormone deficiency in adults, and the growth hormone evaluation process and therapy. It also describes pituitary tumors, prolactinomas, and other diseases related to the pituitary gland, including Cushing disease, acromegaly, and diabetes insipidus.

Part Three: Thyroid and Parathyroid Gland Disorders offers facts about proper thyroid functioning and common dysfunctions, including Hashimoto thyroiditis, hypothyroidism, hyperthyroidism, Graves disease, and congenital hypothyroidism. It also describes disorders of the parathyroid glands and discusses thyroid and parathyroid cancers.

Part Four: Adrenal Gland Disorders provides facts about diseases of adrenal insufficiency, including Addison disease, Cushing syndrome, and pheochromocytoma, along with information about adrenal gland cancer, X-linked adrenal hypoplasia congenita, and congenital adrenal hyperplasia. The management of adrenal insufficiency and the use of laparoscopic techniques for adrenal gland removal are also described.

Part Five: Pancreatic and Diabetic Disorders provides information about pancreas function tests and the management of pancreatitis, insulin resistance and prediabetes, diabetes mellitus, and hypoglycemia. Facts about pancreatic and islet cell cancer and Zollinger–Ellison syndrome are also included.

Part Six: Disorders of the Ovaries and Testes describes problems that result when the sex gland hormone production is not balanced. These include hypogonadism, gynecomastia, menstrual problems, polycystic ovarian syndrome, premature ovarian failure, and disorders of puberty.

Part Seven: Other Disorders of Endocrine and Metabolic Functioning presents information about inherited metabolism storage disorder, inborn errors of metabolism including Gaucher disease, glycogen storage diseases, and other syndromes and diseases that result from, or impact, hormonal and metabolic processes.

Part Eight: Additional Help and Information includes a glossary of related terms and a directory of organizations able to provide more information about endocrine and metabolic disorders.

Bibliographic Note

This volume contains documents and excerpts from publications issued by the following U.S. government agencies: Agency for Healthcare Research and Quality (AHRQ); Centers for Disease Control and Prevention (CDC); *Eunice Kennedy Shriver* National Institute of Child Health and Human Development (NICHD); Genetic and Rare Diseases Information Center (GARD); Genetics Home Reference (GHR); National Cancer Institute (NCI); National Center for Biotechnology Information (NCBI); National Heart, Lung, and Blood Institute (NHLBI); National Human Genome Research Institute (NHGRI); National Institute of Diabetes and Digestive and Kidney Diseases (NIDDK); National Institute of Environmental Health Sciences (NIEHS); National Institute of Neurological Disorders and Stroke (NINDS); National Institutes of Health (NIH); *NIH News in Health*; Office on Women's Health (OWH); U.S. Environmental Protection Agency (EPA); and U.S. Social Security Administration (SSA).

It may also contain original material produced by Omnigraphics and reviewed by medical consultants.

About the Health Reference Series

The *Health Reference Series* is designed to provide basic medical information for patients, families, caregivers, and the general public. Each volume takes a particular topic and provides comprehensive coverage. This is especially important for people who may be dealing with a newly diagnosed disease or a chronic disorder in themselves or in a family member. People looking for preventive guidance, information about disease warning signs, medical statistics, and risk factors for health problems will also find answers to their questions in the *Health Reference Series*. The *Series*, however, is not intended to serve as a tool for diagnosing illness, in prescribing treatments, or as a substitute for the physician/patient relationship. All people concerned about medical symptoms or the possibility of disease are encouraged to seek professional care from an appropriate healthcare provider.

A Note about Spelling and Style

Health Reference Series editors use *Stedman's Medical Dictionary* as an authority for questions related to the spelling of medical terms and *The Chicago Manual of Style* for questions related to grammatical structures, punctuation, and other editorial concerns. Consistent adherence is not always possible, however, because the individual volumes within the *Series* include many documents from a wide variety of different producers, and the editor's primary goal is to present material from each source as accurately as is possible. This sometimes means that information in different chapters or sections may follow other guidelines and alternate spelling authorities. For example, occasionally a copyright holder may require that eponymous terms be shown in possessive forms (Crohn's disease vs. Crohn disease) or that British spelling norms be retained (leukaemia vs. leukemia).

Medical Review

Omnigraphics contracts with a team of qualified, senior medical professionals who serve as medical consultants for the *Health Reference Series*. As necessary, medical consultants review reprinted and originally written material for currency and accuracy. Citations including the phrase "Reviewed (month, year)" indicate material reviewed by this team. Medical consultation services are provided to the *Health Reference Series* editors by:

Dr. Vijayalakshmi, MBBS, DGO, MD
Dr. Senthil Selvan, MBBS, DCH, MD
Dr. K. Sivanandham, MBBS, DCH, MS (Research), PhD

Our Advisory Board

We would like to thank the following board members for providing initial guidance on the development of this series:

- Dr. Lynda Baker, Associate Professor of Library and Information Science, Wayne State University, Detroit, MI

- Nancy Bulgarelli, William Beaumont Hospital Library, Royal Oak, MI

- Karen Imarisio, Bloomfield Township Public Library, Bloomfield Township, MI

- Karen Morgan, Mardigian Library, University of Michigan-Dearborn, Dearborn, MI

- Rosemary Orlando, St. Clair Shores Public Library, St. Clair Shores, MI

Health Reference Series *Update Policy*

The inaugural book in the *Health Reference Series* was the first edition of *Cancer Sourcebook* published in 1989. Since then, the *Series* has been enthusiastically received by librarians and in the medical community. In order to maintain the standard of providing high-quality health information for the layperson the editorial staff at Omnigraphics felt it was necessary to implement a policy of updating volumes when warranted.

Medical researchers have been making tremendous strides, and it is the purpose of the *Health Reference Series* to stay current with the most recent advances. Each decision to update a volume is made on an individual basis. Some of the considerations include how much new information is available and the feedback we receive from people who use the books. If there is a topic you would like to see added to the update list, or an area of medical concern you feel has not been adequately addressed, please write to:

Managing Editor
Health Reference Series
Omnigraphics
615 Griswold St., Ste. 520
Detroit, MI 48226

Part One

Endocrine Functioning and Metabolism

Chapter 1

Introduction to the Endocrine System

What Is the Endocrine System?

Endocrine systems also referred to as "hormone systems," are found in all mammals, birds, fish, and many other types of living organisms. They are made up of:

- Glands located throughout the body

- Hormones that are made by the glands and released into the bloodstream or the fluid surrounding cells

- Receptors in various organs and tissues that recognize and respond to the hormones

Why Are Hormones Important?

Hormones act as chemical messengers that are released into the bloodstream to act on an organ in another part of the body. Although

This chapter contains text excerpted from the following sources: Text under the heading "What Is Endocrine System?" is excerpted from "Endocrine Disruption—What Is the Endocrine System?" U.S. Environmental Protection Agency (EPA), January 24, 2017; Text under the heading "Endocrine Glands: Types and Their Functions" is excerpted from "Endocrine Glands and Their Hormones," Surveillance, Epidemiology, and End Results Program (SEER), National Cancer Institute (NCI), July 1, 2002. Reviewed September 2019.

hormones reach all parts of the body, only target cells with compatible receptors are equipped to respond. Over 50 hormones have been identified in humans and other vertebrates.

Hormones control or regulate many biological processes and are often produced in exceptionally low amounts within the body. Examples of such processes include:

- Blood sugar control (insulin)

- Differentiation, growth, and function of reproductive organs (testosterone (T) and estradiol)

- Body growth and energy production (growth hormone and thyroid hormone)

Much like a lock and key, many hormones act by binding to receptors that are produced within cells. When a hormone binds to a receptor, the receptor carries out the hormone's instructions, either by altering the cell's existing proteins or turning on genes that will build a new protein. The hormone-receptor complex switches on or switches off specific biological processes in cells, tissues, and organs.

Some examples of hormones include:

- **Estrogens** are a group of hormones responsible for female sexual development. They are produced primarily by the ovaries and in small amounts by the adrenal glands.

- **Androgens** are responsible for male sex characteristics. Testosterone, the sex hormone produced by the testicles, is an androgen.

- **Thyroxine and triiodothyronine.** The thyroid gland secretes two main hormones, thyroxine and triiodothyronine, into the bloodstream. These thyroid hormones stimulate all the cells in the body and control biological processes, such as growth, reproduction, development, and metabolism.

The endocrine system, made up of all the body's different hormones, regulates all biological processes in the body from conception through adulthood and into old age, including the development of the brain and nervous system, the growth and function of the reproductive system, as well as the metabolism and blood sugar levels. The female ovaries, male testes, pituitary, thyroid, and adrenal glands are major constituents of the endocrine system.

Where Are Endocrine Glands Located in the Human Body?

- **Hypothalamus.** The hypothalamus links our endocrine and nervous systems together. The hypothalamus drives the endocrine system.

- **Pituitary gland.** The pituitary gland receives signals from the hypothalamus. This gland has two lobes, the posterior and anterior lobes. The posterior lobe secretes hormones that are made by the hypothalamus. The anterior lobe produces its own hormones, several of which act on other endocrine glands.

- **Thyroid gland.** The thyroid gland is critical to the healthy development and maturation of vertebrates and regulates metabolism.

- **Adrenal glands.** The adrenal gland is made up of two glands: the cortex and medulla. These glands produce hormones in response to stress and regulate blood pressure, glucose metabolism, and the body's salt and water balance.

- **Pancreas.** The pancreas is responsible for producing glucagon and insulin. Both hormones help regulate the concentration of glucose (sugar) in the blood.

- **Gonads.** The male reproductive gonads, or testes, and female reproductive gonads, or ovaries, produce steroids that affect growth and development and also regulate reproductive cycles and behaviors. The major categories of gonadal steroids are androgens, estrogens, and progestins, all of which are found in both males and females but at different levels.

How Chemicals Can Affect the Endocrine System

Scientific research on human epidemiology, laboratory animals, and fish and wildlife suggests that environmental contaminants can disrupt the endocrine system and lead to adverse health consequences. It is important to gain a better understanding of what concentrations of chemicals found in the environment may cause an adverse effect. Various types of scientific studies (epidemiology, mammalian toxicology, and ecological toxicology) are necessary to resolve many of the scientific questions and uncertainty surrounding the endocrine-disruptor issue. Many such studies are underway, organized by government agencies, industry, and academia.

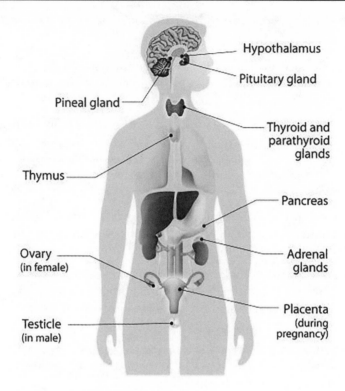

Figure 1.1. *Endocrine System*

Endocrine Glands: Types and Their Functions

The endocrine system is made up of the endocrine glands that secrete hormones. Although there are eight major endocrine glands scattered throughout the body, they are still considered to be one system because they have similar functions, similar mechanisms of influence, and many important interrelationships.

Some glands also have nonendocrine regions that have functions other than hormone secretion. For example, the pancreas has a major exocrine portion that secretes digestive enzymes and an endocrine portion that secretes hormones. The ovaries and testes secrete hormones and also produce the ova and sperm. Some organs, such as the stomach, intestines, and heart, produce hormones, but their primary function is not hormone secretion.

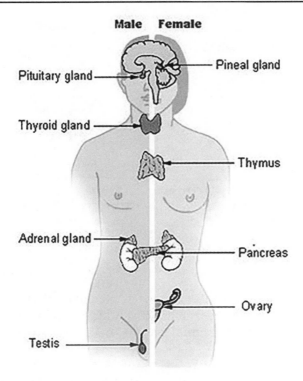

Male **Female**

Pituitary gland

Pineal gland

Thyroid gland

Thymus

Adrenal gland

Pancreas

Ovary

Testis

Figure 1.2. *Major Endocrine Glands in Male and Female*

Pituitary Glands

The pituitary gland or hypophysis is a small gland about one centimeter in diameter or the size of a pea. It is nearly surrounded by bone as it rests in the sella turcica, a depression in the sphenoid bone. The gland is connected to the hypothalamus of the brain by a slender stalk called the "infundibulum."

There are two distinct regions in the gland: the anterior lobe (adenohypophysis) and the posterior lobe (neurohypophysis). The activity of the adenohypophysis is controlled by releasing hormones from the hypothalamus. The neurohypophysis is controlled by nerve stimulation.

Hormones of the Anterior Lobe

Growth hormone (GH) is a protein that stimulates the growth of bones, muscles, and other organs by promoting protein synthesis. This hormone drastically affects the appearance of an individual because it influences height. If there is too little growth hormone in a child, that

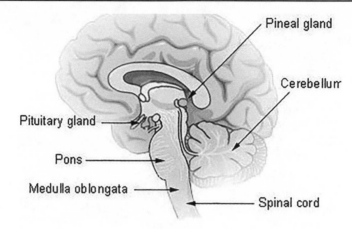

Pineal gland

Cerebellum

Pituitary gland

Pons

Medulla oblongata

Spinal cord

Figure 1.3. *Pituitary and Pineal Glands*

person may become a pituitary dwarf of normal proportions but small stature. An excess of the hormone in a child results in an exaggerated bone growth, and the individual becomes exceptionally tall or a giant.

Thyroid-stimulating hormone (TSH), or thyrotropin, causes the glandular cells of the thyroid to secrete thyroid hormone. When there is a hypersecretion of thyroid-stimulating hormone, the thyroid gland enlarges and secretes too much thyroid hormone.

Adrenocorticotropic hormone (ACTH) reacts with receptor sites in the cortex of the adrenal gland to stimulate the secretion of cortical hormones, particularly cortisol.

Gonadotropic hormones react with receptor sites in the gonads, or ovaries and testes, to regulate the development, growth, and function of these organs.

Prolactin hormone promotes the development of glandular tissue in the female breast during pregnancy and stimulates milk production after the birth of the infant.

Hormones of the Posterior Lobe

Antidiuretic hormone promotes the reabsorption of water by the kidney tubules, with the result that less water is lost as urine. This mechanism conserves water for the body. Insufficient amounts of antidiuretic hormone cause excessive water loss in the urine.

Oxytocin causes contraction of the smooth muscle in the wall of the uterus. It also stimulates the ejection of milk from the lactating breast.

Pineal Gland

The pineal gland, also called "pineal body" or "epiphysis cerebri," is a small cone-shaped structure that extends posteriorly from the third ventricle of the brain. The pineal gland consists of portions of neurons, neuroglial cells, and specialized secretory cells called "pinealocytes." The pinealocytes synthesize the hormone melatonin and secrete it directly into the cerebrospinal fluid (CSF), which takes it into the blood. Melatonin affects reproductive development and daily physiologic cycles.

Thyroid Gland

The thyroid gland is a very vascular organ that is located in the neck. It consists of two lobes, one on each side of the trachea, just below the larynx or voice box. The two lobes are connected by a narrow band of tissue called the "isthmus." Internally, the gland consists of follicles, which produce thyroxine and triiodothyronine hormones. These hormones contain iodine.

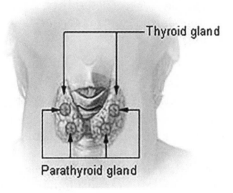

Figure 1.4. *Thyroid Gland*

About 95 percent of the active thyroid hormone is thyroxine, and most of the remaining five percent is triiodothyronine. Both of these require iodine for their synthesis. Thyroid hormone secretion is regulated by a negative feedback mechanism that involves the amount of circulating hormone, hypothalamus, and adenohypophysis.

If there is an iodine deficiency, the thyroid cannot make sufficient hormone. This stimulates the anterior pituitary gland to secrete thyroid-stimulating hormone, which causes the thyroid gland to increase in size in a vain attempt to produce more hormones. But, it cannot produce more hormones because it does not have the necessary raw material, iodine. This type of thyroid enlargement is called "simple goiter" or "iodine deficiency goiter."

Calcitonin is secreted by the parafollicular cells of the thyroid gland. This hormone opposes the action of the parathyroid glands (PTH) by reducing the calcium level in the blood. If blood calcium becomes too high, calcitonin is secreted until calcium ion levels decrease to normal.

Parathyroid Gland

Four small masses of epithelial tissue are embedded in the connective tissue capsule on the posterior surface of the thyroid glands. These are parathyroid glands, and they secrete parathyroid hormone or parathormone. Parathyroid hormone is the most important regulator of blood calcium levels. The hormone is secreted in response to low blood calcium levels, and its effect is to increase those levels.

Hypoparathyroidism, or insufficient secretion of parathyroid hormone, leads to increased nerve excitability. The low blood calcium levels trigger spontaneous and continuous nerve impulses, which then stimulate muscle contraction.

Adrenal Gland

The adrenal, or suprarenal, gland is paired with one gland located near the upper portion of each kidney. Each gland is divided into an outer cortex and an inner medulla. The cortex and medulla of the adrenal gland, like the anterior and posterior lobes of the pituitary gland, develop from different embryonic tissues and secrete different hormones. The adrenal cortex is essential to life, but the medulla may be removed with no life-threatening effects.

The hypothalamus of the brain influences both portions of the adrenal gland but by different mechanisms. The adrenal cortex is regulated by negative feedback involving the hypothalamus and adrenocorticotropic hormone; the medulla is regulated by nerve impulses from the hypothalamus.

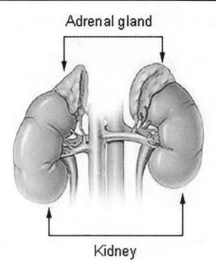

Figure 1.5. *Adrenal Gland*

Hormones of the Adrenal Cortex

The adrenal cortex consists of three different regions, with each region producing a different group or type of hormones. Chemically, all the cortical hormones are steroids.

Mineralocorticoids are secreted by the outermost region of the adrenal cortex. The principal mineralocorticoid is aldosterone, which acts to conserve sodium ions and water in the body. Glucocorticoids are secreted by the middle region of the adrenal cortex. The principal glucocorticoid is cortisol, which increases blood glucose levels.

The third group of steroids secreted by the adrenal cortex is the gonadocorticoids, or sex hormones. These are secreted by the innermost region. Male hormones, androgens, and female hormones, estrogens, are secreted in minimal amounts in both sexes by the adrenal cortex, but their effect is usually masked by the hormones from the testes and ovaries. In females, the masculinization effect of androgen secretion may become evident after menopause, when estrogen levels from the ovaries decrease.

Hormones of the Adrenal Medulla

The adrenal medulla develops from neural tissue and secretes two hormones, epinephrine and norepinephrine. These two hormones are secreted in response to stimulation by sympathetic nerve, particularly during stressful situations. A lack of hormones from the adrenal medulla produces no significant effects. Hypersecretion, usually from a tumor, causes prolonged or continual sympathetic responses.

Pancreas—Islets of Langerhans

The pancreas is a long, soft organ that lies transversely along the posterior abdominal wall, posterior to the stomach, and extends from the region of the duodenum to the spleen. This gland has an exocrine portion that secretes digestive enzymes that are carried through a duct to the duodenum. The endocrine portion consists of the pancreatic islets, which secrete glucagons and insulin.

Alpha cells in the pancreatic islets secrete the hormone glucagon in response to a low concentration of glucose in the blood. Beta cells in the pancreatic islets secrete the hormone insulin in response to a high concentration of glucose in the blood.

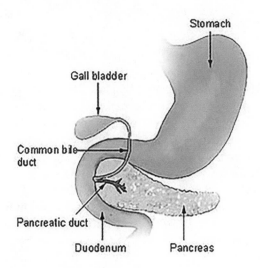

Figure 1.6. *Pancreas*

Gonads

The gonads, the primary reproductive organs, are the testes in the male and the ovaries in the female. These organs are responsible for producing sperm and ova, but they also secrete hormones and are considered to be endocrine glands.

Testes

Male sex hormones, as a group, are called "androgens." The principal androgen is testosterone, which is secreted by the testes. A small amount is also produced by the adrenal cortex. Production of testosterone begins during fetal development, continues for a short time after birth, nearly ceases during childhood, and then resumes at puberty. This steroid hormone is responsible for:

- The growth and development of the male reproductive structures
- Increased skeletal and muscular growth
- Enlargement of the larynx accompanied by voice changes
- Growth and distribution of body hair
- Increased male sexual drive

Testosterone secretion is regulated by a negative feedback system that involves releasing hormones from the hypothalamus and gonadotropins from the anterior pituitary gland.

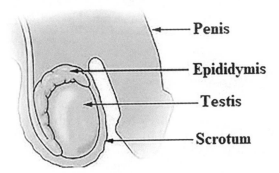

Figure 1.7. *Testes*

Ovaries

Two groups of female sex hormones are produced in the ovaries, the estrogen and progesterone. These steroid hormones contribute to the development and function of the female reproductive organs and sex characteristics. At the onset of puberty, estrogen promotes:

- The development of the breasts
- Distribution of fat evidenced in the hips, legs, and breast
- Maturation of reproductive organs such as the uterus and vagina

Progesterone causes the uterine lining to thicken in preparation for pregnancy. Together, progesterone and estrogen are responsible for the changes that occur in the uterus during the female menstrual cycle.

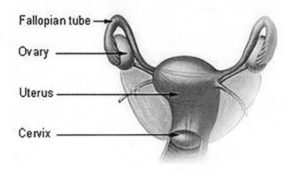

Figure 1.8. *Ovary*

Other Endocrine Glands

In addition to the major endocrine glands, other organs have some hormonal activity as part of their function. These include the thymus, stomach, small intestine, heart, and placenta.

Thymosin, produced by the thymus gland, plays an important role in the development of the body's immune system.

The lining of the stomach, the gastric mucosa, produces a hormone, called "gastrin," in response to the presence of food in the stomach. This hormone stimulates the production of hydrochloric acid and the enzyme pepsin, which are used in the digestion of food.

The mucosa of the small intestine secretes the hormones secretin and cholecystokinin. Secreting stimulates the pancreas to produce a bicarbonate-rich fluid that neutralizes the stomach acid. Cholecystokinin stimulates contraction of the gallbladder, which releases bile. It also stimulates the pancreas to secrete digestive enzymes.

The heart also acts as an endocrine organ in addition to its major role of pumping blood. Special cells in the wall of the upper chambers of the heart, called "atria," produce a hormone called "atrial natriuretic hormone (ANP)," or "atriopeptin."

The placenta develops in the pregnant female as a source of nourishment and gas exchange for the developing fetus. It also serves as a temporary endocrine gland. One of the hormones it secretes is human chorionic gonadotropin (hCG), which signals the mother's ovaries to secrete hormones to maintain the uterine lining so that it does not degenerate and slough off in menstruation.

Chapter 2

Endocrine Gland Hormones

Chapter Contents

Section 2.1

Mechanism of Hormone Action

This section includes text excerpted from "Introduction
to the Endocrine System," National Cancer Institute (NCI),
July 1, 2002. Reviewed September 2019.

Hormones are one of many substances made by glands in the body.
Hormones circulate in the bloodstream and control the actions of certain cells or organs. Some hormones can also be made in the laboratory.

Chemical Nature of Hormones

Chemically, hormones may be classified as either proteins or steroids. All of the hormones in the human body, except the sex hormones
and those from the adrenal cortex, are proteins or protein derivatives.

Mechanism of Hormone

Action hormones are carried by the blood throughout the entire
body, yet they affect only certain cells. The specific cells that respond
to a given hormone have receptor sites for that hormone. This is sort
of a lock-and-key mechanism. If the key fits the lock, then the door will
open. If a hormone fits the receptor site, then there will be an effect. If
a hormone and a receptor site do not match, then there is no reaction.
All the cells that have receptor sites for a given hormone make up
the target tissue for that hormone. In some cases, the target tissue is
localized in a single gland or organ. In other cases, the target tissue
is diffused and scattered throughout the body so that many areas are
affected. Hormones bring about their characteristic effects on target
cells by modifying cellular activity.

Protein hormones react with receptors on the surface of the cell,
and the sequence of events that results in hormone action is relatively
rapid. Steroid hormones typically react with receptor sites inside a cell.
Because this method of action actually involves synthesis of proteins,
it is relatively slow.

Control of Hormone Action

Hormones are very potent substances, which means that very
small amounts of a hormone may have profound effects on metabolic

processes. Because of their potency, hormone secretion must be regulated within very narrow limits in order to maintain homeostasis in the body.

Many hormones are controlled by some form of a negative feedback mechanism. In this type of system, a gland is sensitive to the concentration of a substance that it regulates. A negative feedback system causes a reversal of increases and decreases in body conditions in order to maintain a state of stability or homeostasis. Some endocrine glands secrete hormones in response to other hormones. The hormones that cause secretion of other hormones are called "tropic hormones." A hormone from gland A causes gland B to secrete its hormone. A third method of regulating hormone secretion is by direct nervous stimulation. A nerve stimulus causes gland A to secrete its hormone.

Section 2.2

Hormones Regulate the Digestive Process

"Hormones Regulate the Digestive Process," © 2020 Omnigraphics. Reviewed September 2019.

The brain is the control system for the sensation of feeling hungry or satiated. The response for food starts even before the food enters the mouth. The first phase of food intake, called the "cephalic phase," is controlled by the nervous system response provided by the food stimulus, such as, sight, sense, and smell, which in turn triggers a neural response such as salivation and secretion of gastric juice.

The second phase, which is the "gastric phase," begins once the food enters the stomach. It develops with the stimulation provided by the cephalic phase. Gastric acids and enzymes process the absorbed substance. This phase consists of inhabited hormonal and neural reactions. These responses trigger secretions and powerful contractions.

The last phase, which is the "intestinal phase," starts when the chewed food enters the small intestine, triggering hormonal and neural reactions that coordinate the functioning of the liver, gallbladder, intestinal tract, and pancreas.

What Are Hormones?

Hormones are chemical matters produced by specialized cells present in the body that are known as "endocrine cells." Once hormones are released, they enter the bloodstream and travel to the specific place of action. When the selected cells are triggered, they cause different reactions, such as stimulating or stopping enzymes within the cell or allowing the flow of elements in or out of the cell.

Hormones of the Digestive System

The endocrine system has the power to control the glands in the body and release hormones when needed. For the body to break down and digest the food, along with absorbing the nutrient and spreading the same in the body, the digestive and endocrine systems need to work in harmony.

Digestive hormones are made by the cells lining the stomach and the small intestine. Some of these hormones are explained below.

Gastrin

This is secreted in the stomach during the gastric phase. However, this is produced in the duodenum and pancreas. Gastrin triggers the release of gastric juice, which has a large amount of pepsin and hydrochloric acid (HCL). However, when the stomach is emptied, maintenance of this acidic surrounding is not required, so a hormone called "somatostatin" stops the release of HCL.

Secretin

This is produced in the duodenum (the first segment of the small intestine that plays an essential role in digesting the food that passes through it from the stomach). Secretin is the hormone that is discharged in response to the acid in the small intestine. This triggers the pancreas and gall bladder to discharge bile and pancreatic juice to counterbalance the acid. These secretions also slow down the emptying of the stomach.

Cholecystokinin

This hormone is secreted in the duodenum, which reduces the appetite, thereby slowing down the emptying of the stomach. This also triggers the release of bile from the gall bladder.

Glucagon-Like Peptide 1

This hormone is secreted in the last segment of the small intestine and colon and involves multiple activities, such as resistance of gastric emptying and appetite as well as the activation of insulin release.

Appetite-Regulating Hormones

These hormones are produced by the tissues and organs of the body that travel through the bloodstream to the satiety center, which is the part of the brain that triggers instincts that stimulate our feeling of hunger or help in controlling our appetite. Some of these hormones are explained below.

Ghrelin

This hormone is secreted in the stomach. Its main function is to enhance appetite and slow down the metabolic rate, thereby reducing the level of fat burning. Over secretion of this hormone may contribute to the development of obesity.

Peptide YY

This is secreted in the last segment of the intestine, known as the "ileum," as well as in some parts on the large intestine. This hormone plays a vital role in slowing down the passing of food down the gut, which increases the regulation of digestion and nutrient intake after a meal.

Leptin

This is secreted by the adipose fat tissue and focuses on the hypo-thalamus. Hence, this helps suppress appetite. Thus, the digestive hormones work as chemical messengers to communicate between cells thereby effectively regulating digestion.

References

1. "Digestive System Enzymes," CK-12 Foundation, November 30, 2012.

2. "Hormonal Control of Digestion," The Science Learning Hub, July 13, 2011.

3. "Hormones of the Digestive System," Boundless.com, November 28, 2012.

4. "Digestive System Regulation," Pressbooks, November 4, 2018.

Chapter 3

Metabolism and Its Importance

A biological pathway is a series of actions among molecules in a cell that leads to a certain product or a change in the cell. It can trigger the assembly of new molecules, such as a fat or protein, turn genes on and off, or spur a cell to move.

How Do Biological Pathways Work?

For your body to develop properly and stay healthy, many things must work together at many different levels—from organs to cells to genes.

From both inside and outside the body, cells are constantly receiving chemical cues prompted by such things as injury, infection, stress or even the presence or lack of food. To react and adjust to these cues, cells send and receive signals through biological pathways. The molecules that make up biological pathways interact with signals, as well as with each other, to carry out their designated tasks.

Biological pathways can act over short or long distances. For example, some cells send signals to nearby cells to repair localized damage, such as a scratch on a knee. Other cells produce substances, such as hormones, that travel through the blood to distant target cells.

This chapter includes text excerpted from "Biological Pathways Fact Sheet," National Human Genome Research Institute (NHGRI), August 27, 2015. Reviewed September 2019.

These biological pathways control a person's response to the world. For example, some pathways subtly affect how the body processes drugs, while others play a major role in how a fertilized egg develops into a baby. Other pathways maintain balance while a person is walking, control how and when the pupil in the eye opens or closes in response to light, and affect the skin's reaction to changing temperature.

Biological pathways do not always work properly. When something goes wrong in a pathway, the result can be a disease such as cancer or diabetes.

What Are Some Types of Biological Pathways?

There are many types of biological pathways. Among the most well-known are pathways involved in metabolism, in the regulation of genes and in the transmission of signals.

Metabolic pathways make possible the chemical reactions that occur in our bodies. An example of a metabolic pathway is the process by which cells break down food into energy molecules that can be stored for later use. Other metabolic pathways actually help to build molecules.

Gene-regulation pathways turn genes on and off. Such action is vital because genes provide the recipe by which cells produce proteins,

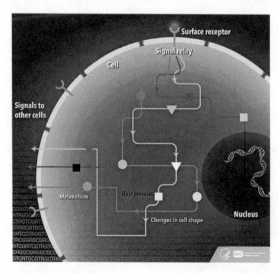

Figure 3.1. *Biological Pathways*

which are the key components needed to carry out nearly every task in our bodies. Proteins make up our muscles and organs, help our bodies move and defend us against germs.

Signal transduction pathways move a signal from a cell's exterior to its interior. Different cells are able to receive specific signals through structures on their surface called "receptors." After interacting with these receptors, the signal travels into the cell, where its message is transmitted by specialized proteins that trigger a specific reaction in the cell. For example, a chemical signal from outside the cell might direct the cell to produce a particular protein inside the cell. In turn, that protein may be a signal that prompts the cell to move.

What Is a Biological Network?

Researchers are learning that biological pathways are far more complicated than once thought. Most pathways do not start at point A and end at point B. In fact, many pathways have no real boundaries, and pathways often work together to accomplish tasks. When multiple biological pathways interact with each other, they form a biological network.

How Do Researchers Find Biological Pathways?

Researchers have discovered many important biological pathways through laboratory studies of cultured cells, bacteria, fruit flies, mice and other organisms. Many of the pathways identified in these model systems are the same as, or are similar to, counterparts in humans.

Still, many biological pathways remain to be discovered. It will take years of research to identify and understand the complex connections among all the molecules in all biological pathways, as well as to understand how these pathways work together.

What Can Biological Pathways Tell Us about Disease?

Researchers are able to learn a lot about human disease from studying biological pathways. Identifying what genes, proteins and other molecules are involved in a biological pathway can provide clues about what goes wrong when a disease strikes.

For example, researchers may compare certain biological pathways in a healthy person to the same pathways in a person with a disease to discover the roots of the disorder. Keep in mind that problems in any number of steps along a biological pathway can often lead to the same disease.

How Can Biological-Pathway Information Improve Health?

Finding out what pathway is involved in a disease—and identifying which step of the pathway is affected in each patient—may lead to more personalized strategies for diagnosing, treating, and preventing disease.

Researchers are using information about biological pathways to develop new and more effective drugs. It likely will take some time before we routinely see specifically designed drugs that are based on information about biological pathways. However, doctors are already beginning to use pathway information to choose and combine existing drugs more effectively.

Why Are Cancer Researchers Excited about Biological Pathways?

Until recently, many researchers hoped that most forms of cancer were driven by single genetic mutations and could be treated by drugs that target those specific mutations. Much of that hope was based on the success of imatinib (Gleevec), a drug that was specifically designed to treat a blood cancer called "chronic myeloid leukemia" (CML). CML occurs because of a single genetic glitch that leads to the production of a defective protein that spurs uncontrolled cell growth. Gleevec binds to that protein, stopping its activity and producing dramatic results in many CML patients.

Unfortunately, the one-target, one-drug approach has not held up for most other types of cancer. Projects that deciphered the genomes of cancer cells have found an array of different genetic mutations that can lead to the same cancer in different patients.

Thus, instead of attempting to discover ways to attack one well-defined genetic enemy, researchers now face the prospect of fighting many enemies.

Fortunately, this complex view can be simplified by looking at which biological pathways are disrupted by the genetic mutations. With further research on biological pathways and the genetic profiles of particular tumors, drug developers might be able to focus their attention on just two or three pathways. Patients could then receive the one or two drugs most likely to repair the pathways affected in their particular tumors.

Chapter 4

Energy Balance

As parents and caregivers, you make a big difference in what your children—and the children you care for—think and do. You are a role model for your family. Eating right and being active can help you maintain a healthy weight. When your kids see you making these choices, there is a good chance that they will do the same. By promoting "energy balance" in your family's life, you can help your family maintain a healthy weight.

What Is Energy Balance?

Energy is another word for "calories." Your energy balance is the balance of calories consumed through eating and drinking compared to calories burned through physical activity. What you eat and drink is ENERGY IN. What you burn through physical activity is ENERGY OUT.

You burn a certain number of calories just by breathing air and digesting food. You also burn a certain number of calories (ENERGY OUT) through your daily routine. For example, children burn calories just being students—walking to their lockers, carrying books,

---

This chapter contains text excerpted from the following sources: Text in this chapter begins with excerpts from "Healthy Weight Basics," National Heart, Lung, and Blood Institute (NHLBI), February 13, 2013. Reviewed September 2019; Text beginning with the heading "What Is Energy Balance?" is excerpted from "Balance Food and Activity," National Heart, Lung, and Blood Institute (NHLBI), February 13, 2013. Reviewed September 2019.

etc.,—and adults burn calories walking to the bus stop, going shopping, etc., A chart of estimated calorie requirements for children and adults is available at the link below; this chart can help you maintain a healthy calorie balance.

An important part of maintaining energy balance is the amount of ENERGY OUT (physical activity) that you do. People who are more physically active burn more calories than those who are not as physically active.

Note:

The same amount of ENERGY IN (calories consumed) and ENERGY OUT (calories burned) over time = weight stays the same
More IN than OUT over time = weight gain
More OUT than IN over time = weight loss

Your ENERGY IN and OUT do not have to balance every day. It is having a balance over time that will help you stay at a healthy weight for the long term. Children need to balance their energy, too, but they are also growing and that should be considered as well. Energy balance in children happens when the amount of ENERGY IN and ENERGY OUT supports natural growth without promoting excess weight gain.

Take a look at the Estimated Calorie Requirement table (Table 4.1), to get a sense of how many calories (ENERGY IN) you and your family need on a daily basis.

Estimated Calorie Requirements

This calorie requirement chart presents the estimated amounts of calories needed to maintain energy balance (and healthy body weight) for various gender and age groups at three different levels of physical activity. The estimates are rounded to the nearest 200 calories and were determined using an equation from the Institute of Medicine (IOM).

Energy Balance in Real Life

Think of it as balancing your "lifestyle budget." For example, if you know you and your family will be going to a party and may eat more high-calorie foods than normal, then you may wish to eat fewer calories for a few days before so that it balances out. Or, you can increase your physical activity level for the few days before or after the party, so that you can burn off the extra energy.

Table 4.1. Estimated Calorie Requirements (in Kilocalories) for Each Gender and Age Group at Three Levels of Physical Activity.

		Activity Level		
Gender	Age (years)	Sedentary	Moderately Active	Active
Child	2 to 3	1,000	1,000 to 1,400	1,000 to 1,400
Female	4 to 8	1,200	1,400 to 1,600	1,400 to 1,800
Female	9 to 13	1,600	1,600 to 2,000	1,800 to 2,000
Female	14 to 18	1,800	2,000	2,400
Female	19 to 30	2,000	2,000 to 2,200	2,400
Female	31 to 50	1,800	2,000	2,200
Female	51+	1,600	1,800	2,000 to 2,200
Male	4 to 8	1,400	1,400 to 1,600	1,600 to 2,000
Male	9 to 13	1,800	1,800 to 2,200	2,000 to 2,600
Male	14 to 18	2,200	2,400 to 2,800	2,800 to 3,200
Male	19 to 30	2,400	2,600 to 2,800	3,000
Male	31 to 50	2,200	2,400 to 2,600	2,800 to 3,000
Male	51+	2,000	2,200 to 2,400	2,400 to 2,800

- *These levels are based on Estimated Energy Requirements (EER) from the IOM Dietary Reference Intakes macronutrients report, 2002, calculated by gender, age, and activity level for reference-sized individuals. "Reference size," as determined by IOM, is based on median height and weight for ages up to age 18 years of age and median height and weight for that height to give a BMI of 21.5 for adult females and 22.5 for adult males.*

- *Sedentary means a lifestyle that includes only the light physical activity associated with typical day-to-day life.*

- *Moderately active means a lifestyle that includes physical activity equivalent to walking about 1.5 to 3 miles per day at 3 to 4 miles per hour, in addition to the light physical activity associated with typical day-to-day life.*

- *Active means a lifestyle that includes physical activity equivalent to walking more than three miles per day at three to four miles per hour, in addition to the light physical activity associated with typical day-to-day life.*

- *The calorie ranges shown are to accommodate the needs of different ages within the group. For children and adolescents, more calories are needed at older ages. For adults, fewer calories are needed at older ages.*

(Source: "Dietary Guidelines for Americans: 2005," U.S. Department of Health and Human Services (HHS)/U.S. Department of Agriculture (USDA).)

The same applies to your kids. If they will be going to a birthday party and eating cake and ice cream—or other foods high in fat and added sugar—help them balance their calories the day before and/or after by providing ways for them to be more physically active.

Here is another way of looking at energy balance in real life.

Eating just 150 calories more a day than you burn can lead to an extra 5 pounds over 6 months. That is a gain of 10 pounds a year. If you do not want this weight gain to happen, or you want to lose the extra weight, you can either reduce your ENERGY IN or increase your ENERGY OUT. Doing both is the best way to achieve and maintain healthy body weight.

- Here are some ways to cut 150 calories (ENERGY IN):
  - Drink water instead of a 12-ounce regular soda.
  - Order a small serving of French fries instead of a medium, or order a salad with dressing on the side instead.
  - Eat an egg-white omelet (with three eggs), instead of whole eggs.
  - Use tuna canned in water (6-ounce can), instead of oil.
- Here are some ways to burn 150 calories (ENERGY OUT), in just 30 minutes (for a 150-pound person):
  - Shoot hoops.
  - Walk two miles.
  - Do yard work (gardening, raking leaves, etc.).
  - Go for a bike ride.
  - Dance with your family or friends.

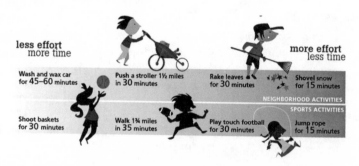

Figure 4.1. *Energy Out Physical Activity* (Source: "Parent Tips: Energy Balance: ENERGY IN and ENERGY OUT," National Heart, Lung, and Blood Institute (NHLBI).)

Chapter 5

Who Is an Endocrinologist?

An endocrinologist is a physician who specializes in diagnosing and treating endocrine and metabolic disorders (such as diabetes or infertility) and thyroid, adrenal, and pituitary-gland problems. They are trained in internal medicine.

Importance of an Endocrinologist
An Endocrinologist Is a True Specialist

If you have been diagnosed with any endocrine or metabolic disorders, it is necessary to identify an endocrinologist who can help you. This is important because an endocrinologist is a specialist in this field. Their knowledge about hormonal conditions and related diseases helps to provide the best possible treatment and most complete diagnosis.

Unlike a general physician, the endocrinologist has in-depth knowledge of this kind of disorder. This is why, even though the general practitioners can diagnose and treat a basic hormonal condition, the help of the endocrinologist is necessary for optimal treatment.

An Endocrinologist Can Help Patients

For some, endocrine and metabolic disease is controlled with standard treatment and procedures that allow them to manage their condition. However, conventional oral and injected medication may not work for some patients for various reasons, including genetic factors and the presence of conditions such as cystic fibrosis, which can influence the way the body reacts to such treatments. The endocrinologist will explore treatment options for such patients, thereby ensuring that they get the finest and most innovative guidance.

An Endocrinologist Knows the Latest Treatments

Medical knowledge and understanding of the endocrine and metabolic disorders are constantly changing. The endocrinologist maintains knowledge or recent advances and developments in this field in order to be up-to-date on the latest treatments available for patients. Hence, patients who regularly see endocrinologists will have access to the latest and most innovative treatment methods available to treat their condition.

An Endocrinologist Works with a Patient's Primary-Care Doctor

Visiting an endocrinologist does not necessarily mean that your general physician has to be replaced. It is best for patients diagnosed with a hormonal condition to visit someone who specializes in their condition, and the endocrinologist will look after your health in addition to your general physician.

Conditions Endocrinologists Treat

The endocrinologists treat people who have an abnormality in hormone secretion, primarily from glands in the endocrine system or certain types of cancers. A few of the conditions that are treated by the endocrinologists are listed below.

- Adrenal disorders

- Osteoporosis and bone health

- Diabetes

- Endocrine dysfunctions (such as deficiency in growth and problems with puberty) in children

- Heart problems (high cholesterol and triglycerides, high blood pressure)

- Pituitary disorders

- Thyroid disorders

- Weight and metabolism

- Women's health (menopause, infertility, and some of the menstrual problems)

- Men's health (infertility, testosterone levels)

The endocrinologist manages various systems within the body. As a result, researchers in the field of endocrinology are always working to better understand how the glands work, which helps them discover new treatments and drugs that treat hormonal disorders.

A proper diagnosis relies on an evaluation of various symptoms and requires specialized knowledge of clinical chemistry and biochemistry. Many laboratory tests are used to make such a diagnosis, including diagnostic imaging. Managing endocrine and metabolic disorders often requires long-term treatment. This may involve treating the patient as a whole as well as observing changes in the patient's cells and molecules.

Tips for Finding the Right Endocrinologist

When diagnosed with an endocrine or metabolic disorder, you may not know where or how to find the right endocrinologist to treat your specific disorder. Some tips for finding the right endocrinologist are outlined below:

- Check with your insurance company to find which endocrinologist covers your disorder.

- Ask your family and friends or check with your local hospital for recommendations.

- If you prefer to visit an academic center, make sure the endocrinologist has a specific interest in your medical condition.

- Ask questions about anything that you need further clarity on to ensure that the treatment you will receive fits you best.

- Check the credentials of the endocrinologist. This includes researching their medical degree, area(s) of specialization, whether she or he is board certified, where she or he completed their fellowship program, etc. This will help you ensure that the physician you choose is knowledgeable and trustworthy.

- Make sure that the physician you choose and you both can communicate well, thereby ensuring a long and comfortable relationship with your physician.

- Be sure to inform your doctor about your lifestyle and health history during your first visit.

The ultimate goal, when diagnosed with an endocrine or metabolic disorder, is to ensure that your disorder is treated as effectively as possible. This outcome is most likely achieved through the help of an endocrinologist; therefore, make sure you find the right endocrinologist who can provide you with the proper medical care you need.

References

1. "Definition of Endocrinologist," National Cancer Institute (NCI), February 10, 2011.

2. "Value of an Endocrinologist," The Hormone Health Network, October 10, 2014.

3. "You and Your Endocrinologist," The Hormone Health Network, June 7, 2019.

4. "Tips for Finding the Right Endocrinologist," Joslin Diabetes Center, November 7, 2008.

Chapter 6

Endocrine Disruptors

Endocrine disruptors are chemicals that may interfere with the body's endocrine system and produce adverse developmental, reproductive, neurological, and immune effects in both humans and wildlife.

A wide range of substances, both natural and manufacturer, are thought to cause endocrine disruption, including pharmaceuticals, dioxin and dioxin-like compounds, polychlorinated biphenyls (PCBs), dichlorodiphenyltrichloroethane (DDT) and other pesticides, and plasticizers such as bisphenol A. Endocrine disruptors may be found in many everyday products—including plastic bottles, metal-food cans, detergents, flame retardants, food, toys, cosmetics, and pesticides.

The National Institute of Environmental Health Sciences (NIEHS) supports studies to determine whether exposure to endocrine disruptors may result in human-health effects including lowered fertility and an increased incidence of endometriosis and some cancers. Research shows that endocrine disruptors may pose the greatest risk during prenatal and early-postnatal development when organ and neural systems are forming.

This chapter contains text excerpted from the following sources: Text in this chapter begins with excerpts from "Endocrine Disruptors," National Institute of Environmental Health Sciences (NIEHS), May 10, 2019; Text under the heading "How Are People Exposed to Endocrine Disruptor?" is excerpted from "Endocrine Disruptors," National Institute of Environmental Health Sciences (NIEHS), May 2010. Reviewed September 2019.

How Do Endocrine Disruptors Work?

From animal studies, researchers have learned much about the mechanisms through which endocrine disruptors influence the endocrine system and alter hormonal functions.

Endocrine disruptors can:

- Mimic or partly mimic naturally occurring hormones in the body such as estrogens (the female sex hormone), androgens (the male sex hormone), and thyroid hormones, potentially producing overstimulation

- Bind to a receptor within a cell and block the endogenous hormone from binding. The normal signal then fails to occur and the body fails to respond properly. Examples of chemicals that block or antagonize hormones are antiestrogens and antiandrogens.

- Interfere or block the way natural hormones or their receptors are made or controlled, for example, by altering their metabolism in the liver

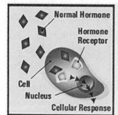 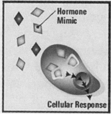 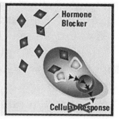

Figure 6.1. *Effect of Endocrine Disruption Chemicals on Hormone Signals*

When absorbed in the body, an endocrine disruptor can decrease or increase normal hormone levels (left), mimic the body's natural hormones (middle), or alter the natural production of hormones (right).

Examples of Endocrine Disruptors

A wide and varied range of substances are thought to cause endocrine disruption.

Chemicals that are known endocrine disruptors include diethylstilbestrol ((DES), the synthetic estrogen), dioxin and dioxin-like compounds, PCBs, DDT, and some other pesticides.

Bisphenol A (BPA) is a chemical produced in large quantities for use primarily in the production of polycarbonate plastics and epoxy resins. The National Toxicology Program's (NTP) Center for the Evaluation of Risks to Human Reproduction (CERHR) completed a review of BPA in September 2008. NTP expressed some concern for effects on the brain, behavior, and prostate gland in fetuses, infants, and children at current human exposures to bisphenol A.

Di(2-ethylhexyl) phthalate (DEHP) is a high production volume chemical used in the manufacture of a wide variety of consumer food packaging, some children's products, and some polyvinyl chloride (PVC) medical devices. In 2006, NTP found that DEHP may pose a risk to human development, especially critically ill male infants.

Phytoestrogens are naturally occurring substances in plants that have hormone-like activity. Examples of phytoestrogens are genistein and daidzein, which can be found in soy-derived products.

How Are People Exposed to Endocrine Disruptors?

People may be exposed to endocrine disruptors through the food and beverages they consume, medicine they take, pesticides they apply, and cosmetics they use. So, exposures may be through the diet, air, skin, and water. Some environmental endocrine disrupting chemicals, such as the pesticide DDT, dioxins, and polychlorinated biphenyls used in electrical equipment, are highly persistent and slow to degrade in the environment making them potentially hazardous over an extended period of time.

Four points about endocrine disruption:

- Low dose matters
- Wide range of health effects
- Persistence of biological effects
- Ubiquitous exposure

Exposures at Low Levels Count

The body's own normal endocrine signaling involves very small changes in hormone levels, yet we know these changes can have significant biological effects. This leads scientists to think that chemical exposures, even at low doses, can disrupt the body's delicate endocrine system and lead to disease.

In 2000, an independent panel of experts convened by the NIEHS and the NTP found that there was "credible evidence" that some hormone-like chemicals can affect test animals' bodily functions at very low levels—well below the "no effect" levels determined by traditional testing.

Health Impact of Endocrine Disrupting Chemicals

Although there is limited evidence to prove that low-dose exposures are causing adverse human health effects, there is a large body of research in experimental animals and wildlife suggesting that endocrine disruptors may cause:

- Reductions in male fertility and declines in the numbers of males born

- Abnormalities in male reproductive organs

- Female reproductive health issues, including fertility problems, early puberty, and early reproductive senescence

- Increases in mammary, ovarian, and prostate cancers

- Increases in immune and autoimmune diseases, and some neurodegenerative diseases

There are data showing that exposure to BPA, as well as other endocrine disrupting chemicals with estrogenic activity, may have effects on obesity and diabetes. These data, while preliminary and only in animals, indicate the potential for endocrine disrupting agents to have effects on other endocrine systems not yet fully examined.

Effects of Endocrine Disruptors

Research shows that endocrine disruptors may pose the greatest risk during prenatal and early-postnatal development when organ and neural systems are developing. In animals, adverse consequences, such as subfertility, premature-reproductive senescence, and cancer, are linked to early exposure, but they may not be apparent until much later in life.

Research from NIEHS researchers have shown that the adverse effects of diethylstilbestrol (DES) in mice can be passed to subsequent generations even though they were not directly exposed. The increased susceptibility for tumors was seen in both the granddaughters and grandsons of mice who were developmentally exposed to DES. Mechanisms involved in the transmission of disease were shown to involve epigenetic events—that is, altering gene function without altering deoxyribonucleic acid (DNA) sequence. Research funded by NIEHS also found that endocrine disruptors may affect not just the offspring of mothers exposed during pregnancy, but future offspring as well. The researchers found that several endocrine disrupting chemicals caused fertility defects in male rats that were passed down to nearly every male in subsequent generations. This study suggests that the compounds may have caused changes in the developing male germ cells and that endocrine disruptors may be able to reprogram or change the expression of genes without mutating DNA.

Chapter 7

Diagnostic Tests and Procedures for Endocrine and Metabolic Disorders

Chapter Contents

Section 7.1

Calcium Blood Test

This section includes text excerpted from "Calcium Blood Test," MedlinePlus, National Institutes of Health (NIH), September 5, 2017.

Calcium is one of the most important minerals in your body. You need calcium for healthy bones and teeth. Calcium is also essential for the proper functioning of your nerves, muscles, and heart. About 99 percent of your body's calcium is stored in your bones. The remaining one percent circulates in the blood. If there is too much or too little calcium in the blood, it may be a sign of bone disease, thyroid disease, kidney disease, or other medical conditions.

A calcium blood test measures the amount of calcium in your blood. It is also know with other names such as total calcium and ionized calcium.

What Is a Calcium Blood Test Used For?

There are two types of calcium blood tests, namely:

- **Total calcium,** which measures the calcium attached to specific proteins in your blood

- **Ionized calcium,** which measures the calcium that is unattached or "free" from these proteins

Total calcium is often part of a routine screening test called a "basic metabolic panel." A basic metabolic panel is a test that measures different minerals and other substances in the blood, including calcium.

Why Do You Need a Calcium Blood Test?

Your healthcare provider may have ordered a basic metabolic panel, which includes a calcium blood test, as part of your regular checkup, or if you have symptoms of abnormal calcium levels.

Symptoms of high calcium levels include:

- Nausea and vomiting

- More frequent urination

- Increased thirst

- Constipation

- Abdominal pain
- Loss of appetite

Symptoms of low calcium levels include:
- Tingling in the lips, tongue, fingers, and feet
- Muscle cramps
- Muscle spasms
- Irregular heartbeat

Many people with high or low calcium levels do not have any symptoms. Your healthcare provider may order a calcium test if you have a preexisting condition that may affect your calcium levels. These include:

- Kidney disease
- Thyroid disease
- Malnutrition
- Certain types of cancer

What Happens during a Calcium Blood Test?

A healthcare professional will take a blood sample from a vein in your arm, using a small needle. After the needle is inserted, a small amount of blood will be collected into a test tube or vial. You may feel a little sting when the needle goes in or out. This usually takes less than five minutes.

Will You Need to Do Anything to Prepare for a Calcium Blood Test?

You do not need any special preparations for a calcium blood test or a basic metabolic panel. If your healthcare provider has ordered more tests on your blood sample, you may need to fast (not eat or drink) for several hours before the test. Your healthcare provider will let you know if there are any special instructions to follow.

Are There Any Risks to a Calcium Blood Test?

There is very little risk of having a blood test. You may have slight pain or bruise at the spot where the needle was put in, but most symptoms go away quickly.

What Do Calcium Blood Test Results Mean?

If your results show higher than normal calcium levels, it may indicate:

- Hyperparathyroidism, a condition in which your parathyroid glands produce too much parathyroid hormone

- Paget disease of the bone, a condition that causes your bones to become too big, weak, and prone to fractures

- Overuse of antacids that contain calcium

- Excessive intake of calcium from vitamin D supplements or milk

- Certain types of cancer

If your results show lower than normal calcium levels, it may indicate:

- Hypoparathyroidism, a condition in which your parathyroid glands produce too little parathyroid hormone

- Vitamin D deficiency

- Magnesium deficiency

- Inflammation of the pancreas (pancreatitis)

- Kidney disease

If your calcium test results are not in the normal range, it does not necessarily mean that you have a medical condition needing treatment. Other factors, such as diet and certain medicines, can affect your calcium levels. If you have questions about your results, talk to your healthcare provider.

Is There Anything Else You Need to Know about a Calcium Blood Test?

A calcium blood test does not tell you how much calcium is in your bones. Bone health can be measured with a type of x-ray called a "bone density scan," or "dexa scan." A dexa scan measures the mineral content, including calcium, and other aspects of your bones.

Section 7.2

Blood Glucose Test

This section includes text excerpted from "Blood
Glucose Test," MedlinePlus, National Institutes of
Health (NIH), September 26, 2017.

A blood glucose test measures the glucose levels in your blood. Glucose is a type of sugar. It is your body's main source of energy. A hormone called "insulin" helps move glucose from your bloodstream into your cells. Too much or too little glucose in the blood can be a sign of a serious medical condition. High blood glucose levels (hyperglycemia) may be a sign of diabetes, a disorder that can cause heart disease, blindness, kidney failure, and other complications. Low blood glucose levels (hypoglycemia) can also lead to major health problems, including brain damage, if not treated.

Blood glucose test is also known with the names such as blood sugar, self-monitoring of blood glucose (SMBG), fasting plasma glucose (FPG), fasting blood sugar (FBS), fasting blood glucose (FBG), glucose challenge test, and oral glucose tolerance test (OGTT).

What Is a Blood Glucose Test Used For?

A blood glucose test is used to find out if your blood sugar levels are in the healthy range. It is often used to help diagnose and monitor diabetes.

Why Do You Need a Blood Glucose Test?

Your healthcare provider may order a blood glucose test if you have symptoms of high glucose levels (hyperglycemia) or low glucose levels (hypoglycemia).

Symptoms of high blood glucose levels include:

- Increased thirst

- More frequent urination

- Blurred vision

- Fatigue

- Wounds that are slow to heal

Symptoms of low blood glucose levels include:

- Anxiety
- Sweating
- Trembling
- Hunger
- Confusion

You may also need a blood glucose test if you have certain risk factors for diabetes. These include:

- Being overweight
- Lack of exercise
- Family member with diabetes
- High blood pressure
- Heart disease

If you are pregnant, you will likely get a blood glucose test between the 24th and 28th week of your pregnancy to check for gestational diabetes. "Gestational diabetes" is a form of diabetes that happens only during pregnancy.

What Happens during a Blood Glucose Test?

A healthcare professional will take a blood sample from a vein in your arm, using a small needle. After the needle is inserted, a small amount of blood will be collected into a test tube or vial. You may feel a little sting when the needle goes in or out. For some types of glucose blood tests, you will need to drink a sugary drink before your blood is drawn.

If you have diabetes, your healthcare provider may recommend a kit to monitor your blood sugar at home. The kit will include a device to prick your finger. You will use this to collect a drop of blood for testing. Read the kit instructions carefully and talk to your healthcare provider to make sure you collect and test your blood correctly.

Will You Need to Do Anything to Prepare for a Blood Glucose Test?

You will probably need to fast (not eat or drink) for eight hours before the test. If you are pregnant and are being checked for gestational diabetes:

- You will drink a sugary liquid one hour before your blood is drawn
- You will not need to fast for this test
- If your results show higher than normal blood glucose levels, you may need another test, which requires fasting
- Talk to your health provider about specific preparations needed for your glucose test

Are There Any Risks to a Blood Glucose Test?

There is very little risk of having a blood test. You may have slight pain or bruise at the spot where the needle was put in, but most symptoms go away quickly.

What Do a Blood Glucose Test Results Mean?

If your results show higher than normal glucose levels, it may mean you have or are at risk for getting diabetes. High glucose levels may also be a sign of:

- Kidney disease
- Hyperthyroidism
- Pancreatitis
- Pancreatic cancer

If your results show lower than normal glucose levels, it may be a sign of:

- Hypothyroidism
- Too much insulin or other diabetes medicine
- Liver disease

If your glucose results are not normal, it does not necessarily mean you have a medical condition needing treatment. High stress and certain medicines can affect glucose levels. To learn what your results mean, talk to your healthcare provider.

Is There Anything Else You Should Know about a Blood Glucose Test?

Many people with diabetes need to check blood glucose levels every day. If you have diabetes, be sure to talk to your healthcare provider about the best ways to manage your disease.

Section 7.3

Glucose Challenge Test

This section contains text excerpted from the following sources: Text in this section begins with excerpts from "Diabetes Tests and Diagnosis," National Institute of Diabetes and Digestive and Kidney Diseases (NIDDK), December 2016. Reviewed September 2019; Text under the heading "What Is an Oral Glucose Challenge Test?" is excerpted from "Screening and Diagnosing Gestational Diabetes Mellitus," Effective Health Care Program, Agency for Healthcare Research and Quality (AHRQ), October 2012. Reviewed September 2019.

If you are pregnant and a healthcare professional is checking you for gestational diabetes, you may first receive the glucose challenge test. Another name for this test is the glucose screening test. In this test, a healthcare professional will draw your blood 1 hour after you drink a sweet liquid containing glucose. You do not need to fast for this test. If your blood glucose is too high—135 to 140 or more—you may need to return for an oral glucose tolerance test while fasting.

What Is an Oral Glucose Tolerance Test?

The oral glucose tolerance test (OGTT) measures blood glucose after you fast for at least eight hours. First, a healthcare professional will draw your blood. Then you will drink the liquid containing glucose. For diagnosing gestational diabetes, you will need your blood drawn every hour for two to three hours.

High blood glucose levels at any two or more blood test times during the OGTT—fasting, one hour, two hours, or three hours—mean you have gestational diabetes. Your healthcare team will explain what your OGTT results mean.

Healthcare professionals also can use the OGTT to diagnose type 2 diabetes and prediabetes in people who are not pregnant. The OGTT helps healthcare professionals detect type 2 diabetes and prediabetes better than the FPG test. However, the OGTT is a more expensive test and is not as easy to give. To diagnose type 2 diabetes and prediabetes, a healthcare professional will need to draw your blood one hour after you drink the liquid containing glucose and again after two hours.

What Is an Oral Glucose Challenge Test?

Typically, a 50g oral glucose challenge test (OGCT) is initially administered between 24 and 28 weeks' gestation in a nonfasting state, in women at moderate risk (i.e., women who do not meet all low-risk criteria but lack two or more risk factors for GDM). The test is administered earlier in gestation for women at high risk of GDM (i.e., multiple risk factors for GDM) and repeated at 24 to 28 weeks' gestation if initial surveillance is normal. Patients who meet or exceed a screening threshold (usually 130mg/dL or 140mg/dL) receive a more involved diagnostic test—the oral glucose tolerance test (OGTT), in which a 75g or 100g oral glucose load is administered in the fasting state, and plasma glucose levels are evaluated after 1, 2, or 3 hours.

A diagnosis of GDM is made in pregnant women when one or more glucose values fall at or above the specified glucose thresholds. Alternatively, a one-step method in which all patients or high-risk patients forego the screening test and proceed directly to the OGTT has been recommended.

Section 7.4

Thyroid Tests

This section includes text excerpted from "Thyroid Tests," National Institute of Diabetes and Digestive and Kidney Diseases (NIDDK), February 2014. Reviewed September 2019.

The thyroid is a two-inch-long, butterfly-shaped gland weighing less than one ounce. Located in the front of the neck below the larynx, or voice box, it has two lobes, one on either side of the windpipe. The thyroid is one of the glands that make up the endocrine system. The glands of the endocrine system produce and store hormones and release them into the bloodstream. The hormones then travel through the body and direct the activity of the body's cells.

What Is the Role of Thyroid Hormones?

Thyroid hormones regulate metabolism—the way the body uses energy—and affect nearly every organ in the body. Thyroid hormones also affect brain development, breathing, heart and nervous system functions, body temperature, muscle strength, skin dryness, menstrual cycles, weight, and cholesterol levels. The thyroid makes two thyroid hormones:

- Thyroxine (T_4)
- Triiodothyronine (T_3)

Only a small amount of T_3 in the blood comes from the thyroid. Most T_3 comes from cells all over the body, where it is made from T_4. Thyroid-stimulating hormone (TSH), which is made by the pituitary gland in the brain, regulates thyroid hormone production. When thyroid hormone levels in the blood are low, the pituitary gland releases more TSH. When thyroid hormone levels are high, the pituitary decreases TSH production.

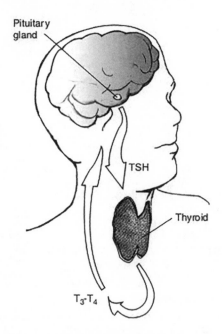

Figure 7.1. *Thyroid-Stimulating Hormone*

When thyroid hormone levels in the blood are low, the pituitary gland releases more TSH. When thyroid hormone levels are high, the pituitary gland decreases TSH production.

Why Do Healthcare Providers Perform Thyroid Tests?

Healthcare providers perform thyroid tests to assess how well the thyroid is working. The tests are also used to diagnose and help find the cause of thyroid disorders, such as hyperthyroidism and hypothyroidism:

- **Hyperthyroidism** is a disorder caused by too much thyroid hormone in the bloodstream, which increases the speed of bodily functions and leads to weight loss, sweating, rapid heart rate, and high blood pressure, among other symptoms.

- **Hypothyroidism** is a disorder that occurs when the thyroid does not make enough thyroid hormone for the body's needs. Without enough thyroid hormone, many of the body's functions slow down. People may have symptoms, such as fatigue, weight gain, and cold intolerance.

What Blood Tests Do Healthcare Providers Use to Check a Person's Thyroid Function?

A healthcare provider may order several blood tests to check thyroid function, including the following:

- TSH test

- T_4 tests

- T_3 test

- Thyroid-stimulating immunoglobulin (TSI) test

- Antithyroid antibody test, also called the "thyroid peroxidase antibody test" (TPOab)

A blood test involves drawing blood at a healthcare provider's office or a commercial facility and sending the sample to a lab for analysis. Blood tests assess thyroid function by measuring TSH and thyroid hormone levels, and by detecting certain autoantibodies present in autoimmune thyroid disease. Autoantibodies are molecules produced by a person's body that mistakenly attack the body's own tissues. Many complex factors affect thyroid function and hormone levels. Healthcare providers take a patient's full medical history into account when interpreting thyroid function tests.

Thyroid-Stimulating Hormone Test

A healthcare provider usually performs the TSH blood test first to check how well the thyroid is working. The TSH test measures the amount of TSH a person's pituitary gland is secreting. The TSH test is the most accurate test for diagnosing both hyperthyroidism and hypothyroidism. Generally, a below-normal level of TSH suggests hyperthyroidism. An abnormally high TSH level suggests hypothyroidism.

The TSH test detects even tiny amounts of TSH in the blood. Normally, the pituitary gland boosts TSH production when thyroid hormone levels in the blood are low. The thyroid responds by making more hormones. Then, when the body has enough thyroid hormone circulating in the blood, TSH output drops. The cycle repeats continuously to maintain a healthy level of thyroid hormone in the body. In people whose thyroid produces too much thyroid hormone, the pituitary gland shuts down TSH production, leading to low or even undetectable TSH levels in the blood.

In people whose thyroid is not functioning normally and produces too little thyroid hormone, the thyroid cannot respond normally to TSH by producing thyroid hormone. As a result, the pituitary gland keeps making TSH, trying to get the thyroid to respond. If results of the TSH test are abnormal, a person will need one or more additional tests to help find the cause of the problem.

T_4 Tests

The thyroid primarily secretes T_4 and only a small amount of T_3. T_4 exists in two forms:

- T_4 that is bound to proteins in the blood and is kept in reserve until needed

- A small amount of unbound or "free" T_4 (FT_4), which is the active form of the hormone and is available to enter body tissues when needed

A high level of total T_4—bound and FT_4 together—or FT_4 suggests hyperthyroidism, and a low level of total T_4 or FT_4 suggests hypothyroidism. Both pregnancy and taking oral contraceptives increase levels of binding protein in the blood. In either of these cases, although a woman may have a high total T_4 level, she may not have hyperthyroidism. Severe illness or the use of corticosteroids—a class of medications that treat asthma, arthritis, and skin conditions, among other health problems—can decrease binding protein levels. Therefore, in these cases, the total T_4 level may be low, yet the person does not have hypothyroidism.

T_3 Test

If a healthcare provider suspects hyperthyroidism in a person who has a normal FT_4 level, a T_3 test can be useful to confirm the condition. In some cases of hyperthyroidism, FT_4 is normal yet free T_3 (FT_3) is elevated, so measuring both T_4 and T_3 can be useful if a healthcare provider suspects hyperthyroidism. The T_3 test is not useful in diagnosing hypothyroidism because levels are not reduced until the hypothyroidism is severe.

Thyroid-Stimulating Immunoglobulin Test

Thyroid-stimulating immunoglobulin is an autoantibody present in Graves disease. TSI mimics TSH by stimulating the thyroid cells, causing the thyroid to secrete extra hormone. The TSI test detects TSI circulating in the blood and is usually measured:

- In people with Graves disease when the diagnosis is obscure

- During pregnancy

- To find out if a person is in remission, or no longer has hyperthyroidism and its symptoms

Antithyroid Antibody Test

Antithyroid antibodies are markers in the blood that are extremely helpful in diagnosing Hashimoto disease. Two principal types of antithyroid antibodies are:

- Anti-TG antibodies, which attack a protein in the thyroid called "thyroglobulin"

- Anti-thyroperoxidase, or anti-TPO, antibodies, which attack an enzyme in thyroid cells called "thyroperoxidase"

Table 7.1. Hyperthyroidism Function Test Results

Cause	Test			
	TSH	T_3/T_4	TSI	Radioactive Iodine Uptake Test
Graves disease	↓	↑	+	↑
Thyroiditis (with hyperthyroidism)	↓	↑	–	↓
Thyroid nodules (hot, or toxic)	↓	↑	–	↑ or Normal

Key: ↑ = Above normal, + = Positive, ↓ = Below normal, – = Negative

Table 7.2. Hypothyroidism Function Test Results

Cause	Test		
	TSH	T_3/T_4	Antithyroid Antibody
Hashimoto disease (thyroiditis, early stage)	↑	↓ or Normal	+
Hashimoto disease (thyroiditis, later stage)	↑	↓	+
Pituitary gland abnormality	↓	↓	–

Key: ↑ = Above normal, + = Positive, ↓ = Below normal, – = Negative

What Imaging Tests Do Healthcare Providers Use to Diagnose and Find the Cause of Thyroid Disorders?

A healthcare provider may use one or a combination of imaging tests, such as an ultrasound of the thyroid, a computerized tomography (CT) scan, or nuclear medicine tests, to diagnose and find the cause of thyroid disorders.

- **Ultrasound.** Ultrasound uses a device called a "transducer," that bounces safe, painless sound waves off organs to create an image of their structure. A specially trained technician performs the procedure in a healthcare provider's office, an outpatient center, or a hospital, and a radiologist—a doctor who specializes in medical imaging—interprets the images; a patient does not need anesthesia. The images can show the size and texture of the thyroid, as well as a pattern of typical autoimmune inflammation. The images can also show nodules or growths within the gland that suggest a malignant tumor.

- **Computed tomography (CT).** CT scans use a combination of x-rays and computer technology to create images. For a CT scan, a healthcare provider may give the patient a solution to drink and an injection of a special dye, called "contrast medium." CT scans require the patient to lie on a table that slides into a tunnel-shaped device where the x-rays are taken. An x-ray technician performs the procedure in an outpatient center or a hospital, and a radiologist interprets the images. The patient does not need anesthesia. CT scans are usually not needed to diagnose thyroid disease; however, healthcare providers will use them to view a large goiter. Also, a CT scan will often show a thyroid nodule when a person is having the scan for other health problems.

- **Nuclear medicine tests.** Nuclear medicine tests of the thyroid include a thyroid scan and a radioactive iodine uptake test. People often have to follow a low iodine diet prior to having the tests.

- **Thyroid scan.** A thyroid scan is a type of nuclear medicine imaging. Nuclear medicine uses small amounts of radioactive material to create a picture of an organ and give information about the organ's structure and function. A thyroid scan is used to look at the size, shape, and position of the gland. This test can help find the cause of hyperthyroidism and check for thyroid nodules. The scan also can help a healthcare provider evaluate thyroid nodules; however, it does not confirm whether the nodules are cancerous or benign. A specially trained technician performs the procedure in an outpatient center or a hospital, and a radiologist interprets the images; a patient does not need anesthesia. For the scan, radioactive iodine or radioactive technetium is injected into the patient's vein or swallowed in liquid or capsule form. The scan takes place 30 minutes after an injection or 6 to 24 hours after the radioactive substance is swallowed. The patient lies on an exam table for the scan, which takes about 30 minutes. A device called a "gamma camera" is suspended over the table or may be located within a large, tunnel-shaped device that resembles a CT scanner. The gamma camera detects the radioactive material and sends images to a computer that show how and where the radioactive substance has been distributed in the thyroid. Nodules that produce too much thyroid hormone—called "hot," or "toxic," nodules—show up clearly because they absorb more radioactive material than normal thyroid tissue. Graves disease shows up as a spread-out, overall increase in radioactivity rather than an increase in a localized spot. Even though the amount of radiation used in this test is small, women who are pregnant or breastfeeding should not have this test because of the risks of exposing the fetus or the baby to radiation.

• **Radioactive iodine uptake test.** The radioactive iodine uptake test, also known as a "thyroid uptake," is a nuclear medicine test used to evaluate the function of the thyroid and find the cause of a patient's hyperthyroidism. A whole-body thyroid scan is used for people who have had thyroid cancer. The test measures the amount of iodine the thyroid collects from the bloodstream in a given time period. The thyroid uptake is not used to assess hypothyroidism. A specially trained technician performs the test in an outpatient center or a hospital, and a radiologist interprets the images; a patient does not need anesthesia. For this test, the patient swallows a small amount of radioactive iodine in liquid or capsule form. After 4 to 6 hours and again at 24 hours, the patient returns to the testing center, where the technician measures the amount of radioactive iodine taken up by the thyroid. The measurement is taken with a small device called a "gamma probe," which resembles a microphone. The gamma probe is positioned near the patient's neck over the thyroid. Measurement takes only a few minutes and is painless. In the diagnosis of hyperthyroidism, a high thyroid uptake reading usually indicates an overactive thyroid that produces too much thyroid hormone, as seen in Graves disease or a condition called "toxic nodular goiter," an enlargement of the thyroid. A low thyroid uptake reading suggests the thyroid is not overactive. Several thyroid disorders that cause inflammation of the thyroid, or thyroiditis, may cause leakage of thyroid hormone and iodine out of the thyroid into the bloodstream, which can lead to high T_4 levels. When the thyroid is inflamed, it does not take up the radioactive iodine given as part of the thyroid uptake test. For example, hyperthyroidism seen in Graves disease would be marked by high blood T_4 and a high thyroid uptake reading. In thyroiditis, temporary hyperthyroidism may exist because of the release of T_4 into the blood; however, the thyroid uptake reading is low because of the inflammation. Temporary hyperthyroidism in thyroiditis is often followed by a period of hypothyroidism before the thyroid heals. Even though the amount of radiation used in this test is small, women who are pregnant or breastfeeding should not have this test because of the risks of exposing the fetus or infant to radiation.

What Tests Do Healthcare Providers Use If a Thyroid Nodule Is Found?

If a healthcare provider feels a nodule in a patient's neck during a physical exam or detects one during imaging tests of the thyroid, a fine needle aspiration biopsy may be done to confirm whether the nodule is cancerous or benign. A fine needle aspiration biopsy of the thyroid involves taking cells from the thyroid for examination with a microscope. The healthcare provider with experience in needle aspirations performs the biopsy in her or his office, an outpatient center, or a hospital; she or he may use medication to numb the area. The patient may feel mild discomfort during the test and the biopsy site may be tender for one to two days. For this test, the patient lies back with support under the shoulders so the neck can be extended and bent back slightly. The healthcare provider inserts a small, thin needle attached to a syringe into the thyroid nodule and uses ultrasound to guide its insertion. Samples of the cells in the nodule are drawn through the needle and sent to a lab to be examined by a pathologist—a doctor who specializes in diagnosing diseases. The healthcare provider may need to take several samples. Once the biopsy is complete, a bandage is placed on the area to lower the chance of bleeding.

Chapter 8

Prenatal Tests

Tests are used during pregnancy to check your and your baby's health. At your first prenatal visit, your doctor will use tests to check for a number of things, such as:

- Your blood type and Rh factor

- Anemia

- Infections, such as toxoplasmosis and sexually transmitted infections (STIs), including hepatitis B, syphilis, chlamydia, and human immunodeficiency virus (HIV)

- Signs that you are immune to rubella (German measles) and chicken pox

Throughout your pregnancy, your doctor or midwife may suggest a number of other tests, too. Some tests are suggested for all women, such as screenings for gestational diabetes, Down syndrome, and HIV. Other tests might be offered based on your:

- Age

- Personal or family health history

- Ethnic background

- Results of routine tests

This chapter includes text excerpted from "Prenatal Care and Tests," Office on Women's Health (OWH), U.S. Department of Health and Human Services (HHS), January 30, 2019.

Some tests are screening tests. They detect risks for or signs of possible health problems in you or your baby. Based on screening test results, your doctor might suggest diagnostic tests. Diagnostic tests confirm or rule out health problems in you or your baby.

Table 8.1. Common Prenatal Tests

Test	What It Is	How It Is Done
Amniocentesis	This test can diagnosis certain birth defects, including: • Down syndrome • Cystic fibrosis (CF) • Spina bifida It is performed at 14 to 20 weeks. It may be suggested for couples at higher risk for genetic disorders. It also provides deoxyribonucleic acid (DNA) for paternity testing.	A thin needle is used to draw out a small amount of amniotic fluid and cells from the sac surrounding the fetus. The sample is sent to a lab for testing.
Biophysical profile (BPP)	This test is used in the third trimester to monitor the overall health of the baby and to help decide if the baby should be delivered early.	Biophysical profile involves an ultrasound exam along with a nonstress test. The BPP looks at the baby's breathing, movement, muscle tone, heart rate, and the amount of amniotic fluid.
Chorionic villus sampling (CVS)	A test done at 10 to 13 weeks to diagnose certain birth defects, including: • Chromosomal disorders, including Down syndrome • Genetic disorders, such as CF CVS may be suggested for couples at higher risk for genetic disorders. It also provides DNA for paternity testing.	A needle removes a small sample of cells from the placenta to be tested.

Table 8.1. Continued

Test	What It Is	How It Is Done
First trimester screen	A screening test done at 11 to 14 weeks to detect higher risk of: • Chromosomal disorders, including Down syndrome and trisomy 18 • Other problems, such as heart defects also can reveal multiple births. Based on test results, your doctor may suggest other tests to diagnose a disorder.	This test involves both a blood test and an ultrasound exam called "nuchal translucency screening." The blood test measures the levels of certain substances in the mother's blood. The ultrasound exam measures the thickness at the back of the baby's neck. This information, combined with the mother's age, help doctors determine risk to the fetus.
Glucose challenge screening	A screening test done at 26 to 28 weeks to determine the mother's risk of gestational diabetes. Based on test results, your doctor may suggest a glucose tolerance test.	First, you consume a special sugary drink from your doctor. A blood sample is taken one hour later to look for high blood sugar levels.
Glucose tolerance test	This test is done at 26 to 28 weeks to diagnose gestational diabetes.	Your doctor will tell you what to eat a few days before the test. Then, you cannot eat or drink anything but sips of water for 14 hours before the test. Your blood is drawn to test your "fasting blood glucose level." Then, you will consume a sugary drink. Your blood will be tested every hour for 3 hours to see how well your body processes sugar.
Group B Streptococcus infection	This test is done at 36 to 37 weeks to look for bacteria that can cause pneumonia or serious infection in newborn.	A swab is used to take cells from your vagina and rectum to be tested.

Table 8.1. Continued

Test	What It Is	How It Is Done
Maternal serum screen (also called quad screen, triple test, triple screen, multiple marker screen, or AFP)	A screening test done at 15 to 20 weeks to detect higher risk of: • Chromosomal disorders, including Down syndrome and trisomy 18 • Neural tube defects, such as spina bifida Based on test results, your doctor may suggest other tests to diagnose a disorder.	Blood is drawn to measure the levels of certain substances in the mother's blood.
Nonstress test (NST)	This test is performed after 28 weeks to monitor your baby's health. It can show signs of fetal distress, such as your baby not getting enough oxygen.	A belt is placed around the mother's belly to measure the baby's heart rate in response to its own movements.
Ultrasound exam	An ultrasound exam can be performed at any point during the pregnancy. Ultrasound exams are not routine. But it is not uncommon for women to have a standard ultrasound exam between 18 and 20 weeks to look for signs of problems with the baby's organs and body systems and confirm the age of the fetus and proper growth. It also might be able to tell the sex of your baby. Ultrasound exam is also used as part of the first trimester screen and BPP. Based on exam results, your doctor may suggest other tests or other types of ultrasound to help detect a problem.	Ultrasound uses sound waves to create a "picture" of your baby on a monitor. With a standard ultrasound, a gel is spread on your abdomen. A special tool is moved over your abdomen, which allows your doctor and you to view the baby on a monitor.

Table 8.1. Continued

Test	What It Is	How It Is Done
Urine test	A urine sample can look for signs of health problems, such as: • Urinary tract infection (UTI) • Diabetes • Preeclampsia If your doctor suspects a problem, the sample might be sent to a lab for more in-depth testing.	You will collect a small sample of clean, midstream urine in a sterile plastic cup. Testing strips that look for certain substances in your urine are dipped in the sample. The sample also can be looked at under a microscope.

Understanding Prenatal Tests and Test Results

If your doctor suggests certain prenatal tests, do not be afraid to ask lots of questions. Learning about the test, why your doctor is suggesting it for you, and what the test results could mean can help you cope with any worries or fears you might have. Keep in mind that screening tests do not diagnose problems. They evaluate risk. So, if a screening test comes back abnormal, this does not mean there is a problem with your baby. More information is needed. Your doctor can explain what the test results mean and possible next steps.

Avoid Keepsake Ultrasounds

You might think a keepsake ultrasound is a must-have for your scrapbook. But, doctors advise against ultrasound when there is no medical need to do so. Some companies sell "keepsake" ultrasound videos and images. Although ultrasound is considered safe for medical purposes, exposure to ultrasound energy for a keepsake video or image may put a mother and her unborn baby at risk. Do not take that chance.

Chapter 9

Newborn Screening for Metabolic Disorders

What Is the Purpose of Newborn Screening?

The purpose of newborn screening is to detect potentially fatal or disabling conditions in newborns as early as possible, often before the infant displays any signs or symptoms of a disease or condition. Such early detection allows treatment to begin immediately, which reduces or even eliminates the effects of the condition. Many of the conditions detectable in newborn screening, if left untreated, have serious symptoms and effects, such as lifelong nervous system damage; intellectual, developmental, and physical disabilities; and even death.

What Disorders Are Newborns Screened for in the United States?

The Advisory Committee on Heritable Disorders in Newborns and Children (ACHDNC) issues a Recommended Universal Screening Panel (RUSP) that identifies a number of core conditions—those for which screening is highly recommended—and secondary conditions, for

This chapter includes text excerpted from "What Is the Purpose of Newborn Screening?" *Eunice Kennedy Shriver* National Institute of Child Health and Human Development (NICHD), September 1, 2017.

which screening is optional. As of November 2016, the RUSP included 34 core conditions and 26 secondary conditions.

The committee's recommendations are based on the Newborn Screening: Towards a Uniform Screening Panel and System and on current research evidence, which means that the number of core and secondary conditions may change.

Phenylketonuria

Phenylketonuria (PKU) is a metabolic disorder that is detected by newborn screening. In PKU, the body cannot digest or process one of the building blocks of proteins, an amino acid called "phenylalanine," or "Phe." Phe is found naturally in many foods, especially high-protein foods.

Phenylketonuria was the first condition for which a screening test was developed, and the first condition for which widespread newborn testing was implemented in the 1960s.

If PKU is left untreated, the Phe builds up in the body and brain. By three to six months of age, infants with untreated PKU begin to show symptoms of intellectual and developmental disabilities. These disabilities can become severe if Phe remains at high levels.

Fortunately, PKU is treatable. The treatment consists of a diet containing little or no Phe and higher levels of other amino acids. If children with the condition are placed on this diet at birth, they grow normally and usually show no symptoms or health problems. The *Eunice Kennedy Shriver* National Institute of Child Health and Human Development (NICHD)-sponsored research has shown that people with PKU should stay on the restricted diet as they enter adulthood and, in fact, throughout their lives. This is especially important for women of childbearing age who wish to or who might become pregnant.

Before newborn screening programs could detect PKU in the first few hours after birth, PKU was one of the leading causes of intellectual and developmental disabilities (IDD) in the United States. Nowadays, as a result of newborn screening programs that allow for almost immediate treatment of the condition, PKU has been virtually eliminated as a cause of IDD in this country.

Galactosemia

Another metabolic disorder included in newborn screening is galactosemia, which means being unable to use galactose. Galactose is one of two simple sugars that make up lactose, the sugar in milk. People with galactosemia cannot have any milk or milk products.

If someone with galactosemia consumes milk or milk products (human or animal), the galactose builds up in their blood and causes serious damage to their liver, brain, kidneys, and eyes. Infants with untreated galactosemia can die of serious blood infection or of liver failure. Those that may survive usually have IDD and other damage to the brain and nervous system. Even milder forms of galactosemia still require treatment to prevent early cataracts, an unsteady gait, and delays in learning, talking, and growth.

The treatment for galactosemia is not to consume any milk or milk products and to avoid other foods that contain this sugar. If this disease is diagnosed very early and the infant is placed on a strict galactose-free diet, she or he is likely to live a relatively normal life, although mild IDD may still develop. If not placed on a galactose-free diet immediately, an infant will develop symptoms in the first few days after birth.

Before it could be detected either before birth or through a newborn screening program, galactosemia was a frequent cause of IDD and early death. Oregon began screening newborns for galactosemia 50 years ago, and all states now screen for this condition. Screening has identified more than 2,500 infants with the condition, many of whom would have died without the screening.

Chapter 10

Chromosome Abnormalities

What Are Chromosomes?

Chromosomes are the structures that hold genes. Genes are the individual instructions that tell our bodies how to develop and function; they govern physical and medical characteristics, such as hair color, blood type and susceptibility to disease.

Many chromosomes have two segments, called "arms," separated by a pinched region known as the "centromere." The shorter arm is called the "p" arm. The longer arm is called the "q" arm.

Where Are Chromosomes Found in the Body?

The body is made up of individual units called "cells." Your body has many different kinds of cells, such as skin cells, liver cells and blood cells. In the center of most cells is a structure called the "nucleus." This is where chromosomes are located.

How Many Chromosomes Do Humans Have?

The typical number of chromosomes in a human cell is 46:23 pairs, holding an estimated total of 20,000 to 25,000 genes. One set of 23

This chapter includes text excerpted from "Chromosome Abnormalities Fact Sheet," National Human Genome Research Institute (NHGRI), January 6, 2016. Reviewed September 2019.

chromosomes is inherited from the biological mother (from the egg), and the other set is inherited from the biological father (from the sperm).

Of the 23 pairs of chromosomes, the first 22 pairs are called "autosomes." The final pair is called the "sex chromosomes." Sex chromosomes determine an individual's sex: females have two X chromosomes (XX), and males have an X and a Y chromosome (XY). The mother and father each contribute one set of 22 autosomes and one sex chromosome.

How Do Scientists Study Chromosomes?

For a century, scientists studied chromosomes by looking at them under a microscope. In order for chromosomes to be seen this way, they need to be stained. Once stained, the chromosomes look like strings with light and dark "bands," and their picture can be taken. A picture, or chromosome map, of all 46 chromosomes is called a "karyotype." The karyotype can help identify abnormalities in the structure or the number of chromosomes.

To help identify chromosomes, the pairs have been numbered from 1 to 22, with the 23rd pair labeled "X" and "Y." In addition, the bands that appear after staining are numbered; the higher the number, the farther that area is from the centromere.

In the past decade, newer techniques have been developed that allow scientists and doctors to screen for chromosomal abnormalities without using a microscope. These newer methods compare the patient's deoxyribonucleic acid (DNA) to a normal DNA sample. The comparison can be used to find chromosomal abnormalities where the two samples differ.

One such method is called "noninvasive prenatal testing." This is a test to screen a pregnancy to determine whether a baby has an increased chance of having specific chromosome disorders. The test examines the baby's DNA in the mother's blood.

What Are Chromosome Abnormalities?

There are many types of chromosome abnormalities. However, they can be organized into two basic groups: numerical abnormalities and structural abnormalities.

Numerical abnormalities. When an individual is missing one of the chromosomes from a pair, the condition is called "monosomy." When an individual has more than two chromosomes instead of a pair, the condition is called "trisomy." An example of a condition caused by numerical abnormalities is Down syndrome, which is marked by mental retardation, learning difficulties, a characteristic facial appearance and poor muscle tone (hypotonia) in infancy. An individual with Down syndrome has three copies of chromosome 21 rather than two; for that reason, the condition is also known as "Trisomy 21." An example of monosomy, in which an individual lacks a chromosome, is Turner syndrome. In Turner syndrome, a female is born with only one sex chromosome, an X, and is usually shorter than average and unable to have children, among other difficulties.

Structural abnormalities. A chromosome's structure can be altered in several ways.

- **Deletions:** A portion of the chromosome is missing or deleted.

- **Duplications:** A portion of the chromosome is duplicated, resulting in extra genetic material.

- **Translocations:** A portion of one chromosome is transferred to another chromosome. There are two main types of translocation. In a reciprocal translocation, segments from two different chromosomes have been exchanged. In a Robertsonian translocation, an entire chromosome has attached to another at the centromere.

- **Inversions:** A portion of the chromosome has broken off, turned upside down, and reattached. As a result, the genetic material is inverted.

- **Rings:** A portion of a chromosome has broken off and formed a circle or ring. This can happen with or without loss of genetic material.

Most chromosome abnormalities occur as an accident in the egg or sperm. In these cases, the abnormality is present in every cell of the body. Some abnormalities, however, happen after conception; then some cells have the abnormality and some do not.

Chromosome abnormalities can be inherited from a parent (such as a translocation) or be "de novo" (new to the individual). This is why, when a child is found to have an abnormality, chromosome studies are often performed on the parents.

Chapter 11

Genetic Counseling

Who Are Genetic Professionals?

Genetics professionals are healthcare professionals with specialized degrees and experience in medical genetics and counseling. Genetics professionals include geneticists, genetic counselors, and genetics nurses.

What Is Genetic Counseling and Evaluation?

Genetic professionals work as members of healthcare teams, providing information and support to individuals or families who have genetic disorders or may be at risk for inherited conditions. Genetic professionals:

- Assess the risk of a genetic disorder by researching a family's history, evaluating medical records, and conducting a physical examination of the patient and other family members when indicated

- Weigh the medical, social and ethical decisions surrounding genetic testing

This chapter contains text excerpted from the following sources: Text beginning with the heading "Who Are Genetic Professionals?" is excerpted from "Genetic Counseling FAQ," National Human Genome Research Institute (NHGRI), November 20, 2013. Reviewed September 2019; Text under the heading "Reasons for Genetic Counseling" is excerpted from "Genetic Counseling," Centers for Disease Control and Prevention (CDC), October 4, 2018.

- Provide support and information to help a person make a decision about testing

- Interpret the results of genetic tests and medical data

- Provide counseling or refer individuals and families to support services

- Serve as patient advocates

- Explain possible treatments or preventive measures

- Discuss reproductive options

How You Can Find a Genetic Professional

Your healthcare provider may refer you to a genetic professional. Universities and medical centers also often have affiliated genetic professionals, or can provide referrals to a genetic professional or genetics clinic.

As more has been learned about genetics, genetic professionals have grown more specialized. For example, they may specialize in a particular disease (such as cancer genetics), an age group (such as adolescents) or a type of counseling (such as prenatal).

How Do You Decide Whether to See a Geneticist?

Your healthcare provider may refer you to a geneticist—a medical doctor or medical researcher—who specializes in your disease or disorder. A medical geneticist has completed a fellowship or has other advanced training in medical genetics. While a genetic counselor or genetic nurse may help you with testing decisions and support issues, a medical geneticist will make the actual diagnosis of a disease or condition. Many genetic diseases are so rare that only a geneticist can provide the most complete and current information about your condition.

Along with a medical geneticist, you may also be referred to a physician who is a specialist in the type of disorder you have. For example, if a genetic test is positive for colon cancer, you might be referred to an oncologist. For a diagnosis of Huntington disease, you may be referred to a neurologist.

Reasons for Genetic Counseling

Based on your personal and family health history, your doctor can refer you for genetic counseling. There are different stages in your life when you might be referred for genetic counseling:

- **Planning for pregnancy.** Genetic counseling before you become pregnant can address concerns about factors that might affect your baby during infancy or childhood or your ability to become pregnant, including:

  - Genetic conditions that run in your family or your partner's family

  - History of infertility, multiple miscarriages, or stillbirth

  - Previous pregnancy or child affected by a birth defect or genetic condition

  - Assisted Reproductive Technology (ART) options

- **During pregnancy.** Genetic counseling while you are pregnant can address certain tests that may be done during your pregnancy, any detected problems, or conditions that might affect your baby during infancy or childhood, including:

  - History of infertility, multiple miscarriages, or stillbirth

  - Previous pregnancy or child affected by a birth defect or genetic condition

  - Abnormal test results, such as a blood test, ultrasound, chorionic villus sampling (CVS), or amniocentesis

  - Maternal infections, such as cytomegalovirus (CMV), and other exposures such as medications, drugs, chemicals, and x-rays

  - Genetic screening that is recommended for all pregnant women, which includes cystic fibrosis, sickle cell disease, and any conditions that run in your family or your partner's family

- **Caring for children.** Genetic counseling can address concerns if your child is showing signs and symptoms of a disorder that might be genetic, including:

  - Abnormal newborn screening results

  - Birth defects

  - Intellectual disability or developmental disabilities

  - Autism spectrum disorders (ASD)

  - Vision or hearing problems

- **Managing your health.** Genetic counseling for adults includes specialty areas such as cardiovascular, psychiatric, and cancer. Genetic counseling can be helpful if you have symptoms of a condition or have a family history of a condition that makes you more likely to be affected with that condition, including:

  - Hereditary breast and ovarian cancer (HBOC) syndrome

  - Lynch syndrome (hereditary colorectal and other cancers)

  - Familial hypercholesterolemia

  - Muscular dystrophy and other muscle diseases

  - Inherited movement disorders such as Huntington disease

  - Inherited blood disorders such as sickle cell disease

Following your genetic counseling session, you might decide to have genetic testing. Genetic counseling after testing can help you better understand your test results and treatment options, help you deal with emotional concerns, and refer you to other healthcare providers and advocacy and support groups.

Part Two

The Pituitary Gland and Growth Disorders

Chapter 12

Common Growth Disorders in Children

Does your child seem much shorter—or much taller—than other kids her or his age? It could be normal. Some children may be small for their age but still be developing normally. Some children are short or tall because their parents are.

But, some children have growth disorders. Growth disorders are problems that prevent children from developing normal height, weight, sexual maturity or other features.

Very slow or very fast growth can sometimes signal a gland problem or disease.

The pituitary gland makes growth hormone, which stimulates the growth of bone and other tissues. Children who have too little of it may be very short. Treatment with growth hormone can stimulate growth.

People can also have too much growth hormone. Usually, the cause is a pituitary-gland tumor, which is not cancer. Too much growth hormone can cause gigantism in children, where their bones and their body grow too much. In adults, it can cause acromegaly, which makes

This chapter contains text excerpted from the following sources: Text in this chapter begins with excerpts from "Growth Disorders," MedlinePlus, National Institutes of Health (NIH), November 30, 2016. Reviewed September 2019; Text under the heading "Constitutional Growth Delay" is © 2017 Omnigraphics. Reviewed September 2019; Text under the heading "Idiopathic Short Stature" is © 2017 Omnigraphics. Reviewed September 2019.

the hands, feet and faces larger than normal. Possible treatments include surgery to remove the tumor, medicines, and radiation therapy.

Constitutional Growth Delay

Constitutional growth delay is a relatively common condition in which physical development and maturation occurs at a much later age than average. Children with this condition are sometimes called "late bloomers" because they grow more slowly than their peers and reach puberty several years later. Although, children with constitutional growth delay tend to be short in stature during their teen years, in most cases the condition is temporary. Once the growth spurt associated with puberty finally occurs, they continue growing after their peers have stopped and eventually reach an adult height similar to that of their parents. As a result, constitutional growth delay is not considered a disease. Rather, it is viewed as a variant of normal growth patterns in otherwise healthy teenagers.

Although constitutional growth delay can occur in either sex, it is more common among boys than girls. Children who are diagnosed with the condition tend to have a characteristic pattern of growth. After being born at a normal weight and length, they typically have a slow growth rate during the first two years of life. Their growth rate usually returns to normal around age three, however, so children with constitutional growth delay typically will be small for their age but keep pace with their peers. This situation changes when peers' growth rate accelerates upon reaching puberty. For children with congenital growth delay, the onset of puberty—and the associated growth spurt— may not occur for several more years. Consequently, their growth and physical maturation fall significantly behind at this time, sometimes resulting in social and psychological challenges.

Causes of Constitutional Growth Delay

Experts believe that constitutional growth delay has a genetic component, since between 60 and 90 percent of children affected by the condition have a family member who was also affected. Heredity may account for delays in the release of hormones that are responsible for initiating the changes associated with puberty, such as the maturation of the ovaries and testicles.

In children with constitutional growth delay, the pattern of development of secondary sexual characteristics is normal, but the age at which it begins is much later than average. The absence or disruption of this normal pattern may indicate hormonal deficiencies that warrant further investigation. The growth that is delayed or slower than expected can also result from other medical conditions, such as chronic diseases or infections, endocrine disorders, autoimmune disorders, inflammatory bowel disease, or poor nutrition. Some of the syndromes that can mimic constitutional growth delay include Turner syndrome, Noonan syndrome, Kallmann syndrome, and Russell-Silver syndrome. These conditions must be ruled out in order to form a diagnosis of constitutional growth delay.

Diagnosis of Constitutional Growth Delay

In diagnosing constitutional growth delay, a doctor will begin by taking a complete medical history of the child. The doctor is likely to inquire about the child's growth pattern over time, eating habits or feeding schedule, and any medications or supplements they might take. The doctor is also likely to ask about any other symptoms that might be present, especially delays in social interactions or other skill development. Finally, the doctor will likely inquire about the child's biological parents, including their height, weight, and age upon reaching puberty.

Next, the doctor will perform a physical examination that includes measurements of the child's height, weight, and head circumference. The doctor may order additional laboratory tests as well, including blood tests, urine tests, and stool samples to rule out infections, diseases, and nutritional deficiencies. In addition, an x-ray will typically be conducted on the child's left hand and wrist to determine the child's "bone age," or degree of skeletal maturation. The growth plates in long bones in the forearm remain open until the growth spurt that accompanies puberty. Afterward, the bones begin to fuse, meaning that further growth will be limited. The extent of skeletal maturation provides valuable clues about whether a child's growth is merely delayed or is being limited by some other biological factor.

Social and Psychological Effects of Constitutional Growth Delay

Once other causes of growth delay have been ruled out, the main priority is helping the child cope with the social and psychological challenges that often accompany the condition. Children with constitutional growth delay are likely to be quite short for their age and appear much younger than their friends. As their peers reach puberty and show signs of sexual maturation, they may feel self-conscious, left out, and anxious about their future sexual function and fertility.

Since adolescence is fraught with social changes, concerns surrounding delayed growth can create a serious emotional or psychological disturbance for some teenagers. Some may respond by behaving immaturely, or acting the age they appear rather than their chronological age. Others may respond to teasing or bullying with aggressive, antisocial behavior. Under most circumstances, constitutional growth delay does not require treatment. Doctors merely provide reassurance that children with the condition are developing normally, will experience the onset of puberty soon, and will eventually reach appropriate adult height. But children who have trouble coping with the condition may need therapeutic help to accelerate the timing of puberty and growth.

Treatment of Constitutional Growth Delay

While medical treatment is not necessary for most cases of constitutional growth delay, it may be indicated for patients who experience psychological distress due to their slow patterns of growth and development. Short courses of therapy with growth hormones or sex hormones can accelerate growth and advance the onset of puberty. Although hormone therapy does not increase adult height, it does help speed up the process so that teenagers feel less different than their peers.

One potential benefit of medical treatment for constitutional growth delay is that it may help protect adult bone mass. Because of the activity of sex hormones and growth hormones, puberty is the peak period for bone mineralization. In fact, more than half of all bone calcium accumulates between the ages of 11 and 14 for girls, and 14 and 17 for boys. As a result, delays in the circulation of these hormones may increase the risk of osteopenia, or reduced bone mass, in adulthood. Hormone therapy thus has the potential to increase adult bone mass in children with constitutional growth delay.

References

1. Alter, Craig, and Sue Smith. "Constitutional Delay of Growth," MAGIC Foundation, n.d.

2. Clark, Pamela A. "Constitutional Growth Delay Clinical Presentation," Medscape, July 28, 2016.

3. "Delayed Growth," Agency for Healthcare Research and Quality (AHRQ), U.S. Department of Health and Human Services (HHS), 2016.

4. Stanhope, Richard. "Constitutional Delay of Growth and Puberty," Child Growth Foundation (CGF), September 2000.

Idiopathic Short Stature

Idiopathic short stature (ISS) is the term used to describe a child who is considerably shorter than others of the same age, sex, and genetic background when there is no known medical cause for the condition. ("Idiopathic" refers to a condition that arises spontaneously with no discernible origin.) Although ISS is not itself considered a disease, children who fit the definition need to be evaluated by a growth specialist in order to rule out the numerous diseases and disorders that can cause short stature before a diagnosis of ISS can be made.

When to See a Growth Specialist

Accurate height measurement is an ongoing process that should be charted by a pediatrician or family doctor throughout a child's growth years. The American Academy of Pediatrics (AAP) recommends measuring height and weight at birth, at age 2 to 4 days, periodically from 1 to 24 months, and then yearly until age 21. In this way, growth can be monitored and compared to established standards, and if there is significant deviation further evaluation and testing can be initiated.

If parents suspect that their child is small for her or his age, or if the child appears to have stopped growing, the regular physician should be consulted first for an opinion. The doctor will compare the child's height and rate of growth to demographic standards, perform a physical examination, and perhaps order some preliminary tests, such as blood work. If appropriate, the physician may then refer the child to a specialist, such as a pediatric endocrinologist.

Diagnosis of Idiopathic Short Stature

One of the first things a specialist will do is confirm that the child is actually of short stature, beginning with measurements of height, weight, and arm and leg lengths. Technically, that would mean that she or he is two standard deviations (SD) or more below average for someone of the same age, race, ethnic background, and geographical origin. The doctor will also take a thorough family history, both to learn about the height of close relatives and to ask about genetic disorders that might affect growth.

If short stature is confirmed, the next step is to determine whether it is idiopathic or the result of a medical condition. Beginning with a physical examination, the doctor would then likely order a series of tests that might include:

- Complete blood count (CBC), an indicator of overall health
- Other blood work to check kidney, liver, and immune system function
- Thyroid function tests, blood tests that ensure the thyroid gland is working properly
- Growth hormone stimulation, which tests the function of the pituitary gland
- Insulin growth factor 1 test to identify growth hormone deficiency
- Bone tests, including x-rays and scans, such as magnetic resonance imaging (MRI)

Because short stature can be the result of such a wide variety of diseases or genetic disorders, diagnosing the underlying pathology, if any, can be a lengthy process. Eliminating possible causes can take weeks, or even months, depending on the condition and the individual child.

Causes of Short Stature

Since growth rate and height are the results of so many factors, ranging from genetic traits to nutrition to disease, the causes of short stature are numerous and varied. Some possible causes include:

- Growth hormone deficiency
- Thyroid disorders, such as Cushing disease and hypothyroidism
- Juvenile rheumatoid arthritis
- Celiac disease
- Kidney disorders
- Genetic conditions, such as Turner syndrome and Down syndrome
- Sickle cell anemia
- Gastrointestinal disease
- Rickets
- Malnutrition

If no specific medical cause of short stature can be determined, then it may be diagnosed as ISS. In that case, assuming all relevant tests have been completed and the conditions are not judged to be dangerous, the physician may recommend regular follow-up examinations, testing, and measurement to monitor the child's condition and growth patterns.

Treatment of Idiopathic Short Stature

If testing reveals an underlying medical cause of short stature, then treatment will be based on that disease or disorder. For example, hypothyroidism is normally treated with thyroid hormone replacement pills; juvenile rheumatoid arthritis could be treated with nonsteroidal anti-inflammatory drugs, such as ibuprofen or naproxen; and celiac disease would be addressed with a gluten-free diet.

Children for whom testing reveals growth hormone deficiency are commonly treated with growth hormone (GH) injections. These can be given at home, usually once per day, and have proven effective, particularly when treatment is begun at least five years before the onset of puberty.

In 2003, the use of GH was approved by the U.S. Food and Drug Administration (FDA) for the treatment of children with ISS, if a doctor predicts that they will attain a very short final height (under 4 feet 11 inches for a girl, and under 5 feet 4 inches for a boy). Again, the treatments, when started well before puberty, have been shown to aid growth and increase final height. But the use of GH to treat ISS is not without controversy.

For one thing, children with ISS, by definition, have normal GH levels, and some healthcare professionals are not comfortable administering medicine that tests indicate is not required. Others feel it unwise to administer hormone treatments—or any medication—when the condition is not physically harmful and the underlying cause is unknown. Another point of contention is that response to GH is highly variable, with some children experiencing only a moderate increase in height.

In addition, GH treatments can be very expensive and, if low hormone levels have not been supported by tests, some insurance plans will not cover the cost. And although GH is generally considered a safe treatment, its benefits must be weighed against the possible side effects, which can include allergic reactions, headaches, blurred vision, nervousness, and, in rare cases, chest pain, abdominal pain, rash, nausea, and vomiting.

References

1. "Childhood Growth and Height Issues," Children's Hospital of Philadelphia, n.d.

2. "Controversies in the Definition and Treatment of Idiopathic Short Stature (ISS)," National Center for Biotechnology Information (NCBI), February 1, 2009.

3. Geffner, Mitchell, MD. "Idiopathic Short Stature," MAGIC Foundation, n.d Lee, Kimberly G., MD, MSc, IBCLC. "Short Stature," University of Maryland Medical Center (UMMC), December 12, 2014.

4. Rogol, Alan D., MD, PhD. "Causes of Short Stature," UpToDate.com, August 16, 2016.

5. Rosenbloom, Arlan L., MD. " Idiopathic Short Stature: Conundrums of Definition and Treatment," National Center for Biotechnology Information (NCBI), March 12, 2009.

6. Sinha, Sunil, MD. "Short Stature," Medscape, June 17, 2016.

Chapter 13

Growth Hormone Deficiency in Adults

Growth hormone deficiency (GHD) is characterized by abnormally short height due to lack (or shortage) of growth hormone. It can be congenital (present at birth) or acquired. Most cases are identified in children. Although it is uncommon, GHD may also be diagnosed in adults. Too little growth hormone can cause short stature in children, and changes in muscle mass, cholesterol levels, and bone strength in adults. Most of the time, no single clear cause can be identified but several genetic causes of GHD have been described, such as mutations in the *POU1F1/Pit1, PROP1 GHRH,* and *GH1* genes. In adolescents, puberty may be delayed or absent. Treatment involves growth-hormone injections.

Treatment of Growth Hormone Deficiency in Adults

The medication(s) listed below have been approved by the U.S. Food and Drug Administration (FDA) as orphan products for the treatment of this condition.

This chapter includes text excerpted from "Growth Hormone Deficiency," Genetic and Rare Diseases Information Center (GARD), National Center for Advancing Translational Sciences (NCATS), June 3, 2016. Reviewed September 2019.

- **Somatropin (r-DNA) for injection (Brand name: Genotropin).** Manufactured by Pfizer, Inc. FDA-approved indication for long-term treatment of growth failure in children born small for gestational age who fail to manifest catch-up growth by two years of age. It is also used as a treatment for adults with growth hormone deficiency.

- **Macimorelin acetate (Brand name: Macrilen).** Manufactured by Strongbridge Biopharma and FDA-approved (December 2017), is used for the diagnosis of adult growth hormone deficiency (AGHD). Note: This product is used for diagnosis and is not a medical treatment.

- **Somatropin (r-DNA) for injection (Brand name: Norditropin).** Manufactured by Novo Nordisk Pharmaceuticals and is FDA-approved. It is used as long-term treatment of children who have growth failure due to inadequate secretion of endogenous growth hormone.

- **Somatropin (r-DNA) for injection (Brand name: Nutropin AQ).** Manufactured by Genentech, Inc. and is FDA-approved. It is used for long-term treatment of children who have growth failure due to a lack of adequate endogenous growth hormone secretion. It is also used for the treatment of children with growth failure associated with chronic renal insufficiency and as replacement therapy for growth hormone deficiency in adults after epiphyseal closure.

- **Somatropin (r-DNA) for injection (Brand name: Saizen).** Manufactured by EMD Serono, Inc., and FDA-approved. It is used for the long-term treatment of children with growth failure due to inadequate secretion of endogenous growth hormone. It is also used for the treatment of adults with GHD that started as a child or as an adult.

Finding a Specialist

If you need medical advice, you can look for doctors or other health-care professionals who have experience with this disease. You may find these specialists through advocacy organizations, clinical trials, or articles published in medical journals. You may also want to contact a university or tertiary medical center in your area, because these centers tend to see more complex cases and have the latest technology and treatments.

If you cannot find a specialist in your local area, try contacting national or international specialists. They may be able to refer you to someone they know through conferences or research efforts. Some specialists may be willing to consult with you or your local doctors over the phone or by e-mail if you cannot travel to them for care.

Chapter 14

Growth Hormone Evaluation Process

Growth hormone (GH), sometimes called "human growth hormone" (HGH) or "somatotropin," is a substance secreted by the pituitary gland that controls functions such as growth, cell reproduction, cell regeneration, and a healthy balance of fat, muscle, and bone. In children, too little GH can cause abnormal shortness, and too much can cause gigantism (acromegaly). In adults, an excess of GH can cause bones to thicken, those in the extremities and face to increase in size, and the person's appearance to change significantly, while a GH deficiency can result in issues such as excess fat in the abdomen, weakened muscle tone, osteoporosis, and high cholesterol levels. Of the two disorders, GH deficiency is by far the more common, and acromegaly is very rare in children.

Growth hormone disorders in children are usually the result of a problem with the hypothalamus—the part of the brain that, among other functions, controls the endocrine system—causing it to fail to stimulate the pituitary gland. An underactive hypothalamus is also possible in adults, but it is quite rare. More commonly, GH abnormalities in adults are caused by damage to the pituitary gland, such as might be caused by brain surgery, radiation treatment for a brain tumor, surgery to remove a pituitary tumor, or a traumatic head injury.

"Growth Hormone Evaluation Process," © 2017 Omnigraphics. Reviewed September 2019.

Testing for GH disorders primarily measures pituitary-gland function and blood hormone levels. The examinations and test procedures, which are similar for children and adults, typically begin with a physical examination, in which the doctor will evaluate the patient's height, weight, and overall body proportions. If a visual examination raises concerns, measurements may be taken and compared to age-appropriate standards. But, the primary way GH is tested is through a variety of blood tests and other evaluative procedures that are usually overseen by an endocrinologist, a physician who specializes in the endocrine system, which controls hormones.

Blood Tests for Growth Hormone Levels

Blood for GH testing is generally drawn in a doctor's office or clinic. No special preparation is normally required, although, depending on the specific tests, the patient may be asked to fast prior to the test or to stop taking regularly prescribed medication for a certain period beforehand. GH blood tests can include:

- **GH stimulation test.** This test, done after a 10 to 12-hour fast, checks for growth hormone deficiency by measuring the level of GH in the blood after the injection of substances, such as arginine, clonidine, and glucagon, which trigger the pituitary gland to release GH. By taking blood samples at timed intervals over several hours before, during, and after these injections are given, medical professionals are able to test accurately for GH levels.

- **GH suppression test.** Used to diagnose acromegaly, or an excess of GH, this test entails taking a blood sample after the patient has fasted for 10 to 12 hours. She or he is then given a large amount of glucose (sugar) solution, and blood samples are drawn at intervals. When tested for GH levels, these can help determine how much the pituitary gland has been suppressed from producing growth hormone.

- **Binding protein levels tests.** Generally done prior to GH testing, these tests (IGF-1 and IGFBP-3) evaluate pituitary-gland function by measuring the amount of insulin-like growth factor (IGF) in the blood. Fasting is not required, and samples can be taken in a single blood draw. Unlike GH, whose levels fluctuate throughout the day, IGF tends to remain stable, making it reliable for gauging average GH levels. Low readings indicate GH deficiency and high levels are an indication of GH overproduction.

- **Insulin tolerance test.** Used in GH evaluation to measure pituitary-gland function, this test involves injecting the patient with insulin through an intravenous therapy (IV) to induce hypoglycemia, or low blood sugar. In response to this condition, among other bodily reactions, the pituitary gland releases GH. Measuring this response, facilitated by drawing blood at intervals, provides a means of assessing the gland's health. Note that hypoglycemia carries some risk, so this test is generally performed in a hospital setting so the patient can be monitored continuously and treated if necessary.

A number of other blood tests may be performed to evaluate the function of the pituitary and thyroid glands. Most of these are done before GH testing is ordered and may include checking the levels of various hormones, such as free luteinizing hormone (LH), thyroxine (T_4), thyroid-stimulating hormone (TSH), cortisol, and testosterone. If abnormalities are found, the conditions indicated by these tests are normally treated with medication prior to proceeding to GH testing.

Other Tests Used to Evaluate Growth Hormone Issues

Although blood testing is the most common way to evaluate GH disorders, a number of other tests may be ordered to help in the diagnosis or to rule out other conditions. These may include:

- **Head x-rays.** By taking an x-ray of the patient's head, a doctor may be able to detect any problems related to growth of the skull, such as enlarged sinuses, thickening of the calvaria (skull cap), or enlarged sella turcica (the skull cavity that holds the pituitary gland).

- **Hand x-rays.** X-rays of the hand can reveal bone-development issues. By comparing hand and wrist radiographs to established standards, and comparing apparent bone age to the patient's chronological age, the doctor may be able to begin the diagnosis of GH problems or other disorders.

- **Brain magnetic resonance imaging (MRI) or computerized tomography (CT) scan.** A clear picture of the brain can help the doctor assess abnormalities in the pituitary gland and hypothalamus. An MRI does this with a magnetic field, radio waves, and a computer, while a CT (computerized tomography) scan creates pictures using x-ray images and a computer.

- **Dual x-ray absorptiometry (DXA).** It is a method of measuring bone density, which can be an indication of GH disorders. It works by scanning the patient with two x-ray beams, one high energy and one low energy. By comparing the level of radiation that passes through the bone from each beam, an accurate determination of bone density can be made.

Risks Involved in Tests Used for Growth Hormone Evaluation

There are very few risks associated with most tests for GH disorders. And scans, such as x-rays, MRIs, and CTs, carry virtually no risk and generally cause no discomfort to the patient. There are, however, some slight risks with blood testing that may include:

- **Minor discomfort.** An injection or the insertion of an IV needle may cause discomfort in some patients. This is especially true in cases in which the medical professional has difficulty locating a suitable blood vessel.

- **Bruising.** Some patients experience bruising, or hematoma, at the site of the injection or IV. This can be minimized by keeping pressure on the site for a short time.

- **Fainting.** Occasionally patients may faint or feel light-headed during the testing procedures. Lying quietly for several minutes usually provides relief.

- **Excessive bleeding.** Certain blood-thinning medications, such as aspirin and warfarin, can increase the risk of bleeding. If a patient is taking such medicine, or if she or he has a bleeding disorder, the doctor should be informed prior to the blood draw.

- **Infection.** Any time the skin is broken, as when a needle is inserted for blood testing, there is at least a slight risk of infection. The individual administering the test will take appropriate precautions, but patients should be made aware of proper after-care procedures to guard against infection.

- **Phlebitis.** This is the inflammation of a vein caused by a blood clot. In rare instances, this can occur after a blood draw. It can usually be treated with warm compresses, although in some cases the doctor may prescribe anti-inflammatory medication to help relieve the symptoms.

- **Medication issues.** Some of the drugs in testing, such as those used to stimulate the pituitary gland, can cause side effects. For instance, the medication used in the insulin tolerance may, in very rare cases, cause heart palpitations or even loss of consciousness. In addition, some prescription drugs can interfere with GH test results. Examples include dopamine and estrogens, which can increase GH levels, and corticosteroids and phenothiazines, which can decrease GH levels.

References

1. Carmichael, Kim A., MD, FACP. "Growth Hormone Testing," Mount Sinai Hospital, December 2014.

2. Cook, David, MD. "Adult Growth Hormone Deficiency," The Magic Foundation, n.d.

3. Gentile, Julie M. "Growth Hormone Deficiency Diagnosis," EndocrineWeb.com, May 27, 2014.

4. "Growth Hormone," Lab Tests Online, March 23, 2015.

5. Romito, Kathleen, MD. "Growth Hormone," WebMD.com, November 20, 2015.

Chapter 15

Growth Hormone Therapy

The human growth hormone (GH) is produced by a pea-sized endocrine gland present in the brain that fuels childhood growth and helps to maintain tissues and organs throughout our lives. Initially, GHs were used medically to increase the height of children who had growth deficiency. However, these days, they are used medically to treat several other conditions, including:

- GH deficiency

- Turner syndrome

- Idiopathic short stature

- Noonan syndrome

- Prader-Willi syndrome

- Children who did not undergo "catch-up" growth

In adults, GH therapy is used in a muscle-wasting disease that is associated with human immunodeficiency virus (HIV) or acquired immunodeficiency syndrome (AIDS). However, it is not approved by the U.S. Food and Drug Administration (FDA).

"Growth Hormone Therapy," © 2020 Omnigraphics. Reviewed September 2019.

Facts about Growth Hormone Therapy

Following are a few facts related to growth hormone therapy:

- Growth hormone treatment has been used to treat children who have a GH deficiency and other conditions that cause short stature.

- Some medical tests are performed to confirm GH deficiency. Magnetic resonance imaging (MRI), stimulation tests, and x-rays are few of the tests used to detect a pituitary tumor, which secretes GH.

- Growth hormone therapy is considered to be an effective and safe method for the treatment of GH deficiency, Turner syndrome, and other conditions associated with short stature.

- Growth hormone therapy has few side effects.

How Growth Works

The main organ involved in the growth of a child is the pituitary gland. GH is produced by the pituitary gland during deep sleep. A number of factors can affect the release of GH, however, including nutrition, sleep, stress, blood-glucose level, exercise, medication, and other hormones present in the body. When GH is not released properly growth is either slow or there is no growth at all. This does not affect the intelligence of a child, but will result is low self-esteem and the development of mature social skills. Hence, GH therapy is used for growth and for personal development.

How Growth Hormone Works

Once the doctor determines GH deficiency, Turner syndrome, or other such conditions treatable with GH deficiency, an endocrinologist will explain the pros and cons of this treatment. The GH that is used for the treatment is prepared at the laboratory to match the natural GH produced by the pituitary gland. Hence, this method is safe and effective. This laboratory-prepared GH is injected through a subcutaneous injection, which goes into the fatty tissue just beneath the skin. A special injection device that looks like a pen is also used to inject the GH hormone. It is a shallow injection and the needle is too small to hurt much.

Results of Growth Hormone Therapy

A child undergoing GH treatment will definitely grow in height. However, it takes around three to six months to determine any height differences in the child. You will probably notice a few other differences within the first six months of the treatment:

- The foot growth of the child will occur once in six to eight weeks.

- The child will experience an increased appetite and the child will want to eat more during the treatment.

- The child may look lean as there will be an increase in lean body mass and a decrease in fat body mass.

Growth hormone therapy is a long process and that usually occurs over a number of years until a child attains an adult height. Routine consultation with your pediatric endocrinologist and periodic blood tests and x-rays should be continued to monitor the child's progress. Although the treatment takes a long period of time, the child should continue with it:

- Until they attain their full adult height

- Until their bones are completely matured

- Until there is a growth of fewer than two centimeters in the last year

Getting and Giving Growth Hormone Injections

Getting GH injected is quite simple and almost painless. Children age 10 and older can inject it themselves (with parent supervision to ensure that the child gives the right amount of dosage). For children below 10 years of age, a parent should give the injection. Bedtime is the right time for GH treatment, since it works effectively during night hours and because natural hormones are released during our sleeping hours.

Possible Side Effects of Growth Hormone Therapy

Growth hormone therapy is an effective method that helps to treat GH deficiency. Fortunately, serious side effects are rare, yet there are a few common side effects that one should be aware of. They are:

- A temporary rise in blood sugar levels during the course of treatment. The blood-sugar level becomes normal as soon as the treatment stops

- A progression of spine curvature for patients with scoliosis

- Hip, knee, and other joint pain

- Allergic reactions, such as swelling at the injection site, rashes, or hives

- Headache

Call the endocrinology clinic or office if the headache is severe or if you have doubts or questions about a reaction that your child is undergoing.

Psychiatric Treatment

Along with GH therapy, psychiatric treatment may be given to the child as well. For instance, if a child is too short, this will likely affect his or her self-esteem, which may affect them mentally and emotionally. The psychiatric therapy will help the child cope.

References

1. "Growth Hormone Treatment," University of Pittsburgh Medical Center (UPMC), September 17, 2010.

2. "Growth Hormone Therapy," Cincinnati Children's, December 29, 2013.

3. "Growth Hormone Therapy," Remedy Health Media & EndocrineWeb, August 4, 2011.

Chapter 16

Acromegaly

What Is Acromegaly?

Acromegaly is a hormonal disorder that results from too much growth hormone (GH) in the body. The pituitary gland, a small gland in the brain, makes GH. In acromegaly, the pituitary produces excessive amounts of GH. Usually, the excess GH comes from benign, or noncancerous, tumors on the pituitary. These benign tumors are called "adenomas."

Acromegaly is most often diagnosed in middle-aged adults, although symptoms can appear at any age. If not treated, acromegaly can result in serious illness and premature death. Acromegaly is treatable in most patients, but because of its slow and often "sneaky" onset, it often is not diagnosed early or correctly. The most serious health consequences of acromegaly are type 2 diabetes, high blood pressure, increased risk of cardiovascular disease (CVD), and arthritis. Patients with acromegaly are also at increased risk for colon polyps, which may develop into colon cancer if not removed.

When GH-producing tumors occur in childhood, the disease that results is called "gigantism" rather than acromegaly. A child's height is determined by the length of the so-called "long bones" in the legs. In response to GH, these bones grow in length at the growth plates—areas near either end of the bone. Growth plates fuse after puberty, so the

This chapter includes text excerpted from "Acromegaly," National Institute of Diabetes and Digestive and Kidney Diseases (NIDDK), April 2012. Reviewed September 2019.

excessive GH production in adults does not result in increased height. However, prolonged exposure to excess GH before the growth plates fuse causes increased growth of the long bones and thus increased height. Pediatricians may become concerned about this possibility if a child's growth rate suddenly and markedly increases beyond what would be predicted by previous growth and how tall the child's parents are.

What Are the Symptoms of Acromegaly?

The name "acromegaly" comes from the Greek words for "extremities" and "enlargement," reflecting one of its most common symptoms—the abnormal growth of the hands and feet. Swelling of the hands and feet is often an early feature, with patients noticing a change in ring or shoe size, particularly shoe width. Gradually, bone changes alter the patient's facial features: The brow and lower jaw protrude, the nasal bone enlarges, and the teeth space out.

Overgrowth of bone and cartilage often leads to arthritis. When tissue thickens, it may trap nerves, causing carpal tunnel syndrome, which results in numbness and weakness of the hands. Body organs, including the heart, may enlarge.

Other symptoms of acromegaly include:

- Joint aches
- Thick, coarse, oily skin
- Skin tags
- Enlarged lips, nose, and tongue
- Deepening of the voice due to enlarged sinuses and vocal cords
- Sleep apnea—breaks in breathing during sleep due to obstruction of the airway
- Excessive sweating and skin odor
- Fatigue and weakness
- Headaches
- Impaired vision
- Abnormalities of the menstrual cycle and sometimes breast discharge in women
- Erectile dysfunction (ED) in men
- Decreased libido

What Causes Acromegaly

Acromegaly is caused by prolonged overproduction of GH by the pituitary gland. The pituitary gland produces several important hormones that control body functions such as growth and development, reproduction, and metabolism. But, hormones never seem to act simply and directly. They usually "cascade" or flow in a series, affecting each other's production or release into the bloodstream.

The GH is part of a cascade of hormones that, as the name implies, regulates the physical growth of the body. This cascade begins in a part of the brain called the "hypothalamus." The hypothalamus makes hormones that regulate the pituitary gland. One of the hormones in the GH series, or "axis," is growth hormone-releasing hormone (GHRH), which stimulates the pituitary gland to produce GH.

The secretion of GH by the pituitary gland into the bloodstream stimulates the liver to produce another hormone called "insulin-like growth factor I" (IGF-I). IGF-I is what actually causes tissue growth in the body. High levels of IGF-I, in turn, signal the pituitary gland to reduce GH production.

The hypothalamus makes another hormone called "somatostatin," which inhibits GH production and release. Normally, GHRH, somatostatin, GH, and IGF-I levels in the body are tightly regulated by each other and by sleep, exercise, stress, food intake, and blood sugar levels. If the pituitary gland continues to make GH independent of the normal regulatory mechanisms, the level of IGF-I continues to rise, leading to bone overgrowth and organ enlargement. High levels of IGF-I also cause changes in glucose (sugar) and lipid (fat) metabolism and can lead to diabetes, high blood pressure, and heart disease.

Pituitary Tumors

In more than 95 percent of people with acromegaly, a benign tumor of the pituitary gland called an "adenoma," produces excess GH. Pituitary tumors are labeled either micro- or macro-adenomas, depending on their size. Most GH-secreting tumors are macro-adenomas, meaning they are larger than 1 centimeter. Depending on their location, these larger tumors may compress surrounding brain structures. For example, a tumor growing upward may affect the optic chiasm—where the optic nerves cross—leading to visual problems and vision loss. If the tumor grows to the side, it may enter an area of the brain called the "cavernous sinus" where there are many nerves, potentially damaging them.

Compression of the surrounding normal pituitary tissue can alter the production of other hormones. These hormonal shifts can lead to changes in menstruation and breast discharge in women and erectile dysfunction in men. If the tumor affects the part of the pituitary gland that controls the thyroid—another hormone-producing gland—then thyroid hormones may decrease. Too little thyroid hormone can cause weight gain, fatigue, and hair and skin changes. If the tumor affects the part of the pituitary gland that controls the adrenal gland, the hormone cortisol may decrease. Too little cortisol can cause weight loss, dizziness, fatigue, low blood pressure, and nausea.

Some GH-secreting tumors may also secrete too much of other pituitary hormones. For example, they may produce prolactin, the hormone that stimulates the mammary glands to produce milk. Rarely, adenomas may produce thyroid-stimulating hormone. Doctors should assess all pituitary hormones in people with acromegaly.

Rates of GH production and the aggressiveness of the tumor vary greatly among people with adenomas. Some adenomas grow slowly and symptoms of GH excess are often not noticed for many years. Other adenomas grow more rapidly and invade surrounding brain areas or the venous sinuses, which are located near the pituitary gland. Younger patients tend to have more aggressive tumors. Regardless of size, these tumors are always benign.

Most pituitary tumors develop spontaneously and are not genetically inherited. They are the result of a genetic alteration in a single pituitary cell, which leads to increased cell division and tumor formation. This genetic change, or mutation, is not present at birth but happens later in life. The mutation occurs in a gene that regulates the transmission of chemical signals within pituitary cells. It permanently switches on the signal that tells the cell to divide and secrete GH. The events within the cell that cause disordered pituitary gland cell growth and GH oversecretion are the subject of intensive research.

Nonpituitary Tumors

Rarely, acromegaly is caused not by pituitary tumors but by tumors of the pancreas, lungs, and other parts of the brain. These tumors also lead to excess GH, either because they produce GH themselves or, more frequently, because they produce GHRH, the hormone that stimulates the pituitary gland to make GH. When these nonpituitary tumors are surgically removed, GH levels fall and the symptoms of acromegaly improve.

In patients with GHRH-producing, nonpituitary tumors, the pituitary gland still may be enlarged and may be mistaken for a tumor.

Physicians should carefully analyze all "pituitary tumors" removed from patients with acromegaly so they do not overlook the rare possibility that a tumor elsewhere in the body is causing the disorder.

How Common Is Acromegaly

Small pituitary adenomas are common, affecting about 17 percent of the population. However, research suggests most of these tumors do not cause symptoms and rarely produce excess GH. Scientists estimate that 3 to 4 out of every million people develop acromegaly each year and about 60 out of every million people suffer from the disease at any time. Because the clinical diagnosis of acromegaly is often missed, these numbers probably underestimate the frequency of the disease.

How Is Acromegaly Diagnosed?
Blood Tests

If acromegaly is suspected, a doctor must measure the GH level in a person's blood to determine if it is elevated. However, a single measurement of an elevated blood GH level is not enough to diagnose acromegaly: Because GH is secreted by the pituitary gland in impulses, or spurts, its concentration in the blood can vary widely from minute to minute. At a given moment, a person with acromegaly may have a normal GH level, whereas a GH level in a healthy person may even be five times higher.

More accurate information is obtained when GH is measured under conditions that normally suppress GH secretion. Healthcare professionals often use the oral glucose tolerance test to diagnose acromegaly because drinking 75 to 100 grams of glucose solution lowers blood GH levels to less than 1 nanogram per milliliter (ng/ml) in healthy people. In people with GH overproduction, this suppression does not occur. The oral glucose tolerance test is a highly reliable method for confirming a diagnosis of acromegaly.

Physicians also can measure IGF-I levels, which increase as GH levels go up, in people with suspected acromegaly. Because IGF-I levels are much more stable than GH levels over the course of the day, they are often a more practical and reliable screening measure. Elevated IGF-I levels almost always indicate acromegaly. However, a pregnant woman's IGF-I levels are two to three times higher than normal. In addition, physicians must be aware that IGF-I levels decline with age and may also be abnormally low in people with poorly controlled diabetes, or liver, or kidney disease.

Imaging

After acromegaly has been diagnosed by measuring GH or IGF-I levels, a magnetic resonance imaging (MRI) scan of the pituitary gland is used to locate and detect the size of the tumor causing GH overproduction. MRI is the most sensitive imaging technique, but computerized tomography (CT) scans can be used if the patient should not have an MRI. For example, people who have pacemakers or other types of implants containing metal should not have an MRI scan because MRI machines contain powerful magnets.

If a head scan fails to detect a pituitary tumor, the physician should look for nonpituitary "ectopic" tumors in the chest, abdomen, or pelvis as the cause of excess GH. The presence of such tumors usually can be diagnosed by measuring GHRH in the blood and by a CT scan of possible tumor sites.

Rarely, a pituitary tumor secreting GH may be too tiny to detect even with a sensitive MRI scan.

How Is Acromegaly Treated?

Treatment options include surgical removal of the tumor, medical therapy, and radiation therapy of the pituitary gland.

Goals of treatment are to:

- Reduce excess hormone production to normal levels

- Relieve the pressure that the growing pituitary tumor may be exerting on the surrounding brain areas

- Preserve normal pituitary gland function or treat hormone deficiencies

- Improve the symptoms of acromegaly

Surgery

Surgery is the first option recommended for most people with acromegaly, as it is often a rapid and effective treatment. The surgeon reaches the pituitary gland via an incision through the nose or inside the upper lip and, with special tools, removes the tumor tissue in a procedure called "transsphenoidal surgery." This procedure promptly relieves the pressure on the surrounding brain regions and leads to a rapid lowering of GH levels. If the surgery is successful, facial appearance and soft tissue swelling improve within a few days.

Surgery is most successful in patients with blood GH levels below 45 ng/ml before the operation and with pituitary tumors no larger than 10 millimeters (mm) in diameter. Success depends in large part on the skill and experience of the surgeon, as well as the location of the tumor. Even with the most experienced neurosurgeon, the chance of a cure is small if the tumor has extended into critical brain structures or into the cavernous sinus where surgery could be risky.

The success rate also depends on what level of GH is defined as a cure. The best measure of surgical success is the normalization of GH and IGF-I levels. The overall rate of remission—control of the disease—after surgery ranges from 55 to 80 percent.

A possible complication of surgery is damage to the surrounding normal pituitary tissue, which requires lifelong use of pituitary hormone replacement. The part of the pituitary gland that stores antidiuretic hormone (ADH)—a hormone important in water balance—may be temporarily or, rarely, permanently damaged and the patient may require medical therapy. Other potential problems include cerebrospinal fluid (CSF) leaks and, rarely, meningitis. CBF bathes the brain and can leak from the nose if the incision area does not heal well. Meningitis is a bacterial or viral infection of the meninges, the outer covering of the brain.

Even when surgery is successful and hormone levels return to normal, people with acromegaly must be carefully monitored for years for possible recurrence of the disease. More commonly, hormone levels improve but do not return to normal. Additional treatment, usually medications, may be required.

Medical Therapy

Medical therapy is most often used if the surgery does not result in a cure and sometimes to shrink large tumors before surgery. Three medication groups are used to treat acromegaly.

Somatostatin analogs (SSAs) are the first medication group used to treat acromegaly. They shut off GH production and are effective in lowering GH and IGF-I levels in 50 to 70 percent of patients. SSAs also reduce tumor size in around 0 to 50 percent of patients but only to a modest degree. Several studies have shown that SSAs are safe and effective for long-term treatment and in treating patients with acromegaly caused by nonpituitary tumors. Long-acting SSAs are given by intramuscular injection once a month.

Digestive problems—such as loose stools, nausea, and gas—are a side effect in about half of people taking SSAs. However, the effects are usually temporary and rarely severe. About 10 to 20 percent of patients develop gallstones, but the gallstones do not usually cause symptoms. In rare cases, treatment can result in elevated blood glucose levels. More commonly, SSAs reduce the need for insulin and improve blood glucose control in some people with acromegaly who already have diabetes.

The second medication group is the GH receptor antagonists (GHRAs), which interfere with the action of GH. They normalize IGF-I levels in more than 90 percent of patients. They do not, however, lower GH levels. Given once a day through injection, GHRAs are usually well-tolerated by patients. The long-term effects of these drugs on tumor growth are still under study. Side effects can include headaches, fatigue, and abnormal liver function.

Dopamine agonists make up the third medication group. These drugs are not as effective as the other medications at lowering GH or IGF-I levels, and they normalize IGF-I levels in only a minority of patients. Dopamine agonists are sometimes effective in patients who have mild degrees of excess GH and have both acromegaly and hyperprolactinemia—too much of the hormone prolactin. Dopamine agonists can be used in combination with SSAs. Side effects can include nausea, headache, and lightheadedness.

Radiation Therapy

Radiation therapy is usually reserved for people who have some tumor remaining after surgery and do not respond to medications. Because radiation leads to a slow lowering of GH and IGF-I levels, these patients often also receive medication to lower hormone levels. The full effect of this therapy may not occur for many years.

The two types of radiation delivery are conventional and stereotactic. Conventional radiation delivery targets the tumor with external beams but can damage surrounding tissue. The treatment delivers small doses of radiation multiple times over four to six weeks, giving normal tissue time to heal between treatments.

Stereotactic delivery allows precise targeting of a high-dose beam of radiation at the tumor from varying angles. The patient must wear a rigid head frame to keep the head still. The types of stereotactic radiation delivery available are proton beam, linear accelerator (LINAC), and gamma knife. With stereotactic delivery, the tumor must be at least 5 mm from the optic chiasm to prevent radiation damage. This treatment can sometimes be done in a single session, reducing the risk of damage to surrounding tissue.

All forms of radiation therapy cause a gradual decline in the production of other pituitary hormones over time, resulting in the need for hormone replacement in most patients. Radiation also can impair a patient's fertility. Vision loss and brain injury are rare complications. Rarely, secondary tumors can develop many years later in areas that were in the path of the radiation beam.

Which Treatment for Acromegaly Is Most Effective

No single treatment is effective for all patients. Treatment should be individualized, and often combined, depending on patient characteristics such as age and tumor size.

If the tumor has not yet invaded surrounding nonpituitary tissues, removal of the pituitary adenoma by an experienced neurosurgeon is usually the first choice. Even if a cure is not possible, surgery may be performed if the patient has symptoms of neurological problems such as loss of peripheral vision or cranial nerve problems. After surgery, hormone levels are measured to determine whether a cure has been achieved. This determination can take up to eight weeks because IGF-I lasts a long time in the body's circulation. If cured, a patient must be monitored for a long time for increasing GH levels.

If surgery does not normalize hormone levels or a relapse occurs, an endocrinologist should recommend additional drug therapy. With each medication, long-term therapy is necessary because their withdrawal can lead to rising GH levels and tumor reexpansion.

Radiation therapy is generally reserved for patients whose tumors are not completely removed by surgery, who are not good candidates for surgery because of other health problems, or who do not respond adequately to surgery and medication.

Chapter 17

Pituitary Cushing Disease

Cushing disease (CD) is caused by elevated levels of a hormone called "cortisol," which leads to a wide variety of signs and symptoms. This condition usually occurs in adults between the ages of 20 and 50; however, children may also be affected.

The first sign of this condition is usually weight gain around the trunk and in the face. Affected individuals may get stretch marks (striae) on their thighs and abdomen and bruise easily. Individuals with CD can develop a hump on their upper back caused by abnormal deposits of fat. People with this condition can have muscle weakness, severe tiredness, and progressively thin and brittle bones that are prone to fracture (osteoporosis). They also have a weakened immune system and are at an increased risk of infections. CD can cause mood disorders such as anxiety, irritability, and depression. This condition can also affect a person's concentration and memory. People with CD have an increased chance of developing high blood pressure (hypertension) and diabetes. Women with CD disease may experience irregular menstruation and have excessive hair growth (hirsutism) on their face, abdomen, and legs. Men with CD may have erectile dysfunction (ED). Children with CD typically experience slow growth.

This chapter includes text excerpted from "Cushing Disease," Genetics Home Reference (GHR), National Institutes of Health (NIH), June 2012. Reviewed September 2019.

Frequency of Cushing Disease

Cushing disease is estimated to occur in 10 to 15 per million people worldwide. For reasons that are unclear, CD affects females more often than males.

Causes of Cushing Disease

The genetic cause of CD is often unknown. In only a few instances, mutations in certain genes have been found to lead to CD. These genetic changes are called "somatic mutations." They are acquired during a person's lifetime and are present only in certain cells. The genes involved often play a role in regulating the activity of hormones.

Cushing disease is caused by an increase in the hormone cortisol, which helps maintain blood sugar levels, protects the body from stress, and stops (suppresses) inflammation. Cortisol is produced by the adrenal glands, which are small glands located at the top of each kidney. The production of cortisol is triggered by the release of a hormone called "adrenocorticotropic hormone" (ACTH) from the pituitary gland, located at the base of the brain. The adrenal and pituitary glands are part of the hormone-producing (endocrine) system in the body that regulates development, metabolism, mood, and many other processes.

Cushing disease occurs when a noncancerous (benign) tumor called an "adenoma" forms in the pituitary gland, causing excessive release of ACTH and, subsequently, elevated production of cortisol. Prolonged exposure to increased cortisol levels results in the signs and symptoms of CD: changes to the amount and distribution of body fat, decreased muscle mass leading to weakness and reduced stamina, thinning skin causing stretch marks and easy bruising, thinning of the bones resulting in osteoporosis, increased blood pressure, impaired regulation of blood sugar leading to diabetes, a weakened immune system, neurological problems, irregular menstruation in women, and slow growth in children. The overactive adrenal glands that produce cortisol may also produce increased amounts of male sex hormones (androgens), leading to hirsutism in females. The effect of the excess androgens in males is unclear.

Most often, CD occurs alone, but rarely, it appears as a symptom of genetic syndromes that have pituitary adenomas as a feature, such as multiple endocrine neoplasia type 1 (MEN1) or familial isolated pituitary adenoma (FIPA).

Cushing disease is a subset of a larger condition called "Cushing syndrome," which results when cortisol levels are increased by one of a number of possible causes. Sometimes adenomas that occur in organs or tissues other than the pituitary gland, such as adrenal gland adenomas, can also increase cortisol production, causing Cushing syndrome. Certain prescription drugs can result in an increase in cortisol production and lead to Cushing syndrome. Sometimes prolonged periods of stress or depression can cause an increase in cortisol levels; when this occurs, the condition is known as "pseudo-Cushing syndrome." Not accounting for increases in cortisol due to prescription drugs, pituitary adenomas cause the vast majority of Cushing syndrome in adults and children.

Inheritance Pattern of Cushing Disease

Most cases of CD are sporadic, which means they occur in people with no history of the disorder in their family. Rarely, the condition has been reported to run in families; however, it does not have a clear pattern of inheritance.

The various syndromes that have CD as a feature can have different inheritance patterns. Most of these disorders are inherited in an autosomal dominant pattern, which means one copy of the altered gene in each cell is sufficient to cause the disorder.

Chapter 18

Diabetes Insipidus

What Is Diabetes Insipidus?

Diabetes insipidus is a rare disorder that occurs when a person's kidneys pass an abnormally large volume of urine that is insipid—dilute and odorless. In most people, the kidneys pass about 1 to 2 quarts of urine a day. In people with diabetes insipidus, the kidneys can pass 3 to 20 quarts of urine a day. As a result, a person with diabetes insipidus may feel the need to drink large amounts of liquids.

Diabetes insipidus and diabetes mellitus (DM)—which includes both type 1 and type 2 diabetes—are unrelated, although both conditions cause frequent urination and constant thirst. Diabetes mellitus causes high blood glucose, or blood sugar, resulting from the body's inability to use blood glucose for energy. People with diabetes insipidus have normal blood glucose levels; however, their kidneys cannot balance fluid in the body.

What Are the Kidneys and What Do They Do?

The kidneys are two bean-shaped organs, each about the size of a fist. They are located just below the rib cage, one on each side of the spine. Every day, the kidneys normally filter about 120 to 150 quarts of blood to produce about 1 to 2 quarts of urine, composed of wastes and

This chapter includes text excerpted from "Diabetes Insipidus," National Institute of Diabetes and Digestive and Kidney Diseases (NIDDK), October 2015. Reviewed September 2019.

extra fluid. The urine flows from the kidneys to the bladder through tubes called "ureters." The bladder stores urine. When the bladder empties, urine flows out of the body through a tube called the "urethra," located at the bottom of the bladder.

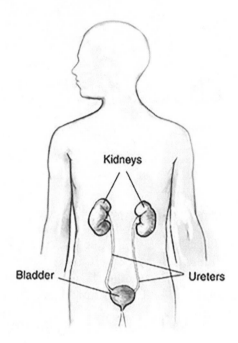

Figure 18.1. *Kidneys*

How Is Fluid Regulated in the Body?

A person's body regulates fluid by balancing liquid intake and removing extra fluid. Thirst usually controls a person's rate of liquid intake, while urination removes most fluid, although people also lose fluid through sweating, breathing, or diarrhea. The hormone vasopressin also called "antidiuretic hormone" (ADH) controls the fluid removal rate through urination. The hypothalamus, a small gland located at the base of the brain, produces vasopressin. The nearby pituitary gland stores the vasopressin and releases it into the bloodstream when the body has a low fluid level. Vasopressin signals the kidneys to absorb less fluid from the bloodstream, resulting in less urine. When the body has extra fluid, the pituitary gland releases smaller amounts of vasopressin, and sometimes none, so the kidneys remove more fluid from the bloodstream and produce more urine.

What Are the Types of Diabetes Insipidus?

The types of diabetes insipidus include:

- Central
- Nephrogenic
- Dipsogenic
- Gestational

Each type of diabetes insipidus has a different cause.

Central Diabetes Insipidus

Central diabetes insipidus happens when damage to a person's hypothalamus or pituitary gland causes disruptions in the normal production, storage, and release of vasopressin. The disruption of vasopressin causes the kidneys to remove too much fluid from the body, leading to an increase in urination. Damage to the hypothalamus or pituitary gland can result from the following:

- Surgery
- Infection
- Inflammation
- A tumor
- Head injury

Central diabetes insipidus can also result from an inherited defect in the gene that produces vasopressin, although this cause is rare. In some cases, the cause is unknown.

Nephrogenic Diabetes Insipidus

Nephrogenic diabetes insipidus occurs when the kidneys do not respond normally to vasopressin and continue to remove too much fluid from a person's bloodstream. Nephrogenic diabetes insipidus can result from inherited gene changes, or mutations, that prevent the kidneys from responding to vasopressin. Other causes of nephrogenic diabetes insipidus include:

- Chronic kidney disease (CKD)
- Certain medications, particularly lithium

- Low potassium levels in the blood
- High calcium levels in the blood
- Blockage of the urinary tract

The causes of nephrogenic diabetes insipidus can also be unknown.

Dipsogenic Diabetes Insipidus

A defect in the thirst mechanism, located in a person's hypothalamus, causes dipsogenic diabetes insipidus. This defect results in an abnormal increase in thirst and liquid intake that suppresses vasopressin secretion and increases urine output. The same events and conditions that damage the hypothalamus or pituitary gland—surgery, infection, inflammation, a tumor, head injury—can also damage the thirst mechanism. Certain medications or mental-health problems may predispose a person to dipsogenic diabetes insipidus.

Gestational Diabetes Insipidus

Gestational diabetes insipidus occurs only during pregnancy. In some cases, an enzyme made by the placenta—a temporary organ joining the mother and baby—breaks down the mother's vasopressin. In other cases, pregnant women produce more prostaglandin, a hormone-like chemical that reduces kidney sensitivity to vasopressin. Most pregnant women who develop gestational diabetes insipidus have a mild case that does not cause noticeable symptoms. Gestational diabetes insipidus usually goes away after the mother delivers the baby; however, it may return if the mother becomes pregnant again.

What Are the Complications of Diabetes Insipidus?

The main complication of diabetes insipidus is dehydration if fluid loss is greater than liquid intake. Signs of dehydration include:

- Thirst
- Dry skin
- Fatigue
- Sluggishness
- Dizziness

- Confusion

- Nausea

Severe dehydration can lead to seizures, permanent brain damage, and even death.

Seek Immediate Care

Usually, people can prevent dehydration by increasing the amount of liquids they drink. However, some people may not realize they need to drink more liquids, which can lead to dehydration. People should seek immediate care if they experience symptoms of more severe dehydration, such as:

- Confusion

- Dizziness

- Sluggishness

How Is Diabetes Insipidus Diagnosed?

A healthcare provider can diagnose a person with diabetes insipidus based on the following:

- Medical and family history
- Physical exam
- Urinalysis
- Blood tests
- Fluid deprivation test
- Magnetic resonance imaging (MRI)

Medical and Family History

Taking a medical and family history can help a healthcare provider diagnose diabetes insipidus. A healthcare provider will ask the patient to review her or his symptoms and ask whether the patient's family has a history of diabetes insipidus or its symptoms.

Physical Exam

A physical exam can help diagnose diabetes insipidus. During a physical exam, a healthcare provider usually examines the patient's skin and appearance, checking for signs of dehydration.

Urinalysis

Urinalysis tests a urine sample. A patient collects the urine sample in a special container at home, in a healthcare provider's office, or at a commercial facility. A healthcare provider tests the sample in the same location or sends it to a lab for analysis. The test can show whether the urine is dilute or concentrated. The test can also show the presence of glucose, which can distinguish between diabetes insipidus and DM. The healthcare provider may also have the patient collect urine in a special container over a 24-hour period to measure the total amount of urine produced by the kidneys.

Blood Tests

A blood test involves drawing a patient's blood at a healthcare provider's office or a commercial facility and sending the sample to a lab for analysis. The blood test measures sodium levels, which can help diagnose diabetes insipidus, and in some cases determine the type.

Fluid Deprivation Test

A fluid deprivation test measures changes in a patient's body weight and urine concentration after restricting liquid intake. A healthcare provider can perform two types of fluid deprivation tests:

- **A short form of deprivation test.** A healthcare provider instructs the patient to stop drinking all liquids for a specific period of time, usually during dinner. The next morning, the patient will collect a urine sample at home. The patient then returns the urine sample to her or his healthcare provider or takes it to a lab where a technician measures the concentration of the urine sample.

- **A formal fluid deprivation test.** A healthcare provider performs this test in a hospital to continuously monitor the patient for signs of dehydration. Patients do not need anesthesia. A healthcare provider weighs the patient and analyzes a urine sample. The healthcare provider repeats the tests and measures the patient's blood pressure every one to two hours until one of the following happens:

    - The patient's blood pressure drops too low or the patient has a rapid heartbeat when standing.

- The patient loses five percent or more of her or his initial body weight.

- Urine concentration increases only slightly in two to three consecutive measurements.

At the end of the test, a healthcare provider will compare the patient's blood sodium, vasopressin levels, and urine concentration to determine whether the patient has diabetes insipidus. Sometimes, the healthcare provider may administer medications during the test to see if they increase a patient's urine concentration. In other cases, the healthcare provider may give the patient a concentrated sodium solution intravenously at the end of the test to increase the patient's blood sodium level and determine if she or he has diabetes insipidus.

Magnetic Resonance Imaging

Magnetic resonance imaging (MRI) is a test that takes pictures of the body's internal organs and soft tissues without using x-rays. A specially trained technician performs the procedure in an outpatient center or a hospital, and a radiologist—a doctor who specializes in medical imaging—interprets the images. A patient does not need anesthesia, although people with a fear of confined spaces may receive light sedation. An MRI may include an injection of a special dye, called "contrast medium." With most MRI machines, the person lies on a table that slides into a tunnel-shaped device that may be open-ended or closed at one end. Some MRI machines allow the patient to lie in a more open space. MRIs cannot diagnose diabetes insipidus. Instead, an MRI can show if the patient has problems with her or his hypothalamus or pituitary gland or help the healthcare provider determine if diabetes insipidus is the possible cause of the patient's symptoms.

How Is Diabetes Insipidus Treated?

The primary treatment for diabetes insipidus involves drinking enough liquid to prevent dehydration. A healthcare provider may refer a person with diabetes insipidus to a nephrologist—a doctor who specializes in treating kidney problems—or to an endocrinologist—a doctor who specializes in treating disorders of the hormone-producing glands. Treatment for frequent urination or constant thirst depends on the patient's type of diabetes insipidus:

- **Central diabetes insipidus.** A synthetic, or manufactured, a hormone called "desmopressin" treats central diabetes insipidus.

The medication comes as an injection, a nasal spray, or a pill. The medication works by replacing the vasopressin that a patient's body normally produces. This treatment helps a patient manage symptoms of central diabetes insipidus; however, it does not cure the disease.

- **Nephrogenic diabetes insipidus.** In some cases, nephrogenic diabetes insipidus goes away after treatment of the cause. For example, switching medications or taking steps to balance the amount of calcium or potassium in the patient's body may resolve the problem. Medications for nephrogenic diabetes insipidus include diuretics, either alone or combined with aspirin or ibuprofen. Healthcare providers commonly prescribe diuretics to help patients' kidneys remove fluid from the body. Paradoxically, in people with nephrogenic diabetes insipidus, a class of diuretics called "thiazides" reduces urine production and helps patients' kidneys concentrate urine. Aspirin or ibuprofen also helps reduce urine volume.

- **Dipsogenic diabetes insipidus.** Researchers have not yet found an effective treatment for dipsogenic diabetes insipidus. People can try sucking on ice chips or sour candies to moisten their mouths and increase saliva flow, which may reduce the desire to drink. For a person who wakes multiple times at night to urinate because of dipsogenic diabetes insipidus, taking a small dose of desmopressin at bedtime may help. Initially, the healthcare provider will monitor the patient's blood sodium levels to prevent hyponatremia or low sodium levels in the blood.

- **Gestational diabetes insipidus.** A healthcare provider can prescribe desmopressin for women with gestational diabetes insipidus. An expecting mother's placenta does not destroy desmopressin as it does vasopressin. Most women will not need treatment after delivery.

Most people with diabetes insipidus can prevent serious problems and live a normal life if they follow the healthcare provider's recommendations and keep their symptoms under control.

Eating, Diet, and Nutrition for Diabetes Insipidus

Researchers have not found that eating, diet, and nutrition play a role in causing or preventing diabetes insipidus.

Chapter 19

Prolactinomas

What Is a Prolactinoma?

A prolactinoma is a benign noncancerous tumor of the pituitary gland that produces a hormone called "prolactin." Prolactinomas are the most common type of pituitary tumor. Symptoms of prolactinoma are caused by hyperprolactinemia—too much prolactin in the blood—or by the pressure of the tumor on surrounding tissues.

Prolactin stimulates the breast to produce milk during pregnancy. After giving birth, a mother's prolactin levels fall unless she breast-feeds her infant. Each time the baby nurses, prolactin levels rise to maintain milk production.

What Is the Pituitary Gland?

The pituitary gland, sometimes called the "master gland," plays a critical role in regulating growth and development, metabolism, and reproduction. It produces prolactin and other key hormones including:

- **Growth hormone (GH)**, which regulates growth

- **Adrenocorticotropin (ACTH)**, which stimulates the adrenal glands to produce cortisol, a hormone important in metabolism and the body's response to stress

This chapter includes text excerpted from "Prolactinoma," National Institute of Diabetes and Digestive and Kidney Diseases (NIDDK), April 2019.

- **Thyrotropin**, which signals the thyroid gland to produce thyroid hormone, also involved in metabolism and growth

- **Luteinizing hormone (LH)** and **follicle-stimulating hormone (FSH)**, which regulate ovulation and estrogen and progesterone production in women and sperm formation and testosterone production in men

The pituitary gland sits in the middle of the head in a bony box called the "sella turcica." The optic nerves sit directly above the pituitary gland. Enlargement of the gland can cause symptoms such as headaches or visual disturbances. Pituitary tumors may also impair the production of one or more pituitary hormones, causing reduced pituitary function, also called "hypopituitarism."

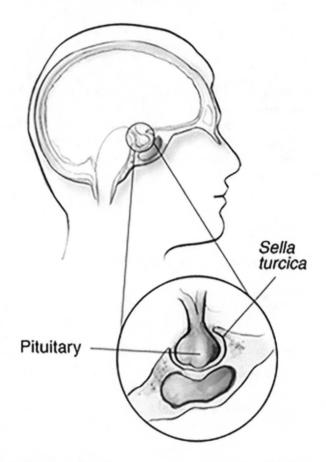

Figure 19.1. *Pituitary Gland*

How Common Is Prolactinoma

Although small-benign pituitary tumors are fairly common in the general population, symptomatic prolactinomas are uncommon. Prolactinomas occur more often in women than men and rarely occur in children.

What Are the Symptoms of Prolactinoma?

In women, high levels of prolactin in the blood often cause infertility and changes in menstruation. In some women, periods may stop. In others, periods may become irregular or menstrual flow may change. Women who are not pregnant or nursing may begin producing breast milk. Some women may experience a loss of libido-interest in sex. Intercourse may become painful because of vaginal dryness.

In men, the most common symptom of prolactinoma is erectile dysfunction. Because men have no reliable indicator such as changes in menstruation to signal a problem, many men delay going to the doctor until they have headaches or eye problems caused by the enlarged pituitary gland pressing against nearby optic nerves. They may not recognize a gradual loss of sexual function or libido. Only after treatment do some men realize they had a problem with sexual function.

What Causes Prolactinoma

The cause of pituitary tumors remains largely unknown. Most pituitary tumors are sporadic, meaning they are not genetically passed from parents to their children.

What Else Causes Prolactin to Rise

In some people, high blood levels of prolactin can be traced to causes other than prolactinoma. Some of these causes are discussed below.

Prescription drugs. Prolactin secretion in the pituitary gland is normally suppressed by the brain chemical dopamine. Drugs that block the effects of dopamine at the pituitary gland or deplete dopamine stores in the brain may cause the pituitary to secrete prolactin. These drugs include older antipsychotic medications such as trifluoperazine (Stelazine®) and haloperidol (Haldol®); the newer antipsychotic drugs risperidone (Risperdal®) and molindone (Moban®); metoclopramide (Reglan®), used to treat gastroesophageal reflux and the nausea caused by certain cancer drugs; and less often, verapamil, alpha-methyldopa

(Aldochlor®, Aldoril®), and reserpine (Serpalan®, Serpasil®), used to control high blood pressure. Some antidepressants may cause hyperprolactinemia, but further research is needed.

Other pituitary tumors. Other tumors arising in or near the pituitary gland may block the flow of dopamine from the brain to the prolactin-secreting cells. Such tumors include those that cause acromegaly, a condition caused by too much growth hormone, and Cushing syndrome, caused by too much cortisol. Other pituitary tumors that do not result in excess hormone production may also block the flow of dopamine.

Hypothyroidism. Increased prolactin levels are often seen in people with hypothyroidism, a condition in which the thyroid does not produce enough thyroid hormone. Doctors routinely test people with hyperprolactinemia for hypothyroidism.

Chest involvement. Nipple stimulation also can cause a modest increase in the amount of prolactin in the blood. Similarly, chest wall injury or shingles involving the chest wall may also cause hyperprolactinemia.

How Is Prolactinoma Diagnosed?

A doctor will test for prolactin blood levels in women with unexplained milk secretion, called "galactorrhea," or with irregular menses or infertility and in men with impaired sexual function and, in rare cases, milk secretion. If prolactin levels are high, a doctor will test thyroid function and ask first about other conditions and medications known to raise prolactin secretion. The doctor may also request magnetic resonance imaging (MRI), which is the most sensitive test for detecting pituitary tumors and determining their size. MRI scans may be repeated periodically to assess tumor progression and the effects of therapy. Computerized tomography (CT) scan also gives an image of the pituitary gland but is less precise than the MRI.

The doctor will also look for damage to surrounding tissues and perform tests to assess whether the production of other pituitary hormones is normal. Depending on the size of the tumor, the doctor may request an eye exam with measurement of visual fields.

How Is Prolactinoma Treated?

The goals of treatment are to return prolactin secretion to normal, reduce tumor size, correct any visual abnormalities, and restore normal pituitary function. In the case of large tumors, the only partial achievement of these goals may be possible.

Medical Treatment

Because dopamine is the chemical that normally inhibits prolactin secretion, doctors may treat prolactinoma with the dopamine agonists bromocriptine (Parlodel®) or cabergoline (Dostinex®). Agonists are drugs that act like a naturally occurring substance. These drugs shrink the tumor and return prolactin levels to normal in approximately 80 percent of patients. Both drugs have been approved by the U.S. Food and Drug Administration (FDA) for the treatment of hyperprolactinemia. Bromocriptine is the only dopamine agonist approved for the treatment of infertility. This drug has been in use longer than cabergoline and has a well-established safety record.

Nausea and dizziness are possible side effects of bromocriptine. To avoid these side effects, bromocriptine treatment must be started slowly. A typical starting dose is one-quarter to one-half of a 2.5 milligram (mg) tablet taken at bedtime with a snack. The dose is gradually increased every 3 to 7 days as needed and taken in divided doses with meals or at bedtime with a snack. Most people are successfully treated with 7.5mg a day or less, although some people need 15mg or more each day. Because bromocriptine is short-acting, it should be taken either twice or three times daily.

Bromocriptine treatment should not be stopped without consulting a qualified endocrinologist—a doctor specializing in disorders of the hormone-producing glands. Prolactin levels rise again in most people when the drug is discontinued. In some, however, prolactin levels remain normal, so the doctor may suggest reducing or discontinuing treatment every two years on a trial basis.

Cabergoline is a newer drug that may be more effective than bromocriptine in normalizing prolactin levels and shrinking tumor size. Cabergoline also has less frequent and less severe side effects. Cabergoline is more expensive than bromocriptine and, being newer on the market, its long-term safety record is less well defined. As with bromocriptine therapy, nausea and dizziness are possible side effects but may be avoided if treatment is started slowly. The usual starting dose is 0.25 mg twice a week. The dose may be increased every four weeks as needed, up to 1 mg two times a week. Cabergoline should not be stopped without consulting a qualified endocrinologist.

Studies suggest prolactin levels are more likely to remain normal after discontinuing long-term cabergoline therapy than after discontinuing bromocriptine.

In people taking cabergoline or bromocriptine to treat Parkinson disease at doses more than 10 times higher than those used for prolactinomas, heart valve damage has been reported. Rare cases of valve damage have been reported in people taking low doses of cabergoline to treat hyperprolactinemia. Before starting these medications, the doctor will order an echocardiogram. An echocardiogram is a sonogram of the heart that checks the heart valves and heart function.

Because limited information exists about the risks of long-term, low-dose cabergoline use, doctors generally prescribe the lowest effective dose and periodically reassess the need for continuing therapy. People taking cabergoline who develop symptoms of shortness of breath or swelling of the feet should promptly notify their physician because these may be signs of heart valve damage.

Surgery

Surgery to remove all or part of the tumor should only be considered if medical therapy cannot be tolerated or if it fails to reduce prolactin levels, restore normal reproduction and pituitary function, and reduce tumor size. If medical therapy is only partially successful, it should be continued, possibly combined with surgery or radiation.

Most often, the tumor is removed through the nasal cavity. Rarely, if the tumor is large or has spread to nearby brain tissue, the surgeon will access the tumor through an opening in the skull.

The results of surgery depend a great deal on tumor size and prolactin levels as well as the skill and experience of the neurosurgeon. The higher the prolactin level before surgery, the lower the chance of normalizing serum prolactin. Serum is the portion of the blood used in measuring prolactin levels. In the best medical centers, surgery corrects prolactin levels in about 80 percent of patients with small tumors and a serum prolactin less than 200 nanograms per milliliter (ng/ml). A surgical cure for large tumors is lower, at 30 to 40 percent. Even in patients with large tumors that cannot be completely removed, drug therapy may be able to return serum prolactin to the normal range-20 ng/ml or less-after surgery. Depending on the size of the tumor and how much of it is removed, studies show that 20 to 50 percent will recur, usually within five years.

Because the results of surgery are so dependent on the skill and knowledge of the neurosurgeon, a patient should ask the surgeon about the number of operations she or he has performed to remove pituitary tumors and for success and complication rates in comparison to major medical centers. The best results come from surgeons who have performed hundreds or even thousands of such operations.

Radiation

Rarely, radiation therapy is used if medical therapy and surgery fail to reduce prolactin levels. Depending on the size and location of the tumor, radiation is delivered in low doses over the course of 5 to 6 weeks or in a single high dose. Radiation therapy is effective about 30 percent of the time.

How Does Prolactinoma Affect Pregnancy?

If a woman has a small prolactinoma, she can usually conceive and have a normal pregnancy after effective medical therapy. If she had a successful pregnancy before, the chance of her having more successful pregnancies is high.

A woman with prolactinoma should discuss her plans to conceive with her physician so she can be carefully evaluated prior to becoming pregnant. This evaluation will include an MRI scan to assess the size of the tumor and an eye examination with measurement of visual fields. As soon as a woman is pregnant, her doctor will usually advise her to stop taking bromocriptine or cabergoline. Although these drugs are safe for the fetus in early pregnancy, their safety throughout an entire pregnancy has not been established. Many doctors prefer to use bromocriptine in patients who plan to become pregnant because it has a longer record of safety in early pregnancy than cabergoline.

The pituitary gland enlarges and prolactin production increases during pregnancy in women without pituitary disorders. Women with prolactin-secreting tumors may experience further pituitary enlargement and must be closely monitored during pregnancy. Less than three percent of pregnant women with small prolactinomas have symptoms of tumor growth such as headaches or vision problems. In women with large prolactinomas, the risk of symptomatic tumor growth is greater, and may be as high as 30 percent.

Most endocrinologists see patients every two months throughout the pregnancy. A woman should consult her endocrinologist promptly if she develops symptoms of tumor growth, particularly headaches, vision changes, nausea, vomiting, excessive thirst or urination, or extreme lethargy. Bromocriptine or, less often, cabergoline treatment may be reinitiated and additional treatment may be required if the woman develops symptoms during pregnancy.

129

How Do Oral Contraceptives and Hormone Replacement Therapy Affect Prolactinoma?

Oral contraceptives are not thought to contribute to the development of prolactinomas, although some studies have found increased prolactin levels in women taking these medications. Because oral contraceptives may produce regular menstrual bleeding in women who would otherwise have irregular menses due to hyperprolactinemia, prolactinoma may not be diagnosed until women stop oral contraceptives and find their menses are absent or irregular. Women with prolactinoma treated with bromocriptine or cabergoline may safely take oral contraceptives. Similarly, postmenopausal women treated with medical therapy or surgery for prolactinoma may be candidates for estrogen replacement therapy.

Is Osteoporosis a Risk in Women with High Prolactin Levels?

Women whose ovaries produce inadequate estrogen are at increased risk for osteoporosis. Hyperprolactinemia can reduce estrogen production. Although estrogen production may be restored after treatment for hyperprolactinemia, even a year or two without estrogen can compromise bone strength. Women should protect themselves from osteoporosis by increasing exercise and calcium intake through diet or supplements and by not smoking. Women treated for hyperprolactinemia may want to have periodic bone density measurements and discuss estrogen replacement therapy or other bone-strengthening medications with their doctor.

Chapter 20

Pituitary Tumors and Treatment Options

What Is a Pituitary Tumor?

A pituitary tumor is a growth of abnormal cells in the tissues of the pituitary gland.

Pituitary tumors form in the pituitary gland, a pea-sized organ in the center of the brain, just above the back of the nose. The pituitary gland is sometimes called the "master endocrine gland" because it makes hormones that affect the way many parts of the body work. It also controls hormones made by many other glands in the body.

Pituitary tumors are divided into three groups:

- **Benign pituitary adenomas** are the tumors that are not cancer. These tumors grow very slowly and do not spread from the pituitary gland to other parts of the body.

- **Invasive pituitary adenomas** are benign tumors that may spread to bones of the skull or the sinus cavity below the pituitary gland.

- **Pituitary carcinomas** are tumors that are malignant (cancer). These pituitary tumors spread into other areas of the central

---

This chapter includes text excerpted from "Pituitary Tumors Treatment (PDQ®)—Patient Version," National Cancer Institute (NCI), May 21, 2019.

nervous system (CNS) or outside of the CNS. Very few pituitary tumors are malignant.

Pituitary tumors may be either nonfunctioning or functioning.

- **Nonfunctioning pituitary tumors** do not make extra amounts of hormones.

- **Functioning pituitary tumors** make more than the normal amount of one or more hormones. Most pituitary tumors are functioning tumors. The extra hormones made by pituitary tumors may cause certain signs or symptoms of disease.

The Pituitary-Gland Hormones

Hormones made by the pituitary gland include:

- **Prolactin** is a hormone that causes a woman's breasts to make milk during and after pregnancy.

- **Adrenocorticotropic hormone (ACTH)** causes the adrenal glands to make a hormone called "cortisol." Cortisol helps control the use of sugar, protein, and fats in the body and helps the body deal with stress.

- **Growth hormone (GH)** helps control body growth and the use of sugar and fat in the body. Growth hormone is also called "somatotropin."

- **Thyroid-stimulating hormone (TSH)** causes the thyroid gland to make other hormones that control growth, body temperature, and heart rate. Thyroid-stimulating hormone is also called "thyrotropin."

- **Luteinizing hormone (LH)** and **follicle-stimulating hormone (FSH)** control the menstrual cycle in women and the making of sperm in men.

Risk Factors of Pituitary Tumors

Anything that increases your risk of getting a disease is called a "risk factor." Having a risk factor does not mean that you will get cancer; not having risk factors does not mean that you will not get cancer. Talk with your doctor if you think you may be at risk. Risk factors for pituitary tumors include having the following hereditary diseases:

- Multiple endocrine neoplasia type 1 (MEN1) syndrome
- Carney complex
- Isolated familial acromegaly

Signs and Symptoms of Pituitary Tumors

Signs and symptoms can be caused by the growth of the tumor and/or by hormones the tumor makes or by other conditions. Some tumors may not cause signs or symptoms. Check with your doctor if you have any of these problems.

Signs and Symptoms of a Nonfunctioning Pituitary Tumor

Sometimes, a pituitary tumor may press on or damage parts of the pituitary gland, causing it to stop making one or more hormones. Too little of a certain hormone will affect the work of the gland or organ that the hormone controls. The following signs and symptoms may occur:

- Headache
- Some loss of vision
- Loss of body hair
- In women, less frequent or no menstrual periods or no milk from the breasts
- In men, loss of facial hair, growth of breast tissue, and impotence
- In women and men, lower sex drive
- In children, slowed growth and sexual development

Most of the tumors that make LH and FSH do not make enough extra hormone to cause signs and symptoms. These tumors are considered to be nonfunctioning tumors.

Signs and Symptoms of a Functioning Pituitary Tumor

When a functioning pituitary tumor makes extra hormones, the signs and symptoms will depend on the type of hormone being made.
Too much prolactin may cause:

- Headache
- Some loss of vision

133

- Less frequent or no menstrual periods or menstrual periods with a very light flow
- Trouble becoming pregnant or an inability to become pregnant
- Impotence in men
- Lower sex drive
- Flow of breast milk in a woman who is not pregnant or breast-feeding

Too much ACTH may cause:

- Headache
- Some loss of vision
- Weight gain in the face, neck, and trunk of the body, and thin arms and legs
- A lump of fat on the back of the neck
- Thin skin that may have purple or pink stretch marks on the chest or abdomen
- Easy bruising
- Growth of fine hair on the face, upper back, or arms
- Bones that break easily
- Anxiety, irritability, and depression

Too much growth hormone may cause:

- Headache
- Some loss of vision
- In adults, acromegaly (growth of the bones in the face, hands, and feet). In children, the whole body may grow much taller and larger than normal.
- Tingling or numbness in the hands and fingers
- Snoring or pauses in breathing during sleep
- Joint pain
- Sweating more than usual
- Dysmorphophobia (extreme dislike of or concern about one or more parts of the body)

Too much thyroid-stimulating hormone may cause:

- Irregular heartbeat
- Shakiness
- Weight loss
- Trouble sleeping
- Frequent bowel movements
- Sweating

Other general signs and symptoms of pituitary tumors:

- Nausea and vomiting
- Confusion
- Dizziness
- Seizures
- Runny or "drippy" nose (cerebrospinal fluid (CSF) that surrounds the brain and spinal cord leaks into the nose)

How to Detect and Diagnose a Pituitary Tumor

The following tests and procedures may be used to detect and diagnose a pituitary tumor:

- **Physical examination and history:** An examination of the body to check general signs of health, including checking for signs of disease, such as lumps or anything else that seems unusual. A history of the patient's health habits and past illnesses and treatments will also be taken.

- **Eye examination:** An examination to check vision and the general health of the eyes.

- **Visual field examination:** An examination to check a person's field of vision (the total area in which objects can be seen). This test measures both central vision (how much a person can see when looking straight ahead) and peripheral vision (how much a person can see in all other directions while staring straight ahead). The eyes are tested one at a time. The eye not being tested is covered.

- **Neurological examination:** A series of questions and tests to check the brain, spinal cord, and nerve function. The exam

135

checks a person's mental status, coordination, and ability to walk normally, and how well the muscles, senses, and reflexes work. This may also be called a "neuro examination" or a "neurologic examination."

- **Magnetic resonance imaging (MRI) with gadolinium:** A procedure that uses a magnet, radio waves, and a computer to make a series of detailed pictures of areas inside the brain and spinal cord. A substance called "gadolinium" is injected into a vein. The gadolinium collects around the cancer cells so they show up brighter in the picture. This procedure is also called "nuclear magnetic resonance imaging" (NMRI).

- **Blood chemistry study:** A procedure in which a blood sample is checked to measure the amounts of certain substances, such as glucose (sugar), released into the blood by organs and tissues in the body. An unusual (higher or lower than normal) amount of a substance can be a sign of disease.

- **Blood tests:** Tests to measure the levels of testosterone or estrogen in the blood. A higher or lower than normal amount of these hormones may be a sign of pituitary tumor.

- **Twenty-four-hour urine test:** A test in which urine is collected for 24 hours to measure the amounts of certain substances. An unusual (higher or lower than normal) amount of a substance can be a sign of disease in the organ or tissue that makes it. A higher than normal amount of the hormone cortisol may be a sign of a pituitary tumor and Cushing syndrome.

- **High-dose dexamethasone suppression test:** A test in which one or more high doses of dexamethasone are given. The level of cortisol is checked from a sample of blood or from urine that is collected for three days. This test is done to check if the adrenal gland is making too much cortisol or if the pituitary gland is telling the adrenal glands to make too much cortisol.

- **Low-dose dexamethasone suppression test:** A test in which one or more small doses of dexamethasone are given. The level of cortisol is checked from a sample of blood or from urine that is collected for three days. This test is done to check if the adrenal gland is making too much cortisol.

- **Venous sampling for pituitary tumors:** A procedure in which a sample of blood is taken from veins coming from the pituitary gland. The sample is checked to measure the amount of ACTH released into the blood by the gland. Venous sampling may be done if blood tests show there is a tumor making ACTH, but the pituitary gland looks normal in the imaging tests.

- **Biopsy:** The removal of cells or tissues so they can be viewed under a microscope by a pathologist to check for signs of cancer.

The following tests may be done on the sample of tissue that is removed:

- **Immunohistochemistry:** A test that uses antibodies to check for certain antigens in a sample of tissue. The antibody is usually linked to a radioactive substance or a dye that causes the tissue to light up under a microscope. This type of test may be used to tell the difference between different types of cancer.

- **Immunocytochemistry:** A test that uses antibodies to check for certain antigens in a sample of cells. The antibody is usually linked to a radioactive substance or a dye that causes the cells to light up under a microscope. This type of test may be used to tell the difference between different types of cancer.

- **Light and electron microscopy:** A laboratory test in which cells in a sample of tissue are viewed under regular and high-powered microscopes to look for certain changes in the cells.

Factors Affecting Prognosis and Treatment Options for Pituitary Tumors

The prognosis depends on the type of tumor and whether the tumor has spread into other areas of the CNS (brain and spinal cord) or outside of the CNS to other parts of the body.

Treatment options depend on the following:

- The type and size of the tumor

- Whether the tumor is making hormones

- Whether the tumor is causing problems with vision or other signs or symptoms

- Whether the tumor has spread into the brain around the pituitary gland or to other parts of the body

- Whether the tumor has just been diagnosed or has recurred

137

Stages of Pituitary Tumors

The extent or spread of cancer is usually described as stages. There is no standard staging system for pituitary tumors. Once a pituitary tumor is found, tests are done to find out if the tumor has spread into the brain or to other parts of the body. The following test may be used:

- **Magnetic resonance imaging.** A procedure that uses a magnet, radio waves, and a computer to make a series of detailed pictures of areas inside the body. This procedure is also called "nuclear magnetic resonance imaging" (NMRI).

Pituitary tumors are described by their size and grade, whether or not they make extra hormones, and whether the tumor has spread to other parts of the body. The following sizes are used:

- **Microadenoma.** The tumor is smaller than one centimeter.

- **Macroadenoma.** The tumor is one centimeter or larger.

Most pituitary adenomas are microadenomas.

The grade of a pituitary tumor is based on how far it has grown into the surrounding area of the brain, including the sella (the bone at the base of the skull, where the pituitary gland sits).

Recurrent Pituitary Tumors

A recurrent pituitary tumor is cancer that has recurred after it has been treated. The cancer may come back in the pituitary gland or in other parts of the body.

Treatment Options for Pituitary Tumors

Different types of treatments are available for patients with pituitary tumors. Some treatments are standard (the currently used treatment), and some are being tested in clinical trials. A treatment clinical trial is a research study meant to help improve current treatments or obtain information on new treatments for patients with cancer. When clinical trials show that a new treatment is better than the standard treatment, the new treatment may become the standard treatment. Patients may want to think about taking part in a clinical trial. Some clinical trials are open only to patients who have not started treatment.

Types of Standard Treatment
Surgery

Many pituitary tumors can be removed by surgery using one of the following operations:

- **Transsphenoidal surgery:** A type of surgery in which the instruments are inserted into part of the brain by going through an incision (cut) made under the upper lip or at the bottom of the nose between the nostrils and then through the sphenoid bone (a butterfly-shaped bone at the base of the skull) to reach the pituitary gland. The pituitary gland lies just above the sphenoid bone.

- **Endoscopic transsphenoidal surgery:** A type of surgery in which an endoscope is inserted through an incision (cut) made at the back of the inside of the nose and then through the sphenoid bone to reach the pituitary gland. An endoscope is a thin, tube-like instrument with a light, a lens for viewing, and a tool for removing tumor tissue.

- **Craniotomy:** Surgery to remove the tumor through an opening made in the skull.

After the doctor removes all the cancer that can be seen at the time of the surgery, some patients may be given chemotherapy or radiation therapy after surgery to kill any cancer cells that are left. Treatment given after the surgery, to lower the risk that the cancer will come back, is called "adjuvant therapy."

Radiation Therapy

Radiation therapy is a cancer treatment that uses high-energy x-rays or other types of radiation to kill cancer cells or keep them from growing. There are two types of radiation therapy:

- **External radiation therapy** uses a machine outside the body to send radiation toward the cancer. Certain ways of giving radiation therapy can help keep radiation from damaging nearby healthy tissue. This type of radiation therapy may include the following:

  - **Stereotactic radiosurgery:** A rigid head frame is attached to the skull to keep the head still during the radiation treatment. A machine aims a single large dose of radiation directly at the tumor. This procedure does not involve surgery. It is also called "stereotaxic radiosurgery," "radiosurgery," and "radiation surgery."

- **Internal radiation therapy** uses a radioactive substance sealed in needles, seeds, wires, or catheters that are placed directly into or near the cancer.

The way the radiation therapy is given depends on the type of the cancer being treated. External radiation therapy is used to treat pituitary tumors.

Drug Therapy

Drugs may be given to stop a functioning pituitary tumor from making too many hormones.

Chemotherapy

Chemotherapy may be used as palliative treatment for pituitary carcinomas, to relieve symptoms and improve the patient's quality of life (QOL). Chemotherapy uses drugs to stop the growth of cancer cells, either by killing the cells or by stopping them from dividing. When chemotherapy is taken by mouth or injected into a vein or muscle, the drugs enter the bloodstream and can reach cancer cells throughout the body (systemic chemotherapy). When chemotherapy is placed directly into the cerebrospinal fluid (CBF), an organ, or a body cavity such as the abdomen, the drugs mainly affect cancer cells in those areas (regional chemotherapy). The way the chemotherapy is given depends on the type of the cancer being treated.

Follow-Up Tests May Be Needed

Some of the tests that were done to diagnose the cancer or to find out the stage of the cancer may be repeated. Some tests will be repeated in order to see how well the treatment is working. Decisions about whether to continue, change, or stop treatment may be based on the results of these tests.

Some of the tests will continue to be done from time to time after treatment has ended. The results of these tests can show if your condition has changed or if the cancer has recurred. These tests are sometimes called "follow-up tests" or "check-ups."

Chapter 21

Pituitary Disorders and Treatment Options

The pituitary gland, also known as "master gland," is a pea-sized organ producing hormones that are responsible for regulating a wide range of biological functions including:

- Metabolism

- Growth

- Blood pressure

- Sexual maturation and function

Parts of a Pituitary Gland

The pituitary gland controls the function of the other endocrine glands and is comprised of three parts:

- Anterior lobe

- Intermediate lobe

- Posterior lobe

The Anterior Lobe

The anterior lobe comprises about 80 percent of the pituitary gland and secretes hormones such as:

- **Adrenocorticotropic hormone (ACTH).** This helps the adrenal gland to secrete hormones, chiefly cortisol.

- **Growth hormone (GH).** This helps to regulate the body's growth, metabolism, and composition.

- **Thyroid-stimulating hormone (TSH).** This causes the thyroid gland to secrete hormones.

- **Gonadotropins**—luteinizing hormone (LH) and follicle-stimulating hormone (FSH). This helps the ovaries and testes in the secretion of sex hormones involved in reproduction.

- **Prolactin.** This helps stimulate milk production in women after childbirth.

The Intermediate Lobe

This part of the pituitary gland produces only one hormone:

- **Melanocyte-stimulating hormone.** This hormone affects skin pigmentation.

The Posterior Lobe

This part of the pituitary gland stores two hormones that are produced by the hypothalamus:

- **Antidiuretic hormone (ADH).** This hormone, also known as "vasopressin," helps in regulating water and electrolyte balance.

- **Oxytocin.** This hormone helps in the production and release of breast milk and is also involved in the uterine contractions during childbirth.

What Are Pituitary-Gland Disorders?

Pituitary-gland disorders are certain conditions that are caused by the overactivity of the pituitary gland and the excessive or low secretion of few hormones. This occurs due to the presence of a noncancerous tumor known as a "benign tumor."

Pituitary disorders include:

- Cushing syndrome (hypercortisolism)
- Acromegaly
- Prolactinoma
- Hyperthyroidism

Diagnosis of Pituitary-Gland Disorders

Pituitary-gland disorders are diagnosed through a physical examination that includes:

- **Blood and urine tests.** Overproduction or deficiency of hormones can be determined using this test.
- **Brain imaging.** The location and the size of the tumor can be checked using a magnetic resonance imaging (MRI) or computerized tomography (CT) scan.
- **Vision imaging.** This test helps in determining if the pituitary tumor has affected the peripheral vision or sight.

Treatment Options for Pituitary-Gland Disorders

Treatment methods for pituitary-gland disorders will vary depending on the underlying cause. The treatment options include surgery, medication, and radiotherapy.

Surgical Treatment

Surgical methods used in the treatment of pituitary disorders are discussed below:

Transsphenoidal adenoidectomy. This surgical method is used in the treatment of acromegaly or Cushing syndrome. This method is more effective for small tumors (under 10mm in diameter). The tumor is removed by making a small incision through the upper lip or nose. The success rate of this surgery is more than 80 percent if performed by experienced surgeons. After-effects of this surgery may or do include:

- Long-term dependence on pituitary hormone-replacement therapy
- Cerebrospinal fluid leakage

3-D Endoscopy. This surgical method is performed using a tool that provides three-dimensional stereotypic vision. The optic camera at the end of the narrow endoscopy tube helps the surgeon to view and navigate the delicate area at the base of the brain. After-effects of this surgical method might include:

- Hormone-replacement therapy
- Diabetes insipidus
- Cerebrospinal fluid leakage leading to meningitis, which would require further surgery
- Damage to carotid arteries during surgery may lead to stroke or blood loss.
- Damage in the sinus cavity during surgery can cause nasal deformity or sinus congestion.

Craniotomy. This surgical treatment is used if the tumor growth is large. This method involves the removal of the bone flap from the skull to reach the tumor. After-effects of this surgical method include:

- The same after-effects as those of a 3-D endoscopy
- Blood clots or brain swelling

Radiosurgery. Highly focused beams of radiation are used when a complete tumor cannot be removed using medication or surgery. This method of treatment works gradually. If the symptoms are severe, pituitary doctors will warrant another fast-acting form of treatment. The after-effects of this treatment might include:

- Swelling or edema
- Irritation of the skin, which may later itch, blister, or peel

Medication

Drugs are used when certain conditions do not require surgery, or if the tumor is too large to perform surgery. Certain drugs can be used to reduce prolactin levels and are usually used to treat patients with prolactinoma. Patients suffering from acromegaly can be treated using drugs to lower hormone levels and shrink the size of tumors.

Radiation

Patients who cannot undergo surgery or have residual tumors that are not completely removed after surgery or patients who do not respond to medications are treated using radiation method. There are two types of radiation treatments: conventional radiation therapy and stereotactic therapy

Conventional radiation therapy. Small doses of radiation are given over a period of four to six weeks. This radiation treatment can damage the normal tissue surrounding the tumor.

Stereotactic therapy. This method involves a high dose of radiation that targets the tumor. This therapy is mostly completed in a single session to avoid much damage to the tissues surrounding the tumor. The main after-effect of this therapy is that the patient will require a hormone-replacement therapy after this treatment, as there will be a gradual decline in the secretion of other pituitary hormones.

Treatment for Hormone Deficiency

Growth hormone. Recombinant growth hormone (RGH) is injected under the skin once daily.

Luteinizing hormone (LH) and FSH. For men, testosterone is injected under the skin once daily. For women, estrogen and progesterone are given either in the form of topical patch or pills.

Adrenocorticotropic hormone. Hydrocortisone or prednisone are given as a daily pill.

Thyroid-stimulating hormone (TSH). Levothyroxine is given as a daily pill.

Prolactin. There is no treatment available for prolactin.

Vasopressin. Desmopressin is either given as daily pills or as a nasal spray.

References

1. "Pituitary Gland: Hyperpituitarism (Overactive Pituitary Gland)," Cleveland Clinic, December 2013.

2. "Disorders," Pituitary Network Association, October 27, 2007.

3. "Surgical Treatments," Emory Woodruff Health Sciences Center, December 12, 2010.

4. "Pituitary Tumors," Mayo Foundation for Medical Education and Research (MFMER), March 16, 2019.

Part Three

Thyroid and Parathyroid Gland Disorders

Chapter 22

Overview of Thyroid and Parathyroid Disorders

What Are Thyroid Disorders?

You have probably heard of the thyroid gland, but do you know what it does? You might not give it a second thought unless something goes wrong. Thyroid trouble can cause a range of seemingly unrelated problems, including drastic changes to your weight, energy, digestion, or mood.

The thyroid is a small but powerful butterfly-shaped gland located at the front of your neck. It controls many of your body's most important functions. The thyroid gland makes hormones that affect your breathing, heart rate, digestion, and body temperature. These systems speed up as thyroid hormone levels rise. But problems occur if the thyroid makes too much hormone or not enough.

Nearly 1 in 20 Americans ages 12 and older has an under-active thyroid, or hypothyroidism. When thyroid glands do not produce enough hormones, many body functions slow down. A smaller number

This chapter contains text excerpted from the following sources: Text under the heading "What Are Thyroid Disorders?" is excerpted from "Thinking about Your Thyroid," *NIH News in Health*, National Institutes of Health (NIH), September 2015, Reviewed September 2019; Text under the heading "What Are Parathyroid Disorders?" is excerpted from "Parathyroid Disorders," MedlinePlus, National Institutes of Health (NIH), June 13, 2016. Reviewed September 2019.

of people—about 1 in 100—has an over-active thyroid, called "hyper-thyroidism." Their thyroids release too much hormone.

Thyroid problems are most likely to occur in women or in people over age 60. Having a family history of thyroid disorders also increases the risk.

Learn to recognize signs of thyroid disorder. If you notice signs of thyroid disease, talk with a healthcare provider. Based on your family history, symptoms, and medical exam, your healthcare provider can help you decide if further testing or treatment is needed.

*Types, Diagnosis, and Treatment of Thyroid Disorders**

Thyroid problems include:

- **Goiter** is the enlargement of the thyroid gland.

- **Hyperthyroidism** is when your thyroid gland makes more thyroid hormones than your body needs.

- **Hypothyroidism** is when your thyroid gland does not make enough thyroid hormones.

- **Thyroid cancer**

- **Thyroid nodules** are the lumps in the thyroid gland.

- **Thyroiditis** is the swelling of the thyroid.

To diagnose thyroid diseases, doctors use a medical history, physical exam, and thyroid tests. They sometimes also use a biopsy.

Treatment depends on the problem, but may include medicines, radioiodine therapy, or thyroid surgery.

*Text excerpted from "Thyroid Diseases," MedlinePlus, National Institutes of Health (NIH), June 13, 2018.

What Are Parathyroid Disorders?

Most people have four pea-sized glands, called "parathyroid glands," on the thyroid gland in the neck. Though their names are similar, the thyroid and parathyroid glands are completely different. The parathyroid glands make parathyroid hormone (PTH), which helps your body keep the right balance of calcium and phosphorous.

If your parathyroid glands make too much or too little hormone, it disrupts this balance. If they secrete extra PTH, you have hyperparathyroidism, and your blood calcium rises. In many cases, a benign tumor on a parathyroid gland makes it overactive. Or, the extra hormones can come from enlarged parathyroid glands. Very rarely, the cause is cancer.

If you do not have enough PTH, you have hypoparathyroidism. Your blood will have too little calcium and too much phosphorous. Causes include injury to the glands, endocrine disorders, or genetic conditions. Treatment is aimed at restoring the balance of calcium and phosphorous.

Chapter 23

Thyroid Gland Disorders

Chapter Contents

Section 23.1

Hypothyroidism

This section includes text excerpted from "Hypothyroidism (Underactive Thyroid)," National Institute of Diabetes and Digestive and Kidney Diseases (NIDDK), August 20, 2016. Reviewed September 2019.

What Is Hypothyroidism?

Hypothyroidism, also called "underactive thyroid," is when the thyroid gland does not make enough thyroid hormones to meet your body's needs. The thyroid is a small, butterfly-shaped gland in the front of your neck. Thyroid hormones control the way the body uses energy, so they affect nearly every organ in your body, even the way your heartbeats. Without enough thyroid hormones, many of your body's functions slow down.

How Common Is Hypothyroidism?

About 4.6 percent of the U.S. population ages 12 and older has hypothyroidism, although most cases are mild. That is almost 5 people out of 100.

Who Is More Likely to Develop Hypothyroidism?

Women are much more likely than men to develop hypothyroidism. The disease is also more common among people older than age 60.
You are more likely to have hypothyroidism if you:

- Have had a thyroid problem before, such as a goiter
- Have had surgery to correct a thyroid problem
- Have received radiation treatment to the thyroid, neck, or chest
- Have a family history of thyroid disease
- Were pregnant in the past six months
- Have Turner syndrome, a genetic disorder that affects females
- Have other health problems, including:
  - Sjögren syndrome, a disease that causes dry eyes and mouth
  - Pernicious anemia, a condition caused by a vitamin B_{12} deficiency

- Type 1 diabetes
- Rheumatoid arthritis, an autoimmune disease that affects the joints
- Lupus, a chronic inflammatory condition

Is Hypothyroidism during Pregnancy a Problem?

Hypothyroidism that is not treated can affect both the mother and the baby. However, thyroid medicines can help prevent problems and are safe to take during pregnancy.

What Other Health Problems Could You Have Because of Hypothyroidism?

Hypothyroidism can contribute to high cholesterol, so people with high cholesterol should be tested for hypothyroidism. Rarely, severe, untreated hypothyroidism may lead to myxedema coma, an extreme form of hypothyroidism in which the body's functions slow to the point that it becomes life-threatening. Myxedema coma requires immediate medical treatment.

What Are the Symptoms of Hypothyroidism?

Hypothyroidism has many symptoms that can vary from person to person. Some common symptoms of hypothyroidism include:

- Fatigue
- Weight gain
- A puffy face
- Trouble tolerating cold
- Joint and muscle pain
- Constipation
- Dry skin
- Dry, thinning hair
- Decreased sweating
- Heavy or irregular menstrual periods
- Fertility problems

- Depression
- Slowed heart rate
- Goiter

Because hypothyroidism develops slowly, many people do not notice symptoms of the disease for months or even years.

Many of these symptoms, especially fatigue and weight gain, are common and do not always mean that someone has a thyroid problem.

What Causes Hypothyroidism

Hypothyroidism has several causes, including:

- Hashimoto disease
- Thyroiditis, or inflammation of the thyroid
- Congenital hypothyroidism, or hypothyroidism that is present at birth
- Surgical removal of part or all of the thyroid
- Radiation treatment of the thyroid
- Some medicines

Less often, hypothyroidism is caused by too much or too little iodine in the diet or by pituitary disease.

Hashimoto Disease

Hashimoto disease is the most common cause of hypothyroidism. Hashimoto disease is an autoimmune disorder. With this disease, your immune system attacks the thyroid. The thyroid becomes inflamed and cannot make enough thyroid hormones.

Thyroiditis

Thyroiditis is an inflammation of your thyroid that causes stored thyroid hormone to leak out of your thyroid gland. At first, the leakage increases hormone levels in the blood, leading to hyperthyroidism, a condition in which thyroid hormone levels are too high. The hyperthyroidism may last for up to 3 months, after which your thyroid may become underactive. The resulting hypothyroidism usually lasts 12 to 18 months, but sometimes is permanent.

Several types of thyroiditis can cause hyperthyroidism and then cause hypothyroidism:

- **Subacute thyroiditis.** This condition involves a painfully inflamed and enlarged thyroid. Experts are not sure what causes subacute thyroiditis, but it may be related to an infection caused by a virus or bacteria.

- **Postpartum thyroiditis.** This type of thyroiditis develops after a woman gives birth.

- **Silent thyroiditis.** This type of thyroiditis is called "silent" because it is painless, even though your thyroid may be enlarged. Experts think silent thyroiditis is probably an autoimmune condition.

Congenital Hypothyroidism

Some babies are born with a thyroid that is not fully developed or does not function properly. If untreated, congenital hypothyroidism can lead to intellectual disability and growth failure—when a baby does not grow as expected. Early treatment can prevent these problems, which is why most newborns in the United States are tested for hypothyroidism.

Surgical Removal of Part or All of the Thyroid

When surgeons remove part of the thyroid, the remaining part may produce normal amounts of thyroid hormone, but some people who have this surgery develop hypothyroidism. Removal of the entire thyroid always results in hypothyroidism.

Surgeons may remove part or all of the thyroid as a treatment for:

- Hyperthyroidism

- A large goiter

- Thyroid nodules, which are noncancerous tumors or lumps in the thyroid that can produce too much thyroid hormone

- Thyroid cancer

Radiation Treatment of the Thyroid

Radioactive iodine, a common treatment for hyperthyroidism, gradually destroys the cells of the thyroid. Most people who receive radioactive iodine treatment eventually develop hypothyroidism. Doctors treat people with head or neck cancers with radiation, which can also damage the thyroid.

Medicines

Some medicines can interfere with thyroid hormone production and lead to hypothyroidism, including:

- Amiodarone, a heart medicine
- Interferon-alpha, a cancer medicine
- Lithium, a bipolar disorder medicine
- Interleukin-2, a kidney cancer medicine

How Do Doctors Diagnose Hypothyroidism?

Your doctor will take a medical history and do a physical exam, but also will need to do some tests to confirm a diagnosis of hypothyroidism. Many symptoms of hypothyroidism are the same as those of other diseases, so doctors usually cannot diagnose hyperthyroidism based on symptoms alone.

Because hypothyroidism can cause fertility problems, women who have trouble getting pregnant often get tested for thyroid problems.

Your doctor may use several blood tests to confirm a diagnosis of hypothyroidism and find its cause.

How Is Hypothyroidism Treated?

Hypothyroidism is treated by replacing the hormone that your thyroid can no longer make. You will take levothyroxine, a thyroid hormone medicine that is identical to a hormone the thyroid normally makes. Your doctor may recommend taking the medicine in the morning before eating.

Your doctor will give you a blood test about 6 to 8 weeks after you begin taking thyroid hormone and adjust your dose if needed. Each time your dose is adjusted, you will have another blood test. Once you have reached a dose that is working for you, your healthcare provider will probably repeat the blood test in six months and then once a year.

Your hypothyroidism most likely can be completely controlled with thyroid hormone medicine, as long as you take the recommended dose as instructed. Never stop taking your medicine without talking with your healthcare provider first.

What Should You Eat or Avoid Eating If You Have Hypothyroidism?

The thyroid uses iodine to make thyroid hormones. However, people with Hashimoto disease or other types of autoimmune-thyroid disorders may be sensitive to harmful side effects from iodine. Eating foods that have large amounts of iodine—such as kelp, dulse, or other kinds of seaweed—may cause or worsen hypothyroidism. Taking iodine supplements can have the same effect.

Talk with members of your healthcare team about what foods you should limit or avoid, and let them know if you take iodine supplements. Also, share information about any cough syrups that you take because they may contain iodine.

Women need more iodine when they are pregnant because the baby gets iodine from the mother's diet. If you are pregnant, talk with your healthcare provider about how much iodine you need.

Section 23.2

Congenital Hypothyroidism

This section contains text excerpted from the following sources:
Text in this section begins with excerpts from "Congenital
Hypothyroidism," Genetics Home Reference (GHR), National
Institutes of Health (NIH), September 2015. Reviewed September
2019; Text under the heading "Diagnosis of Congenital
Hypothyroidism" is excerpted from "Congenital Hypothyroidism,"
Genetic and Rare Diseases Information Center (GARD), National
Center for Advancing Translational Sciences (NCATS), February 19,
2016. Reviewed September 2019.

Congenital hypothyroidism is a partial or complete loss of function
of the thyroid gland (hypothyroidism) that affects infants from birth
(congenital). The thyroid gland is a butterfly-shaped tissue in the lower
neck. It makes iodine-containing hormones that play an important
role in regulating growth, brain development, and the rate of chemical
reactions in the body (metabolism). People with congenital hypothyroidism have lower-than-normal levels of these important hormones.

Congenital hypothyroidism occurs when the thyroid gland fails
to develop or function properly. In 80 to 85 percent of cases, the thyroid gland is absent, severely reduced in size (hypoplastic), or abnormally located. These cases are classified as thyroid dysgenesis. In the
remainder of cases, a normal-sized or enlarged thyroid gland (goiter)
is present, but the production of thyroid hormones is decreased or
absent. Most of these cases occur when one of several steps in the
hormone synthesis process is impaired; these cases are classified as
thyroid dyshormonogenesis. Less commonly, reduction or absence of
thyroid hormone production is caused by impaired stimulation of the
production process (which is normally done by a structure at the base
of the brain called the "pituitary gland"), even though the process
itself is unimpaired. These cases are classified as central (or pituitary)
hypothyroidism.

Signs and Symptoms of Congenital Hypothyroidism

Signs and symptoms of congenital hypothyroidism result from the
shortage of thyroid hormones. Affected babies may show no features
of the condition, although some babies with congenital hypothyroidism are less active and sleep more than normal. They may have difficulty feeding and experience constipation. If untreated, congenital

hypothyroidism can lead to intellectual disability and slow growth. In the United States and many other countries, all hospitals test newborns for congenital hypothyroidism. If treatment begins in the first two weeks after birth, infants usually develop normally.

Congenital hypothyroidism can also occur as part of syndromes that affect other organs and tissues in the body. These forms of the condition are described as syndromic. Some common forms of syndromic hypothyroidism include Pendred syndrome, Bamforth-Lazarus syndrome, and brain-lung-thyroid syndrome.

Frequency of Congenital Hypothyroidism

Congenital hypothyroidism affects an estimated 1 in 2,000 to 4,000 newborns. For reasons that remain unclear, congenital hypothyroidism affects more than twice as many females as males.

Causes of Congenital Hypothyroidism

Congenital hypothyroidism can be caused by a variety of factors, only some of which are genetic. The most common cause worldwide is a shortage of iodine in the diet of the mother and the affected infant. Iodine is essential for the production of thyroid hormones. Genetic causes account for about 15 to 20 percent of cases of congenital hypothyroidism.

The cause of the most common type of congenital hypothyroidism, thyroid dysgenesis, is usually unknown. Studies suggest that two to five percent of cases are inherited. Two of the genes involved in this form of the condition are *PAX8* and *TSHR*. These genes play roles in the proper growth and development of the thyroid gland. Mutations in these genes prevent or disrupt the normal development of the gland. The abnormal or missing gland cannot produce normal amounts of thyroid hormones.

Thyroid dyshormonogenesis results from mutations in one of several genes involved in the production of thyroid hormones. These genes include *DUOX2*, *SLC5A5*, *TG*, and *TPO*. Mutations in each of these genes disrupt a step in thyroid hormone synthesis, leading to abnormally low levels of these hormones. Mutations in the *TSHB* gene disrupt the synthesis of thyroid hormones by impairing the stimulation of hormone production. Changes in this gene are the primary cause of central hypothyroidism. The resulting shortage of thyroid hormones disrupts normal growth, brain development, and metabolism, leading to the features of congenital hypothyroidism.

Mutations in other genes that have not been as well character-ized can also cause congenital hypothyroidism. Still, other genes are involved in syndromic forms of the disorder.

Inheritance Pattern of Congenital Hypothyroidism

Most cases of congenital hypothyroidism are sporadic, which means they occur in people with no history of the disorder in their family.

When inherited, the condition usually has an autosomal recessive inheritance pattern, which means both copies of the gene in each cell have mutations. Typically, the parents of an individual with an auto-somal recessive condition each carry one copy of the mutated gene, but they do not show signs and symptoms of the condition.

When congenital hypothyroidism results from mutations in the *PAX8* gene or from certain mutations in the *TSHR* or *DUOX2* gene, the condition has an autosomal dominant pattern of inheritance, which means one copy of the altered gene in each cell is sufficient to cause the disorder. In some of these cases, an affected person inherits the mutation from one affected parent. Other cases result from new (de novo) mutations in the gene that occurs during the formation of reproductive cells (eggs or sperm) or in early embryonic development. These cases occur in people with no history of the disorder in their family.

Diagnosis of Congenital Hypothyroidism

Making a diagnosis for a genetic or rare disease can often be chal-lenging. Healthcare professionals typically look at a person's medical history, symptoms, physical exam, and laboratory test results in order to make a diagnosis. The following resources provide information relat-ing to diagnosis and testing for this condition. If you have questions about getting a diagnosis, you should contact a healthcare professional.

Newborn Screening

- An ACTion (ACT) sheet is available for this condition that describes the short-term actions a health professional should follow when an infant has a positive newborn screening result. ACT sheets were developed by experts in collaboration with the American College of Medical Genetics (ACMG).

- An Algorithm flowchart is available for this condition for determining the final diagnosis in an infant with a positive newborn screening result. Algorithms are developed by experts in collaboration with the ACMG.

- Baby's First Test is the nation's newborn screening education center for families and providers.

- National Newborn Screening and Global Resource Center (NNSGRC) provides information and resources in the area of newborn screening and genetics to benefit health professionals, the public-health community, consumers and government officials.

Section 23.3

Hyperthyroidism

This section includes text excerpted from "Hyperthyroidism (Overactive Thyroid)," National Institute of Diabetes and Digestive and Kidney Diseases (NIDDK), August 24, 2016. Reviewed September 2019.

What Is Hyperthyroidism?

Hyperthyroidism also called "overactive thyroid," is when the thyroid gland makes more thyroid hormones than your body needs. The thyroid is a small, butterfly-shaped gland in the front of your neck. Thyroid hormones control the way the body uses energy, so they affect nearly every organ in your body, even the way your heartbeats.

If left untreated, hyperthyroidism can cause serious problems with the heart, bones, muscles, menstrual cycle, and fertility. During pregnancy, untreated hyperthyroidism can lead to health problems for the mother and baby.

How Common Is Hyperthyroidism?

About 1.2 percent of people in the United States have hyperthyroidism. That is a little more than 1 person out of 100.

Who Is More Likely to Develop Hyperthyroidism?

Women are 2 to 10 times more likely than men to develop hyperthyroidism. You are more likely to have hyperthyroidism if you:

- Have a family history of thyroid disease

- Have other health problems, including:

  - Pernicious anemia, a condition caused by a vitamin B_{12} deficiency

  - Type 1 diabetes

  - Primary adrenal insufficiency, a hormonal disorder

- Eat large amounts of food containing iodine, such as kelp, or use medicines that contain iodine, such as amiodarone, a heart medicine

- Are older than age 60, especially if you are a woman

- Were pregnant within the past 6 months

Is Hyperthyroidism during Pregnancy a Problem?

Thyroid hormone levels that are just a little high are usually not a problem in pregnancy. However, more severe hyperthyroidism that is not treated can affect both the mother and the baby. If you have hyperthyroidism, be sure your disease is under control before becoming pregnant.

What Other Health Problems Could You Have Because of Hyperthyroidism?

If hyperthyroidism is not treated, it can cause some serious health problems, including:

- An irregular heartbeat that can lead to blood clots, stroke, heart failure, and other heart-related problems

- An eye disease called "Graves ophthalmopathy" that can cause double vision, light sensitivity, and eye pain, and rarely can lead to vision loss

- Thinning bones and osteoporosis

What Are the Symptoms of Hyperthyroidism?

Symptoms of hyperthyroidism can vary from person to person and may include:

- Nervousness or irritability
- Fatigue or muscle weakness
- Trouble tolerating heat
- Trouble sleeping
- Shaky hands
- Rapid and irregular heartbeat
- Frequent bowel movements or diarrhea
- Weight loss
- Mood swings
- Goiter

In people over age 60, hyperthyroidism is sometimes mistaken for depression or dementia. Older adults may have different symptoms, such as loss of appetite or withdrawal from people, than younger adults with hyperthyroidism. You may want to ask your healthcare provider about hyperthyroidism if you or your loved one show these symptoms.

What Causes Hyperthyroidism

Hyperthyroidism has several causes, including Graves disease, thyroid nodules, and thyroiditis—inflammation of the thyroid. Rarely, hyperthyroidism is caused by a noncancerous tumor of the pituitary gland located at the base of the brain. Consuming too much iodine or taking too much thyroid hormone medicine also may raise your thyroid hormone levels.

Graves Disease

Graves disease is the most common cause of hyperthyroidism. Graves disease is an autoimmune disorder. With this disease, your immune system attacks the thyroid and causes it to make too much thyroid hormone.

Overactive Thyroid Nodules

Thyroid nodules are lumps in your thyroid. Thyroid nodules are common and usually benign, meaning they are not cancerous. However, one or more nodules may become overactive and produce too much thyroid hormone. The presence of many overactive nodules occurs most often in older adults.

Thyroiditis

Thyroiditis is an inflammation of your thyroid that causes stored thyroid hormone to leak out of your thyroid gland. The hyperthyroidism may last for up to 3 months, after which your thyroid may become underactive, a condition called "hypothyroidism." The hypothyroidism usually lasts 12 to 18 months, but sometimes is permanent.

Several types of thyroiditis can cause hyperthyroidism and then cause hypothyroidism:

- **Subacute thyroiditis.** This condition involves a painfully inflamed and enlarged thyroid. Experts are not sure what causes subacute thyroiditis, but it may be related to an infection caused by a virus or bacteria.

- **Postpartum thyroiditis.** This type of thyroiditis develops after a woman gives birth.

- **Silent thyroiditis.** This type of thyroiditis is called "silent" because it is painless, even though your thyroid may be enlarged. Experts think silent thyroiditis is probably an autoimmune condition.

Too Much Iodine

Your thyroid uses iodine to make thyroid hormone. The amount of iodine you consume affects the amount of thyroid hormone your thyroid makes. In some people, consuming large amounts of iodine may cause the thyroid to make too much thyroid hormone.

Some medicines and cough syrups may contain a lot of iodine. One example is the heart medicine amiodarone. Seaweed and seaweed-based supplements also contain a lot of iodine.

Too Much Thyroid Hormone Medicine

Some people who take thyroid hormone medicine for hypothyroidism may take too much. If you take thyroid hormone medicine, you should see your doctor at least once a year to have your thyroid hormone levels checked. You may need to adjust your dose if your thyroid hormone level is too high.

Some other medicines may also interact with thyroid hormone medicine to raise hormone levels. If you take thyroid hormone medicine, ask your doctor about interactions when starting new medicines.

How Do Doctors Diagnose Hyperthyroidism?

Your doctor will take a medical history and do a physical exam, but also will need to do some tests to confirm a diagnosis of hyperthyroidism. Many symptoms of hyperthyroidism are the same as those of other diseases, so doctors usually cannot diagnose hyperthyroidism based on symptoms alone.

Because hypothyroidism can cause fertility problems, women who have trouble getting pregnant often get tested for thyroid problems.

Your doctor may use several blood tests to confirm a diagnosis of hyperthyroidism and find its cause. Imaging tests, such as a thyroid scan, can also help diagnose and find the cause of hyperthyroidism.

What Treatment Options Are There for Hyperthyroidism?

You may receive medicines, radioiodine therapy, or thyroid surgery to treat your hyperthyroidism. The aim of treatment is to bring thyroid hormone levels back to normal to prevent long-term health problems and to relieve uncomfortable symptoms. No single treatment works for everyone.

Treatment depends on the cause of your hyperthyroidism and how severe it is. When recommending a treatment, your doctor will consider your age, possible allergies to or side effects of the medicines, other conditions such as pregnancy or heart disease, and whether you have access to an experienced thyroid surgeon.

Medicines

Beta-blockers. Beta-blockers do not stop thyroid hormone production, but can reduce symptoms until other treatments take effect. Beta-blockers act quickly to relieve many of the symptoms of hyperthyroidism, such as tremors, rapid heartbeat, and nervousness. Most people feel better within hours of taking beta-blockers.

Antithyroid medicines. Antithyroid therapy is the simplest way to treat hyperthyroidism. Antithyroid medicines cause the thyroid to make less thyroid hormone. These medicines usually do not provide a permanent cure. Healthcare providers most often use the antithyroid medicine methimazole. Healthcare providers more often treat pregnant women with propylthiouracil during the first three months of pregnancy, however, because methimazole can harm the fetus, although this happens rarely.

Once treatment with antithyroid medicine begins, your thyroid hormone levels may not move into the normal range for several weeks or months. The total average treatment time is about one to two years, but treatment can continue for many years. Antithyroid medicines are not used to treat hyperthyroidism caused by thyroiditis.

Antithyroid medicines can cause side effects in some people, including:

- Allergic reactions such as rashes and itching

- A decrease in the number of white blood cells in your body, which can lower resistance to infection

- Liver failure, in rare cases

Call your doctor right away if you have any of the following symptoms:

- Fatigue

- Weakness

- Dull pain in your abdomen

- Loss of appetite

- Skin rash or itching

- Easy bruising

- Yellowing of your skin or whites of your eyes, called "jaundice"

- Constant sore throat

- Fever

Doctors usually treat pregnant and breastfeeding women with antithyroid medicine, since this treatment may be safer for the baby than other treatments.

Radioiodine Therapy

Radioactive iodine is a common and effective treatment for hyperthyroidism. In radioiodine therapy, you take radioactive iodine-131 by mouth as a capsule or liquid. The radioactive iodine slowly destroys the cells of the thyroid gland that produce thyroid hormone. Radioactive iodine does not affect other body tissues.

You may need more than one radioiodine treatment to bring your thyroid hormone levels into the normal range. In the meantime, treatment with beta-blockers can control your symptoms.

Almost everyone who has radioactive iodine treatment later develops hypothyroidism because the thyroid hormone-producing cells have been destroyed. However, hypothyroidism is easier to treat and causes fewer long-term health problems than hyperthyroidism. People with hypothyroidism can completely control the condition with daily thyroid hormone medicine.

Doctors do not use radioiodine therapy in pregnant women or in women who are breastfeeding. Radioactive iodine can harm the fetus' thyroid and can be passed from mother to child in breast milk.

Thyroid Surgery

The least-used treatment for hyperthyroidism is surgery to remove part or most of the thyroid gland. Sometimes doctors use surgery to treat people with large goiters or pregnant women who cannot take antithyroid medicine.

Before surgery, your doctor may prescribe antithyroid medicines to bring your thyroid hormone levels into the normal range. This treatment prevents a condition called "thyroid storm"—a sudden, severe worsening of symptoms—that can occur when people with hyperthyroidism have general anesthesia.

When part of your thyroid is removed, your thyroid hormone levels may return to normal. You may still develop hypothyroidism after surgery and need to take thyroid hormone medicine. If your whole thyroid is removed, you will need to take thyroid hormone medicine for life. After surgery, your doctor will continue to check your thyroid hormone levels.

What Should You Avoid Eating If You Have Hyperthyroidism?

People with Graves disease or other type of autoimmune thyroid disorder may be sensitive to harmful side effects from iodine. Eating foods that have large amounts of iodine—such as kelp, dulse, or other kinds of seaweed—may cause or worsen hyperthyroidism.

Taking iodine supplements can have the same effect. Talk with members of your healthcare team about what foods you should limit or avoid, and let them know if you take iodine supplements. Also, share information about any cough syrups or multivitamins that you take because they may contain iodine.

Section 23.4

Graves Disease

This section includes text excerpted from "Graves' Disease," National Institute of Diabetes and Digestive and Kidney Diseases (NIDDK), September 2017.

What Is Graves Disease?

Graves disease is an autoimmune disorder that causes hyperthyroidism, or overactive thyroid. With this disease, your immune system attacks the thyroid and causes it to make more thyroid hormone than your body needs. The thyroid is a small, butterfly-shaped gland in the front of your neck. Thyroid hormones control how your body uses energy, so they affect nearly every organ in your body—even the way your heartbeats.

If left untreated, hyperthyroidism can cause serious problems with the heart, bones, muscles, menstrual cycle, and fertility. During pregnancy, untreated hyperthyroidism can lead to health problems for the mother and baby. Graves disease also can affect your eyes and skin.

How Common Is Graves Disease

Graves disease is the most common cause of hyperthyroidism in the United States. The disease affects about 1 in 200 people.

Who Is More Likely to Develop Graves Disease?

Graves disease usually affects people between ages 30 and 50, but can occur at any age. The disease is 7 to 8 times more common in women than men. A person's chance of developing Graves disease increases if other family members have the disease.

People with other autoimmune disorders are more likely to develop Graves disease than people without these disorders. Conditions linked with Graves disease include:

- Rheumatoid arthritis (RA), a disorder that affects the joints and sometimes other body systems

- Pernicious anemia, a condition caused by a vitamin B_{12} deficiency

- Lupus, a chronic, or long-term, disorder that can affect many parts of your body

- Addison disease, a hormonal disorder

- Celiac disease, a digestive disorder

- Vitiligo, a disorder in which some parts of the skin are not pigmented

- Type 1 diabetes

What Other Health Problems Could You Develop Because of Graves Disease?

Without treatment, Graves disease can cause some serious health problems, including:

- An irregular heartbeat that can lead to blood clots, stroke, heart failure, and other heart-related problems

- An eye disease called "Graves ophthalmopathy" or "Graves orbitopathy" (GO), which can cause double vision, light sensitivity, and eye pain—and, rarely, can lead to vision loss

- Thinning bones and osteoporosis

Is Graves Disease during Pregnancy a Problem?

Thyroid hormone levels that are just a little high are usually not a problem in pregnancy. However, more severe hyperthyroidism that is not treated can affect both the mother and the baby. If you have Graves disease, be sure your hyperthyroidism is under control before becoming pregnant.

171

What Are the Symptoms of Graves Disease?

You may have common symptoms of hyperthyroidism such as:

- Fast and irregular heartbeat
- Frequent bowel movements or diarrhea
- Goiter
- Heat intolerance
- Nervousness or irritability
- Tiredness or muscle weakness
- Trembling hands
- Trouble sleeping
- Weight loss

Rarely, people with Graves disease develop a reddish thickening of the skin on the shins, a condition called "pretibial myxedema" or "Graves dermopathy." This skin problem is usually painless and mild, but it can be painful for some.

Graves ophthalmopathy can cause retracted eyelids, meaning the eyelids are pulled back from the eye. GO can also cause bulging eyes, double vision, and swelling around the eyes.

What Causes Graves Disease

Researchers are not sure why some people develop autoimmune disorders such as Graves disease. These disorders probably develop from a combination of genes and an outside trigger, such as a virus.

With Graves disease, the immune system makes an antibody called "thyroid-stimulating immunoglobulin" (TSI) that attaches to thyroid cells. TSI acts like a thyroid-stimulating hormone (TSH), a hormone made in the pituitary gland that tells the thyroid how much thyroid hormone to make. TSI causes the thyroid to make too much thyroid hormone.

How Do Healthcare Professionals Diagnose Graves Disease?

Your healthcare provider may suspect Graves disease based on your symptoms and findings during a physical examination. One or more

172

blood tests can confirm that you have hyperthyroidism and may point to Graves disease as the cause.

Other clues that hyperthyroidism is caused by Graves disease are:

- An enlarged thyroid

- Signs of Graves eye disease, present in about one out of three people with Graves disease

- A history of other family members with thyroid or autoimmune problems

If the diagnosis is uncertain, your doctor may order further blood or imaging tests to confirm Graves disease as the cause.

A blood test can detect TSI. However, in mild cases of Graves disease, TSI may not show up in your blood. The next step may be one of two imaging tests that use small, safe doses of radioactive iodine. Your thyroid collects iodine from your bloodstream and uses it to make thyroid hormones; it will collect radioactive iodine in the same way.

- **Radioactive iodine uptake test.** This test measures the amount of iodine the thyroid collects from the bloodstream. If your thyroid collects large amounts of iodine, you may have Graves disease.

- **Thyroid scan.** This scan shows how and where iodine is distributed in the thyroid. With Graves disease, the entire thyroid is involved, so the iodine shows up throughout the gland. With other causes of hyperthyroidism such as nodules—small lumps in the gland—the iodine shows up in a different pattern.

What Treatment Options Are Available for Graves Disease?

You have three treatment options: medicine, radioiodine therapy, and thyroid surgery. Radioiodine therapy is the most common treatment for Graves disease in the United States, but doctors are beginning to use medicine more often than in the past. Based on factors such as your age, whether you are pregnant, or whether you have other medical conditions, your doctor may recommend a specific treatment and can help you decide which one is right for you.

Radioiodine Therapy

For radioiodine therapy, you take radioactive iodine-131 (I-131) by mouth as a capsule or liquid. I-131, at a higher dose than the dose used for imaging tests, slowly destroys the cells of the thyroid gland that produce thyroid hormone. The dose of I-131 usually used for radioiodine therapy does not affect other body tissues.

Although it is unlikely, you may need more than one radioiodine treatment to bring your thyroid hormone levels into the normal range. In the meantime, treatment with medicines called "beta-blockers" can control your symptoms.

Almost everyone who has radioactive iodine treatment later develops hypothyroidism, or underactive thyroid, because the thyroid hormone-producing cells have been destroyed. However, hypothyroidism is easier to treat and causes fewer long-term health problems than hyperthyroidism. People with hypothyroidism can completely control the condition with daily thyroid hormone medicine.

Doctors do not use radioiodine therapy to treat pregnant women or women who are breastfeeding. Radioactive iodine can harm the fetus' thyroid and can be passed from mother to child in breast milk.

Medicines

Beta-blockers. Beta-blockers do not stop your thyroid from producing thyroid hormone but can reduce symptoms until other treatments take effect. These medicines act quickly to relieve many of the symptoms of hyperthyroidism, such as trembling, rapid heartbeat, and nervousness. Most people feel better within hours of taking beta-blockers.

Antithyroid medicines. Antithyroid therapy is the simplest way to treat hyperthyroidism. Antithyroid medicines cause your thyroid to make less thyroid hormone. These medicines usually do not provide a permanent cure, but in some people, the effects last a long time after they stop taking the medicine. Doctors most often use the antithyroid medicine methimazole.

Doctors usually treat pregnant and breastfeeding women with antithyroid medicine, since this treatment may be safer for the baby than other treatments. Doctors use propylthiouracil more often than methimazole during the first three months of pregnancy because methimazole may harm the fetus, although this happens rarely. Also, rarely, propylthiouracil may affect the fetus, but any effects are less harmful than having uncontrolled hyperthyroidism during pregnancy.

Once treatment with antithyroid medicine begins, your thyroid hormone levels may not move into the normal range for several weeks or months. The total average treatment time is about 12 to 18 months, but treatment can continue for many years in people who do not want radioiodine or surgery to treat their Graves disease.

Antithyroid medicines can cause side effects in some people, including:

- Allergic reactions such as rashes and itching
- A decrease in the number of white blood cells (WBCs) in your body, which can lower resistance to infection
- Liver failure, in rare cases

Call your doctor right away if you have any of the following symptoms:

- Fever
- Sore throat
- Tiredness
- Weakness
- Dull pain in your abdomen
- Loss of appetite
- Skin rash or itching
- Easy bruising
- Yellowing of your skin or whites of your eyes, called "jaundice"
- Constant sore throat

Thyroid Surgery

The least-used treatment for Graves disease is surgery to remove the thyroid gland. Sometimes doctors use surgery to treat people with large goiters, or pregnant women who are allergic to or have side effects from antithyroid medicines.

Before surgery, your doctor will prescribe antithyroid medicines to bring your thyroid hormone levels into the normal range. This treatment prevents a condition called "thyroid storm"—a sudden, severe worsening of symptoms—that can occur when people with hyperthyroidism have general anesthesia.

After surgery to remove your thyroid, you will develop hypothyroidism and need to take thyroid hormone medicine every day for life. After surgery, your doctor will continue to check your thyroid hormone levels and adjust your dose as needed.

What Is Graves Ophthalmopathy?

Graves ophthalmopathy is a condition that occurs when the immune system attacks the muscles and other tissues around the eyes. The result is inflammation and a buildup of tissue and fat behind the eye socket, causing the eyeballs to bulge out. Rarely, inflammation is severe enough to compress, or push on, the optic nerve that leads from the eye to the brain, causing vision loss.

Symptoms of Graves Ophthalmopathy

Besides bulging eyes, other GO symptoms are:

- Dry, gritty, and irritated eyes
- Puffy or retracted eyelids
- Double vision
- Light sensitivity
- Pressure or pain in the eyes
- Trouble moving the eyes

About one in three people with Graves disease develop mild GO, and about five percent develop severe GO. This eye condition usually lasts one to two years and often improves on its own.

Graves ophthalmopathy can occur before, at the same time as, or after other symptoms of hyperthyroidism develop. Eye problems sometimes develop long after Graves disease has been treated, but this happens rarely. GO may even occur in people whose thyroid function is normal. Smoking makes GO worse.

Treatment of Graves Ophthalmopathy

The eye problems of Graves disease may not improve after thyroid treatment, so doctors often treat the two problems separately.

Eye drops can relieve dry, gritty, irritated eyes—the most common of the milder symptoms. If pain and swelling occur, your doctor may prescribe a steroid such as prednisone. Other medicines that reduce your body's immune response, such as rituximab, may also provide relief.

Sunglasses can help with light sensitivity. Special eyeglass lenses may help reduce double vision. If you have puffy eyelids, your doctor may advise you to sleep with your head raised to reduce swelling. If your eyelids do not fully close, taping them shut at night can help prevent dry eyes.

Your doctor may recommend surgery to improve bulging of your eyes and correct the vision changes caused by pressure on the optic nerve. A procedure called "orbital decompression" makes the eye socket bigger and gives the eye room to sink back to a more normal position. Eyelid surgery can return retracted eyelids to their normal position.

Rarely, doctors treat Graves eye disease with radiation therapy to the muscles and tissues around the eyes.

What Should You Avoid Eating If You Have Graves Disease?

People with Graves disease may be sensitive to harmful side effects from iodine. Eating foods that have large amounts of iodine—such as kelp, dulse, or other kinds of seaweed—may cause or worsen hyperthyroidism. Taking iodine supplements can have the same effect.

Talk with your healthcare professional about what foods you should limit or avoid, and let her or him know if you take iodine supplements. Also, share information about any cough syrups or multivitamins that you take because they may contain iodine.

Section 23.5

Thyroiditis

"Thyroiditis," © 2020 Omnigraphics.
Reviewed September 2019.

"Thyroiditis" is a term that refers to a group of disorders that causes inflammation of the thyroid gland. The thyroid gland is a butterfly-shaped endocrine gland located in the lower front of the neck. The function of the thyroid gland is to produce thyroid hormones. These hormones help the body stay warm and keep the major organs of the body working as they should.

Causes of Thyroiditis

The causes of thyroiditis depend upon the type of disease you have. Mostly, thyroiditis is caused by an attack on the thyroid gland by antibodies, which causes inflammation and damage to the cells of the thyroid gland.

Thyroiditis is often considered as an autoimmune disease (in which the body attacks itself). It is unclear why certain people develop anti-thyroid antibodies. It can also be caused by an infection, such as those caused by bacteria or a virus. Drugs such as amiodarone or interferon can also damage the cells of the thyroid, leading to thyroiditis.

Symptoms of Thyroiditis

The symptoms of thyroiditis vary based upon the type and phase.

Hyperthyroid Phase

You will have symptoms of hyperthyroidism (overactive thyroid gland) if thyroiditis triggers rapid cell damage, which causes thyroid hormone to leak into your blood, increasing the hormone levels. This phase usually lasts one to three months. The possible symptoms of this phase are as follows:

- Nervousness or anxiety
- Trouble sleeping
- Fatigue
- Muscle weakness
- Weight loss
- Tremors (shaking fingers or hands)

Hypothyroid Phase

You will have symptoms of hypothyroidism (underactive thyroid gland) if the thyroid cells are damaged and cause thyroid hormones to be low in your blood. This phase is slow and can be long-lasting. The symptoms of hypothyroidism are as follows:

- Constipation
- Dry skin
- Unplanned-weight gain

- Depression

- Muscle aches

- Fatigue

Types of Thyroiditis
Hashimoto Thyroiditis

Hashimoto thyroiditis, also called "chronic lymphocytic" or "auto-immune thyroiditis," is the most common form of thyroiditis. During the course of this disease, the thyroid cells become inefficient in converting iodine into the thyroid hormone and thus create a swollen thyroid gland. This disease is more common in women than in men. Hashimoto thyroiditis results in hypothyroidism and requires a thyroid hormone replacement.

Subacute Thyroiditis

Subacute thyroiditis, also called as "De Quervain thyroiditis" or "giant cell thyroiditis," is a painful swelling of the thyroid gland. This disease is thought to be caused by viral infection, such as the flu or mumps. In this disease, the thyroid gland releases an increased number of hormones into your blood (thyrotoxicosis), leading to symptoms of hyperthyroidism.

Postpartum Thyroiditis

Postpartum thyroiditis is an autoimmune condition that sometimes occurs shortly after a woman gives birth. In this condition, the immune system attacks the thyroid gland around six months after she gives birth. After a few weeks, this condition depletes the hormone levels and leads to symptoms of hypothyroidism.

Silent Thyroiditis

Silent (painless) thyroiditis is similar to postpartum thyroiditis. It can occur in both men and women and does not relate to childbirth. This condition increases the hormone levels in your blood and leads to the symptoms of hyperthyroidism. If low hormone levels last for a long period of time, thyroid hormone replacement is required to treat the symptoms.

Drug-Induced Thyroiditis

Some medications can damage the thyroid gland and may cause either symptoms of hypothyroidism or symptoms of hyperthyroidism. Drugs such as interferons, amiodarone, and lithium can cause this condition. Symptoms can improve after you stop the medication. However, always consult with your doctor before stopping a medication.

Acute Thyroiditis

Acute, or infectious, thyroiditis can be triggered by a bacterial infection. This condition is rare and can be associated with a compromised immune system or problems in the development of the thyroid. The common symptoms of acute thyroiditis are pain in the throat and swelling of the thyroid gland, sometimes leading to symptoms of hyperthyroidism or hypothyroidism. Symptoms of acute thyroiditis can usually get better if the infection is treated.

Diagnosis of Thyroiditis
Radioactive Iodine Uptake Test

Radioactive iodine uptake (RAIU) test is a test during which you will be given radioactive iodine in a pill or liquid form. Over the next 24 hours, your doctor will test the amount of iodine that is absorbed by your thyroid. The radioactive iodine uptake will be >60 percent in hyperthyroidism and will be <20 percent in hypothyroidism. The normal uptake will be 20 to 40 percent.

Thyroid-Stimulating Hormone Test

Thyroid-stimulating hormone (TSH) test is a type of blood test used to determine whether the TSH levels in your blood are within range. If the hormone level is found to be either higher or lower than the normal level, this may indicate the presence of thyroiditis.

Thyroid Antibody Tests

Thyroid antibody tests are tests that measure the thyroid antibodies that include thyroid receptor stimulating antibodies (TRAb) or antithyroid antibodies.

Treatment of Thyroiditis

The treatment of thyroiditis depends upon the symptoms, phase, and type of the disease.

- **Thyrotoxic phase.** This phase is temporary. You may either recover over time or it may lead to symptoms of hypothyroid phase. The hypothyroid phase may or may not be temporary. Symptoms need to be treated only when they appear and antithyroid medications are rarely needed.

- **Anxiety/tremors/increased sweating/palpitations.** These symptoms can be treated with beta-blockers.

- **Hypothyroid phase.** Thyroid hormone replacement therapy is used to treat the symptoms of this phase. This therapy lasts for 6 to 12 months. Hashimoto thyroiditis can lead to permanent hypothyroidism and requires continuous treatment.

- **Thyroidal pain.** Anti-inflammatory medications, such as aspirin or ibuprofen, can be used to ease thyroid gland pain. If the pain is severe, undertaking steroid therapy is suggested.

References

1. "Thyroiditis," National Health Service (NHS), September 19, 2017.

2. "Thyroiditis," Cleveland Clinic, October 26, 2018.

3. Milas, Kresimira (Mira). "Hashimoto's Thyroiditis Diagnosis," EndocrineWeb, May 29, 2014.

4. "What Is Thyroiditis?" WebMD, March 1, 2017.

Section 23.6

Hashimoto Thyroiditis

This section includes text excerpted from "Hashimoto's Disease," National Institute of Diabetes and Digestive and Kidney Diseases (NIDDK), September 2017.

Hashimoto disease is an autoimmune disorder that can cause hypothyroidism, or underactive thyroid. With this disease, your immune system attacks your thyroid. The thyroid becomes damaged and cannot make enough thyroid hormones.

The thyroid is a small, butterfly-shaped gland in the front of your neck. Thyroid hormones control how your body uses energy, so they affect nearly every organ in your body—even the way your heart beats. Without enough thyroid hormones, many of your body's functions slow down.

Does Hashimoto Disease Have Another Name?

Hashimoto disease is also called "Hashimoto thyroiditis," "chronic lymphocytic thyroiditis," or "autoimmune thyroiditis."

How Common Is Hashimoto Disease?

Hashimoto disease is the most common cause of hypothyroidism in the United States and affects about five people out of 100.

Who Is More Likely to Develop Hashimoto Disease?

Hashimoto disease is at least eight times more common in women than men. Although the disease may occur in teens or young women, it more often appears between ages 40 and 60. Your chance of developing Hashimoto disease increases if other family members have the disease.

You are more likely to develop Hashimoto disease if you have other autoimmune disorders. Conditions linked to Hashimoto disease include:

- **Addison disease**, a hormonal disorder

- **Autoimmune hepatitis**, a disease in which the immune system attacks the liver

- **Celiac disease**, a digestive disorder

- **Lupus**, a chronic, or long-term, disorder that can affect many parts of your body

- **Pernicious anemia**, a condition caused by a vitamin B_{12} deficiency

- **Rheumatoid arthritis**, a disorder that affects the joints and sometimes other body systems

- **Sjögren syndrome**, a disease that causes dry eyes and mouth

- **Type 1 diabetes**, a disease that occurs when your blood glucose, also called "blood sugar," is too high

- **Vitiligo**, a condition in which some parts of the skin are not pigmented

What Other Health Problems Could You Have Because of Hashimoto Disease?

Many people with Hashimoto disease develop hypothyroidism. Low levels of thyroid hormones can contribute to high cholesterol that can lead to heart disease. Rarely, severe, untreated hypothyroidism may lead to myxedema coma, an extreme form of hypothyroidism in which the body's functions slow to the point that it becomes life-threatening. Myxedema coma requires urgent medical treatment.

Is Hashimoto Disease during Pregnancy a Problem?

Without treatment, hypothyroidism can cause problems for both the mother and the baby. However, thyroid medicines can help prevent problems and are safe to take during pregnancy. Learn about the causes, complications, diagnosis, and treatment of hypothyroidism during pregnancy. Many women taking thyroid hormone medicine need a higher dose during pregnancy, so you should contact your doctor right away if you find out that you are pregnant.

What Are the Symptoms of Hashimoto Disease?

Many people with Hashimoto disease have no symptoms at first. As the disease slowly progresses, the thyroid usually gets larger and may cause the front of the neck to look swollen. The enlarged thyroid called a "goiter," may create a feeling of fullness in your throat, though it is usually not painful. After many years, or even decades, damage to the thyroid causes it to shrink and the goiter to disappear.

The hypothyroidism of Hashimoto disease often is subclinical—mild and without symptoms—especially early in the disease. As hypothyroidism progresses, you may have one or more of the following symptoms:

- Tiredness

- Weight gain

- Trouble tolerating cold

- Joint and muscle pain
- Constipation
- Dry, thinning hair
- Heavy or irregular menstrual periods and problems becoming pregnant
- Depression
- Memory problems
- A slowed heart rate

What Causes Hashimoto Disease

Researchers are not sure why some people develop autoimmune disorders such as Hashimoto disease. These disorders probably result from a combination of genes and an outside trigger, such as a virus.

In Hashimoto disease, your immune system makes antibodies that attack the thyroid gland. Large numbers of white blood cells called "lymphocytes," which are part of the immune system, buildup in the thyroid. Lymphocytes make the antibodies that start the autoimmune process.

How Do Doctors Diagnose Hashimoto Disease?

Your doctor will start with a medical history and physical exam, and will order one or more blood tests to find out if you have hypothyroidism. You may have a goiter, which is common in Hashimoto disease. Your doctor will order more blood tests to look for antithyroid antibodies known as "thyroperoxidase antibodies" (TPO), which almost all people with Hashimoto disease have.

You probably will not need other tests to confirm that you have Hashimoto disease. However, if your doctor suspects Hashimoto disease but you do not have antibodies in your blood, you may have an ultrasound of your thyroid. The images that the ultrasound makes can show the size of your thyroid and other features of Hashimoto disease. The ultrasound also can rule out other causes of an enlarged thyroid, such as thyroid nodules—small lumps in the thyroid gland.

How Do Doctors Treat Hashimoto Disease?

Treatment usually depends on whether your thyroid is damaged enough to cause hypothyroidism. If you do not have hypothyroidism, your doctor may choose to simply monitor you to see if your disease gets worse.

Hypothyroidism is treated by replacing the hormone that your own thyroid can no longer make. You will take levothyroxine, a thyroid hormone medicine that is identical to a hormone the thyroid normally makes. Your doctor may recommend that you take the medicine in the morning before you eat.

Your doctor will give you a blood test about 6 to 8 weeks after you begin taking thyroid hormone and adjust your dose if needed. Each time you change your dose, you will have another blood test. Once you have reached a dose that is working for you, your doctor will probably repeat the blood test in six months and then once a year.

Your hypothyroidism most likely can be completely controlled with thyroid hormone medicine, as long as you take the prescribed dose as instructed. Never stop taking your medicine without talking with your doctor first.

What Should You Avoid Eating If You Have Hashimoto Disease?

The thyroid uses iodine, a mineral in some foods, to make thyroid hormones. However, people with Hashimoto disease or other types of autoimmune thyroid disorders may be sensitive to harmful side effects from iodine. Eating foods that have large amounts of iodine—such as kelp, dulse, or other kinds of seaweed—may cause hypothyroidism or make it worse. Taking iodine supplements can have the same effect.

Talk with your doctor about what foods you should limit or avoid. Let the doctor know if you take iodine supplements. Also, share information about any cough syrups you take, because they may contain iodine.

Women need a little more iodine when they are pregnant because the baby gets iodine from the mother's diet. However, too much iodine can also cause problems, such as goiter in the baby. If you are pregnant, talk with your doctor about how much iodine you need.

Section 23.7

Thyroid Nodule

"Thyroid Nodule," © 2020 Omnigraphics.
Reviewed September 2019.

Thyroid nodules are unusual growth of lumps in the thyroid gland. They are either made up of solid tissues or filled with fluids. Sometimes, the nodules appear as bumps around the throat and can easily be identified. However, if the nodules are hidden deep inside the thyroid gland, it may be hard to feel them. These can be detected only with the help of a healthcare professional. The majority of these nodules do not cause any serious symptoms; but, in rare cases, they may cause pain and even lead to thyroid cancer.

Causes of Thyroid Nodules

The major risk factors for developing thyroid nodules are listed below:

- **Genetics.** Having a family history of thyroid nodules or thyroid cancer may increase the risk of developing thyroid nodules.

- **Gender.** Women are more susceptible to thyroid nodules than men.

- **Age.** The chances of developing thyroid nodules increases with age. The rate of incidence of thyroid nodules is estimated to be higher among people aged 60 and above.

Several health conditions may cause the thyroid gland to develop nodules. These conditions include:

- **Iodine deficiency.** Iodine is an important component that is essential for the secretion of thyroid hormones. Lack of iodine in the diet can sometimes lead to the development of thyroid nodules. However, this condition is not very common in the United States due to the use of iodized salt.

- **Thyroid cyst.** A cyst is a solid component filled with some kind of bodily fluid. It forms due to the degeneration of thyroid adenomas.

- **Thyroid adenoma.** This is a condition in which thyroid tissue overgrows. The exact cause of thyroid adenoma is not known. Some thyroid adenomas may also secrete excess thyroid hormones, resulting in hyperthyroidism.

- **Subacute thyroiditis.** This condition causes enlargement of thyroid glands and is one of the major reasons for the development of thyroid nodules. It usually occurs as a result of viral infections, such as the flu or mumps.

- **Hashimoto thyroiditis.** This is an autoimmune disease where the immune system of the body starts attacking the thyroid gland. It results in hypothyroidism, or reduced secretion of thyroid hormones, and leads to thyroid nodule enlargement.

- **Multinodular goiter.** "Goiter" refers to any kind of enlargement in thyroid glands. Multinodular goiter, as the name suggests, is a condition where multiple nodules are present within a goiter.

In addition, people who are frequently exposed to radiation from medical treatments are considered to be at higher risk of developing thyroid nodules.

Symptoms of Thyroid Nodule

In most cases, thyroid nodules do not cause any kinds of signs or symptoms but occasionally, when the nodules become large, there can be notable symptoms such as:

- Goiter, or enlargement of the thyroid gland
- Tickling sensation in the throat
- Hoarse voice
- Swelling at the base of the neck
- Pain in the neck
- Difficulty in breathing
- Difficulty in swallowing

If the thyroid nodules start producing excess thyroid hormone, then people may also experience the symptoms of hyperthyroidism, such as:

- Anxiety
- Nervousness
- Tremor

- Hyperactivity
- Rapid heartbeat
- Excess sweating
- Hair loss
- Weight loss
- Diarrhea
- Delayed menstrual cycle

The thyroid nodules may also lower the secretion of thyroid hormones, resulting in hypothyroidism. Symptoms of this condition include:

- Depression
- Fatigue
- Weakness
- Dry skin
- Dry hair
- Hair loss
- Hoarse voice
- Forgetfulness
- Excess weight gain
- Constipation
- Frequent menstrual cycle

The most serious complication of thyroid nodule is the development of thyroid cancer, which is very rare.

Diagnosis of Thyroid Nodule

Sometimes, people may feel the presence of a thyroid nodule, but this may not be possible in all cases. Therefore, it is better to seek a diagnosis from a healthcare professional. Some testing methods used by healthcare professionals to diagnose thyroid nodules follow.

- **Physical examination.** During this test, the doctor asks the patient to swallow something and examines the movement of thyroid gland. The doctor also looks for the symptoms of hyperthyroidism and hypothyroidism.

- **Thyroid function test.** It is a blood test, where the doctor looks for the levels of thyroid hormones in the blood. This test can confirm if someone is suffering from hyperthyroidism or hypothyroidism. However, these conditions do not necessarily confirm the presence of thyroid nodules. Therefore, the doctor may order additional tests.

- **Ultrasonography.** This method uses high-frequency sound waves instead of radiation to take images of the thyroid gland. Ultrasonography is very useful in detecting nodules that are present deep inside the thyroid gland. It is also useful to check if the nodule is solid- or fluid-filled.

- **Fine-needle biopsy.** This test involves taking samples of cells from thyroid nodules with the help of a thin needle. The doctor may use ultrasonography to spot the exact position of the nodule during biopsy. These samples are then sent to the laboratory for histopathological analysis to check whether the nodules are cancerous.

- **Thyroid scan.** During this test, the patient is asked to take a small amount of radioactive iodine orally. The doctor analyses the difference in the amount of radioactive iodine absorbed by the nodules and normal thyroid tissue. This test is helpful in determining the likelihood of cancer.

Treatment of Thyroid Nodule

Watchful waiting. If the thyroid nodule is found to be benign, the doctor may suggest waiting and watching for a specific period of time. During this period, the patient needs to visit the doctor at regular intervals and get checked. If the nodules remain benign throughout the process, then no treatment is required. However, if the nodules continue to grow or turns out to be cancerous, then the doctor will recommend other treatment methods.

Radioactive iodine pills. Radioactive iodine pills are used to treat hyperfunctioning thyroid nodules. The nodules absorb the radioactive iodine and shrink. This method is suitable only for noncancerous nodules. There are few side effects associated with this method, but it is not prescribed to pregnant women.

Alcohol ablation. This treatment is better suited for cancerous nodules. The method involves injecting alcohol on thyroid nodules and making them shrink.

Surgery. Surgery is usually recommended when the nodules turn out to be cancerous or grow at a very rapid rate. The surgical procedure is called "near-total thyroidectomy," wherein the malignant nodule is removed, along with the majority of thyroid tissue. After the surgery, the patient may need lifelong treatment and medication in order to secrete a sufficient amount of thyroid hormones.

References

1. "Thyroid Nodules," Mayo Clinic, February 18, 2017.

2. "Thyroid Nodule," Cleveland Clinic, July 30, 2018.

3. Kraft, Sy. "What Are Thyroid Nodules," Medical News Today, September 20, 2018.

4. Brady, Bridget. "Thyroid Nodules: Prevalence, Symptoms, Causes, Diagnosis, and Treatments," EndocrineWeb, February 11, 2015.

Section 23.8

Thyroid Cancer

This section includes text excerpted from "Thyroid Cancer Treatment (Adult) (PDQ®)—Patient Version," National Cancer Institute (NCI), May 16, 2019.

The thyroid is a gland at the base of the throat near the trachea (windpipe). It is shaped like a butterfly, with a right and a left lobe. The isthmus, a thin piece of tissue, connects the two lobes. A healthy thyroid is a little larger than a quarter. It usually cannot be felt through the skin.

The thyroid uses iodine, a mineral found in some foods and in iodized salt, to help make several hormones. Thyroid hormones do the following:

- Control heart rate, body temperature, and how quickly food is changed into energy (metabolism)

- Control the amount of calcium in the blood

Thyroid Nodules Are Common but Usually Are Not Cancer

Your doctor may find a lump (nodule) in your thyroid during a routine medical exam. A thyroid nodule is an abnormal growth of thyroid cells in the thyroid. Nodules may be solid or fluid-filled.

When a thyroid nodule is found, an ultrasound of the thyroid and a fine-needle aspiration biopsy are often done to check for signs of cancer. Blood tests to check thyroid hormone levels and for antithyroid antibodies in the blood may also be done to check for other types of thyroid disease.

Thyroid nodules usually do not cause symptoms or need treatment. Sometimes the thyroid nodules become large enough that it is hard to swallow or breathe and more tests and treatment are needed. Only a small number of thyroid nodules are diagnosed as cancer.

Thyroid Cancer and Its Types

Thyroid cancer can be described as either:

- **Differentiated thyroid cancer,** which includes well-differentiated tumors, poorly differentiated tumors, and undifferentiated tumors

- **Medullary thyroid cancer.** Well-differentiated tumors (papillary thyroid cancer and follicular thyroid cancer) can be treated and can usually be cured. Poorly differentiated and undifferentiated tumors (anaplastic thyroid cancer) are less common. These tumors grow and spread quickly and have a poorer chance of recovery. Patients with anaplastic thyroid cancer should have molecular testing for a mutation in the *BRAF* gene.

Medullary thyroid cancer is a neuroendocrine tumor that develops in C cells of the thyroid. The C cells make a hormone (calcitonin) that helps maintain a healthy level of calcium in the blood.

Risk of Thyroid Cancer

Anything that increases your risk of getting a disease is called a "risk factor." Age, gender, and being exposed to radiation can affect the risk of thyroid cancer. Having a risk factor does not mean that you will get cancer; not having risk factors does not mean that you will not get cancer. Talk with your doctor if you think you may be at risk.

Risk factors for thyroid cancer include the following:

- Being between 25 and 65 years old

- Being female

- Being exposed to radiation to the head and neck as an infant or child or being exposed to radioactive fallout. The cancer may occur as soon as five years after exposure

- Having a history of goiter (enlarged thyroid)

- Having a family history of thyroid disease or thyroid cancer

- Having certain genetic conditions, such as familial medullary thyroid cancer (FMTC), multiple endocrine neoplasia type 2A syndrome (MEN2A), or multiple endocrine neoplasia type 2B syndrome (MEN2B)

- Being Asian

Genetic Causes of Medullary Thyroid Cancer

The genes in cells carry hereditary information from parent to child. A certain change in the *RET* gene that is passed from parent to child (inherited) may cause medullary thyroid cancer.

There is a genetic test that is used to check for the changed gene. The patient is tested first to see if she or he has the changed gene. If the patient has it, other family members may also be tested to find out if they are at increased risk for medullary thyroid cancer. Family members, including young children, who have the changed gene may have a thyroidectomy (surgery to remove the thyroid). This can decrease the chance of developing medullary thyroid cancer.

Signs of Thyroid Cancer

Thyroid cancer may not cause early signs or symptoms. It is sometimes found during a routine physical exam. Signs or symptoms may occur as the tumor gets bigger. Other conditions may cause the same signs or symptoms. Check with your doctor if you have any of the following:

- A lump (nodule) in the neck

- Trouble breathing

- Trouble swallowing

- Pain when swallowing

- Hoarseness

Diagnosis of Thyroid Cancer

Tests that examine the thyroid, neck, and blood are used to detect and diagnose thyroid cancer. The following tests and procedures may be used:

- **Physical exam and history.** An exam of the body to check general signs of health, including checking for signs of disease, such as lumps (nodules) or swelling in the neck, voice box, and lymph nodes, and anything else that seems unusual. A history of the patient's health habits and past illnesses and treatments will also be taken.

- **Laryngoscopy.** A procedure in which the doctor checks the larynx (voice box) with a mirror or a laryngoscope. A laryngoscope is a thin, tube-like instrument with a light and a lens for viewing. A thyroid tumor may press on vocal cords. The laryngoscopy is done to see if the vocal cords are moving normally.

- **Blood hormone studies.** A procedure in which a blood sample is checked to measure the amounts of certain hormones released into the blood by organs and tissues in the body. An unusual (higher or lower than normal) amount of a substance can be a sign of disease in the organ or tissue that makes it. The blood may be checked for abnormal levels of thyroid-stimulating hormone (TSH). TSH is made by the pituitary gland in the brain. It stimulates the release of thyroid hormone and controls how fast follicular thyroid cells grow. The blood may also be checked for high levels of the hormone calcitonin and antithyroid antibodies.

- **Blood chemistry studies.** A procedure in which a blood sample is checked to measure the amounts of certain substances, such as calcium, released into the blood by organs and tissues in the body. An unusual (higher or lower than normal) amount of a substance can be a sign of disease.

- **Ultrasound exam**. A procedure in which high-energy sound waves (ultrasound) are bounced off internal tissues or organs in the neck and make echoes. The echoes form a picture of body tissues called "sonogram." The picture can be printed to be looked at later. This procedure can show the size of a thyroid nodule and whether it is solid or a fluid-filled cyst. Ultrasound may be used to guide a fine-needle aspiration biopsy.

- **Computed tomography (CT) scan.** A procedure that makes a series of detailed pictures of areas inside the body, such as the neck, taken from different angles. The pictures are made by a computer linked to an x-ray machine. A dye may be injected into a vein or swallowed to help the organs or tissues show up more clearly. This procedure is also called "computed tomography," "computerized tomography," or "computerized axial tomography."

- **Fine-needle aspiration biopsy of the thyroid.** The removal of thyroid tissue using a thin needle. The needle is inserted through the skin into the thyroid. Several tissue samples are removed from different parts of the thyroid. A pathologist views the tissue samples under a microscope to look for cancer cells. Because the type of thyroid cancer can be hard to diagnose, patients should ask to have biopsy samples checked by a pathologist who has experience diagnosing thyroid cancer.

- **Surgical biopsy.** The removal of the thyroid nodule or one lobe of the thyroid during surgery so the cells and tissues can be viewed under a microscope by a pathologist to check for signs of cancer. Because the type of thyroid cancer can be hard to diagnose, patients should ask to have biopsy samples checked by a pathologist who has experience diagnosing thyroid cancer.

Factors That Affect Prognosis and Treatment Options

The prognosis and treatment options depend on the following:

- The age of the patient at the time of diagnosis

- The type of thyroid cancer

- The stage of the cancer

- Whether the cancer was completely removed by surgery

- Whether the patient has multiple endocrine neoplasia type 2B (MEN 2B)

- The patient's general health

- Whether the cancer has just been diagnosed or has recurred

Treatment of Thyroid Cancer

Different types of treatment are available for patients with thyroid cancer. Some treatments are standard, and some are being tested in clinical trials. A treatment clinical trial is a research study meant to help improve treatments or obtain information on new treatments for patients with cancer. When clinical trials show that a new treatment is better than the standard treatment, the new treatment may become the standard treatment. Patients may want to think about taking part in a clinical trial. Some clinical trials are open only to patients who have not started treatment.

There are six standard treatment that are used for treating thyroid cancer. They are discussed below.

Surgery

Surgery is the most common treatment for thyroid cancer. One of the following procedures may be used:

- **Lobectomy.** Removal of the lobe in which thyroid cancer is found. Lymph nodes near the cancer may also be removed and checked under a microscope for signs of cancer.

- **Near-total thyroidectomy.** Removal of all but a very small part of the thyroid. Lymph nodes near the cancer may also be removed and checked under a microscope for signs of cancer.

- **Total thyroidectomy.** Removal of the whole thyroid. Lymph nodes near the cancer may also be removed and checked under a microscope for signs of cancer.

- **Tracheostomy.** Surgery to create an opening (stoma) into the windpipe to help you breathe. The opening itself may also be called a "tracheostomy."

Radiation Therapy

Radiation therapy is a cancer treatment that uses high-energy x-rays or other types of radiation to kill cancer cells or keep them from growing. There are two types of radiation therapy:

- **External radiation therapy** uses a machine outside the body to send radiation toward the cancer. Sometimes the radiation is aimed directly at the tumor during surgery. This is called "intraoperative radiation therapy."

- **Internal radiation therapy** uses a radioactive substance sealed in needles, seeds, wires, or catheters that are placed directly into or near the cancer.

Radiation therapy may be given after surgery to kill any thyroid cancer cells that were not removed. Follicular and papillary thyroid cancers are sometimes treated with radioactive iodine (RAI) therapy. RAI is taken by mouth and collects in any remaining thyroid tissue, including thyroid cancer cells that have spread to other places in the body. Since only thyroid tissue takes up iodine, the RAI destroys thyroid tissue and thyroid cancer cells without harming other tissue. Before a full treatment dose of RAI is given, a small test-dose is given to see if the tumor takes up the iodine.

The way the radiation therapy is given depends on the type and stage of the cancer being treated. External radiation therapy and RAI therapy are used to treat thyroid cancer.

Chemotherapy

Chemotherapy is a cancer treatment that uses drugs to stop the growth of cancer cells, either by killing the cells or by stopping them from dividing. When chemotherapy is taken by mouth or injected into a vein or muscle, the drugs enter the bloodstream and can reach cancer cells throughout the body (systemic chemotherapy). When chemotherapy is placed directly into the cerebrospinal fluid, an organ, or a body cavity such as the abdomen, the drugs mainly affect cancer cells in those areas (regional chemotherapy).

The way the chemotherapy is given depends on the type and stage of the cancer being treated.

Thyroid Hormone Therapy

Hormone therapy is a cancer treatment that removes hormones or blocks their action and stops cancer cells from growing. Hormones are substances made by glands in the body and circulated in the bloodstream. In the treatment of thyroid cancer, drugs may be given to prevent the body from making thyroid-stimulating hormone (TSH), a hormone that can increase the chance that thyroid cancer will grow or recur.

Also, because thyroid cancer treatment kills thyroid cells, the thyroid is not able to make enough thyroid hormone. Patients are given thyroid hormone replacement pills.

Targeted Therapy

Targeted therapy is a type of treatment that uses drugs or other substances to identify and attack specific cancer cells without harming normal cells. There are different types of targeted therapy:

- **Tyrosine kinase inhibitor.** Tyrosine kinase inhibitor therapy blocks signals needed for tumors to grow. Sorafenib, lenvatinib, vandetanib, and cabozantinib are used to treat certain types of thyroid cancer. Types of tyrosine kinase inhibitors are being studied to treat advanced thyroid cancer.

- **Protein kinase inhibitor.** Protein kinase inhibitor therapy blocks proteins needed for cell growth and may kill cancer cells. Dabrafenib and trametinib are used to treat anaplastic thyroid cancer in patients with a certain mutation in the *BRAF* gene.

Watchful Waiting

Watchful waiting is closely monitoring a patient's condition without giving any treatment until signs or symptoms appear or change.

Follow-Up Tests May Be Needed

Some of the tests that were done to diagnose the cancer or to find out the stage of the cancer may be repeated. Some tests will be repeated in order to see how well the treatment is working. Decisions about whether to continue, change or stop treatment may be based on the results of these tests.

Some of the tests will continue to be done from time to time after treatment has ended. The results of these tests can show if your condition has changed or if the cancer has recurred (come back). These tests are sometimes called "follow-up tests" or "check-ups."

Chapter 24

Parathyroid Gland Disorders

Chapter Contents

Section 24.1

Hypoparathyroidism

This section includes text excerpted from "Hypoparathyroidism,"
Eunice Kennedy Shriver National Institute of Child Health and
Human Development (NICHD), June 26, 2019.

Hypoparathyroidism is a rare disorder of calcium metabolism.

The body has four parathyroid glands, which are pea-sized and located in the neck behind the thyroid gland. The parathyroid glands make parathyroid hormone (PTH) and are part of the endocrine system. PTH regulates the amount of calcium and phosphorus in the blood through its direct effects on the kidney and bone, where the body stores most of its calcium.

Decreased PTH levels lead to low calcium levels and high phosphorus levels in the blood. This imbalance can lead to problems with muscles, teeth, and nerve endings.

What Are the Symptoms of Hypoparathyroidism?

People with hypoparathyroidism have low or undetectable levels of PTH and low levels of calcium in the blood. Chronic symptoms may include:

- Tingling in the lips, fingers, and toes

- Muscle cramps and spasms (called "tetany") that cause pain in the face, hands, legs, and feet

- Muscle weakness and generalized fatigue

- Problems with the teeth, including weakened enamel

- Calcium deposits in the brain or kidney

- Seizures

- Cataracts

- Increased risk of kidney problems

What Causes Hypoparathyroidism

The most common cause of hypoparathyroidism is an injury to the parathyroid glands during head and neck surgery. For example, thyroid surgery can damage the parathyroid glands or the surrounding tissues.

In adults, the disorder usually is a complication of neck surgery. In children, it is most often due to an inherited disorder. Congenital hypoparathyroidism, which can be present at birth or appear in early childhood, may be caused by a genetic variant or mutation. Some cases of congenital hypoparathyroidism may be part of a syndrome, meaning it is one of several symptoms, while in other instances the problem occurs by itself.

Autoimmune polyglandular failure type 1 (APS-1) is a rare inherited autoimmune disease including hypoparathyroidism. APS-1 is usually diagnosed in early childhood, and hypoparathyroidism is usually the first of several hormonal deficiencies to appear.

How Do Healthcare Providers Diagnose Hypoparathyroidism?

To diagnose hypoparathyroidism, a healthcare provider will usually start with a blood test to determine the levels of the following:

- Parathyroid hormone

- Calcium

- Phosphorus

- Creatinine

- Magnesium

A urine test determines how much calcium the kidneys are releasing.

How Is Hypoparathyroidism Treated?

Unlike most other hormonal deficits, hypoparathyroidism is not treated with replacement of the missing hormone, PTH.

The standard treatment for hypoparathyroidism consists of activated vitamin D (calcitriol) and calcium supplements. Some people may also need magnesium supplementation. Conventional therapy requires many pills taken throughout the day.

Diet recommendations usually include eating foods high in calcium, such as dairy products, breakfast cereals, fortified orange juice, and green, leafy vegetables, or avoiding foods high in phosphorus, such as meat, poultry, fish, nuts, whole grains, and beans.

Conventional therapy with vitamin D and calcium may lead to a buildup of calcium in the kidneys. This buildup may lead to problems, including kidney stones and deposits of calcium, reduced kidney function, tissue damage, or even kidney failure.

The development of PTH as a replacement therapy in patients with hypoparathyroidism was first explored by *Eunice Kennedy Shriver* National Institute of Child Health and Human Development (NICHD) investigators beginning in 1992. Since then, NICHD researchers have conducted a series of classic studies evaluating PTH 1-34 regimens, including once-daily and twice-daily PTH injections without concurrent use of calcitriol or calcium supplements in adults and children. These NICHD researchers also introduced PTH delivery by an insulin pump in two landmark studies in adults and in children. In January 2015, the U.S. Food and Drug Administration (FDA) approved PTH 1-84 for adult hypoparathyroidism patients who do not respond well to standard treatment, as an add-on to that treatment.

Section 24.2

Primary Hyperparathyroidism

This section includes text excerpted from "Primary Hyperparathyroidism," National Institute of Diabetes and Digestive and Kidney Diseases (NIDDK), March 2019.

What Is Primary Hyperparathyroidism?

Primary hyperparathyroidism is a disorder of the parathyroid glands, four pea-sized glands located on or near the thyroid gland in the neck. "Primary" means this disorder begins in the parathyroid glands, rather than resulting from another health problem such as kidney failure. In primary hyperparathyroidism, one or more of the parathyroid glands is overactive. As a result, the gland makes too much parathyroid hormone (PTH).

Too much PTH causes calcium levels in your blood to rise too high, which can lead to health problems, such as bone thinning and kidney stones. Doctors usually catch primary hyperparathyroidism early through routine blood tests, before serious problems occur.

What Do the Parathyroid Glands Do?

The parathyroid glands' only purpose is to make PTH, which helps maintain the right balance of calcium in your body. PTH raises blood calcium levels by:

- Causing bone, where most of your body's calcium is stored, to release calcium into the blood
- Helping your intestines absorb calcium from food
- Helping your kidneys hold on to calcium and return it to your blood instead of flushing it out in urine

When the level of calcium in your blood falls too low, the parathyroid glands release just enough PTH to bring your blood calcium levels back to normal.

You need calcium for good health. This mineral helps build bones and teeth and keep them strong. Calcium also helps your heart, muscles, and nerves work normally. Although their names are similar, the parathyroid glands and the thyroid gland are not related.

How Common Is Primary Hyperparathyroidism?

In the United States, about 100,000 people develop primary hyperparathyroidism each year. Primary hyperparathyroidism is one of the most common hormonal disorders.

Who Is More Likely to Develop Primary Hyperparathyroidism?

Primary hyperparathyroidism most often affects people between age 50 and 60. Women are affected 3 to 4 times more often than men. The disorder was more common in African Americans, followed by Caucasians, in one large study performed in North America.

What Are the Complications of Primary Hyperparathyroidism?

Primary hyperparathyroidism most often affects the bones and kidneys, although it also may play a part in other health problems.

Weakened Bones

High PTH levels trigger the bones to release more calcium than normal into the blood. The loss of calcium from the bones may weaken them.

Kidney Stones

The small intestine may absorb more calcium from food, adding to high levels of calcium in your blood. Extra calcium that is not used by your bones and muscles goes to your kidneys and is flushed out in urine. Too much calcium in your urine can cause kidney stones.

Other Complications

High blood calcium levels might play a part in other problems, such as heart disease, high blood pressure, and trouble concentrating. However, more research is needed to better understand how primary hyperparathyroidism affects the heart, blood vessels, and brain.

What Are the Symptoms of Primary Hyperparathyroidism?

Most people with primary hyperparathyroidism have no symptoms. When symptoms appear, they are often mild and similar to those of many other disorders. Symptoms include:

- Muscle weakness
- Fatigue
- Depression
- Aches and pains in bones and joints

People with more severe disease may have:

- Loss of appetite
- Nausea
- Vomiting
- Constipation
- Confusion
- Increased thirst and urination

What Causes Primary Hyperparathyroidism

In about 8 out of 10 people with primary hyperparathyroidism, a benign, or noncancerous, tumor called an "adenoma" has formed in one of the parathyroid glands. The tumor causes the gland to become overactive. In most other cases, extra PTH comes from two or more adenomas or from hyperplasia, a condition in which all four parathyroid glands are enlarged. People with rare inherited conditions that affect the parathyroid glands, such as multiple endocrine neoplasia type 1 or familial hypocalciuric hypercalcemia, are more likely to have more than one gland affected.

Rarely, primary hyperparathyroidism is caused by cancer of a parathyroid gland.

How Do Doctors Diagnose Primary Hyperparathyroidism?

Doctors diagnose primary hyperparathyroidism when a blood test shows high blood calcium and PTH levels. Sometimes PTH levels are in the upper portion of the normal range, when they should drop to low-normal or below normal in response to high calcium levels. Other conditions can cause high calcium, but elevated PTH is the only source in primary hyperparathyroidism.

Routine blood tests can detect high blood calcium levels. High blood calcium may cause healthcare professionals to suspect hyperparathyroidism, even before symptoms appear.

Sometimes PTH levels are high but calcium levels are not. Doctors do not routinely test for PTH but may do so if you have osteoporosis or another disorder that affects bone strength. In some cases, this may be the first phase of primary hyperparathyroidism, before calcium levels start to rise.

Once doctors diagnose hyperparathyroidism, a 24-hour urine collection can help find the cause. This test measures certain chemicals, such as calcium and creatinine, a waste product that healthy kidneys remove. You will collect your urine over a 24-hour period and your healthcare professional will send it to a lab for analysis. Results of the test may help tell primary hyperparathyroidism from hyperparathyroidism caused by a kidney disorder. The test can also rule out familial hypocalciuric hypercalcemia (FHH), a rare genetic disorder, as a cause.

What Tests Do Doctors Use to Look for Complications of Primary Hyperparathyroidism?

Once doctors diagnose primary hyperparathyroidism, they may use other tests to look for bone weakness, kidney problems, and low levels of vitamin D.

Bone Mineral Density Test

Dual energy x-ray absorptiometry, also called a "DXA" or "DEXA" scan, uses low-dose x-rays to measure bone density. During the test, you will lie on a padded table while a technician moves the scanner over your body. A bone expert or radiologist will read the scan.

Kidney Imaging Tests

Doctors may use one of the following imaging tests to look for kidney stones.

- **Ultrasound.** Ultrasound uses a device called a "transducer" that bounces safe, painless sound waves off organs to create an image of their structure. A specially trained technician does the procedure. A radiologist reads the images, which can show kidney stones.

- **Abdominal x-ray.** An abdominal x-ray is a picture of the abdomen that uses low levels of radiation and is recorded on film or on a computer. During an abdominal x-ray, you lie on a table or stand up. A technician positions the x-ray machine close to your abdomen and asks you to hold your breath so the picture will not be blurry. A radiologist reads the x-ray, which can show the location of kidney stones in the urinary tract. Not all stones are visible on an abdominal x-ray.

- **Computed tomography (CT) scans.** CT scans use a combination of x-rays and computer technology to create images of your urinary tract. CT scans sometimes use a contrast medium—a dye or other substance that makes structures inside your body easier to see. Contrast medium is not usually needed to see kidney stones. For the scan, you will lie on a table that slides into a tunnel-shaped machine that takes the x-rays. A radiologist reads the images, which can show the size and location of a kidney stone.

Vitamin D Blood Test

Healthcare professionals test for vitamin D levels because low levels are common in people with primary hyperparathyroidism. In patients with primary hyperparathyroidism, the low vitamin D level can further stimulate the parathyroid glands to make even more parathyroid hormone. Also, a very low vitamin D level may cause a secondary form of hyperparathyroidism, which resolves when vitamin D levels are returned to normal.

How Do Doctors Treat Primary Hyperparathyroidism?

Guidelines help doctors to decide whether or not parathyroid surgery should be recommended. You might be a candidate for surgery if you meet any of these guidelines:

- Blood calcium > 1 mg/dL above normal

- Bone density by DXA < -2.5 at any site (lumbar spine, hip, or forearm)

- History of kidney stones or evidence of kidney stones or calcifications in the kidney by imaging (e.g., x-ray, ultrasound, CT scan). Evidence for stone risk by 24-hour urine with excessive calcium and other stone risk factors.

- A fracture resulting from relatively little force, such as a fall from a standing or sitting position (a fragility fracture)

- Age < 50

Doctors most often recommend parathyroid surgery, particularly if the patient meets one or more of the guidelines noted above. It is also not inappropriate to recommend surgery in those who do not meet guidelines as long as there are no medical contraindications to surgery. In those who do not meet guidelines or do not choose surgery, the doctor will monitor the patient's condition. If there is evidence for progressive disease (e.g., higher calcium level, lower bone density, a fracture, kidney stone), surgery would be advised. For patients who are not going to have parathyroid surgery, even though guidelines are met, doctors can prescribe medicines to control high blood calcium or improve the bone density.

Surgery

Surgery to remove the overactive parathyroid gland or glands is the only sure way to cure primary hyperparathyroidism. Doctors recommend surgery for people with clear symptoms or complications of the disease. In people without symptoms, doctors follow the above guidelines to identify who might benefit from parathyroid surgery. Surgery can lead to improved bone density and can lower the chance of forming kidney stones.

When performed by experienced surgeons, surgery almost always cures primary hyperparathyroidism.

Surgeons often use imaging tests before surgery to locate the overactive gland or glands to be removed. The tests used most often are sestamibi, ultrasound, and CT scans. In a sestamibi scan, you will get an injection, or shot, of a small amount of radioactive dye in your vein. The overactive parathyroid gland or glands then absorb the dye. The surgeon can see where the dye has been absorbed by using a special camera.

Surgeons use two main types of operations to remove the overactive gland or glands.

- **Minimally invasive parathyroidectomy.** Also called "focused parathyroidectomy" (FP), surgeons use this type of surgery when they think only one of the parathyroid glands is overactive. Guided by a tumor-imaging test, your surgeon will make a small incision, or cut, in your neck to remove the gland. The small incision means you will probably have less pain and a faster recovery than people who have more invasive surgery. You can go home the same day. Your doctor may use regional or general anesthesia during the surgery.

- **Bilateral neck exploration.** This type of surgery uses a larger incision that lets the surgeon find and look at all four parathyroid glands and remove the overactive ones. If you have bilateral neck exploration, you will probably have general anesthesia and may need to stay in the hospital overnight.

Parathyroid surgery is safe. Rarely, problems can occur after surgery. In about 1 out of every 100 people, the nerves controlling the vocal cords are damaged during surgery, which most often results in hoarseness. This condition usually gets better on its own.

Low calcium levels in the blood may occur after surgery but usually return to normal in a few days or weeks. On rare occasions, not enough parathyroid tissue is left to make PTH, which can result in hypoparathyroidism.

Monitoring

Some people who have mild primary hyperparathyroidism may not need surgery right away, or even any surgery, and can be safely monitored.

You may want to talk with your doctor about long-term monitoring if you:

- Do not have symptoms

- Have only slightly high blood calcium levels
- Have normal kidneys and bone density

Long-term monitoring should include regular doctor visits, a yearly blood test to measure calcium levels and check your kidney function, and a bone density test every one to two years.

If you and your doctor choose long-term monitoring, you should:

- Drink plenty of water so you do not get dehydrated
- Get regular physical activity to help keep your bones strong
- Avoid certain diuretics, such as thiazides

Medicines

Cinacalcet is a medicine that decreases the amount of PTH the parathyroid glands make and lowers calcium levels in the blood. Doctors may prescribe cinacalcet to treat very high calcium levels in people with primary hyperparathyroidism who cannot have surgery.

Cinacalcet does not improve bone density. If you have bone loss, your doctor may prescribe alendronate or other medications to help increase bone density.

Should You Change Your Diet If You Have Primary Hyperparathyroidism?

You do not need to change your diet or limit the amount of calcium you get from food and beverages. You will need to take a vitamin D supplement if your vitamin D levels are low. Talk with your healthcare professional about how much vitamin D you should take.

If you lose all your healthy parathyroid tissue and develop lasting low-calcium levels, you will need to take both calcium and vitamin D for life.

Section 24.3

Parathyroid Cancer

This section includes text excerpted from "Parathyroid
Cancer Treatment (PDQ®)—Patient Version," National
Cancer Institute (NCI), April 9, 2019.

What Is Parathyroid Cancer?

Parathyroid cancer is a rare disease in which malignant (cancer)
cells form in the tissues of a parathyroid gland. The parathyroid glands
are four pea-sized organs found in the neck near the thyroid gland.
The parathyroid glands make parathyroid hormone (PTH or parathormone). PTH helps the body use and store calcium to keep the calcium
in the blood at normal levels.

A parathyroid gland may become overactive and make too much
PTH, a condition called "hyperparathyroidism." Hyperparathyroidism
can occur when a benign tumor (noncancer), called an "adenoma,"
forms on one of the parathyroid glands, and causes it to grow and
become overactive. Sometimes hyperparathyroidism can be caused by
parathyroid cancer, but this is very rare.

The extra PTH causes:

• The calcium stored in the bones to move into the blood

• The intestines to absorb more calcium from the food we eat

This condition is called "hypercalcemia" (too much calcium in the
blood). The hypercalcemia caused by hyperparathyroidism is more
serious and life-threatening than parathyroid cancer itself and treating
hypercalcemia is as important as treating the cancer.

What Are the Risk Factors for Parathyroid Cancer?

Having certain inherited disorders can increase the risk of developing parathyroid cancer.

Risk factors for parathyroid cancer include the following rare
disorders that are inherited (passed down from parent to child):

• Familial isolated hyperparathyroidism (FIHP)

• Multiple endocrine neoplasia type 1 (MEN1) syndrome

Treatment with radiation therapy may increase the risk of developing a parathyroid adenoma.

Signs and Symptoms of Parathyroid Cancer

Most parathyroid cancer signs and symptoms are caused by the hypercalcemia that develops. Signs and symptoms of hypercalcemia include the following:

- Weakness
- Feeling very tired
- Nausea and vomiting
- Loss of appetite
- Weight loss for no known reason
- Being much more thirsty than usual
- Urinating much more than usual
- Constipation
- Trouble thinking clearly

Other signs and symptoms of parathyroid cancer include the following:

- Pain in the abdomen, side, or back that does not go away
- Pain in the bones
- A broken bone
- A lump in the neck
- Change in voice such as hoarseness
- Trouble swallowing

Other conditions may cause the same signs and symptoms as parathyroid cancer. Check with your doctor if you have any of these problems.

Diagnosis of Parathyroid Cancer

Tests that examine the neck and blood are used to detect and diagnose parathyroid cancer.

Once blood tests are done and hyperparathyroidism is diagnosed, imaging tests may be done to help find which of the parathyroid glands is overactive. Sometimes the parathyroid glands are hard to find and imaging tests are done to find exactly where they are.

Parathyroid cancer may be hard to diagnose because the cells of a benign parathyroid adenoma and a malignant parathyroid cancer look alike. The patient's symptoms, blood levels of calcium and parathyroid hormone, and characteristics of the tumor are also used to make a diagnosis.

The following tests and procedures may be used:

- **Physical examination and history.** An examination of the body to check general signs of health, including checking for signs of disease, such as lumps or anything else that seems unusual. A history of the patient's health habits and past illnesses and treatments will also be taken.

- **Blood chemistry studies.** A procedure in which a blood sample is checked to measure the amounts of certain substances released into the blood by organs and tissues in the body. An unusual (higher or lower than normal) amount of a substance can be a sign of disease. To diagnose parathyroid cancer, the sample of blood is checked for its calcium level.

- **Parathyroid hormone (PTH) test.** A procedure in which a blood sample is checked to measure the amount of parathyroid hormone released into the blood by the parathyroid glands. A higher than normal amount of parathyroid hormone can be a sign of disease.

- **Sestamibi scan.** A type of radionuclide scan used to find an overactive parathyroid gland. A very small amount of a radioactive substance called "technetium 99" is injected into a vein and travels through the bloodstream to the parathyroid gland. The radioactive substance will collect in the overactive gland and show up brightly on a special camera that detects radioactivity.

- **Computed tomography (CT/CAT) scan.** A procedure that makes a series of detailed pictures of areas inside the body, taken from different angles. The pictures are made by a computer linked to an x-ray machine. A dye may be injected into a vein or swallowed to help the organs or tissues show up more clearly. This procedure is also called "computed tomography," "computerized tomography," or "computerized axial tomography."

- **Single-photon emission computed tomography (SPECT) scan.** A procedure to find malignant tumor cells in the neck. A small amount of a radioactive substance is injected into a vein or inhaled through the nose. As the substance travels through the blood, a camera rotates around the body and takes pictures of the neck. A computer uses the pictures to make a 3-dimensional (3-D) image of the neck. There will be increased blood flow and more activity in areas where cancer cells are growing. These areas will show up brighter in the picture.

- **Ultrasound exam.** A procedure in which high-energy sound waves (ultrasound) are bounced off internal tissues or organs and make echoes. The echoes form a picture of body tissues called a "sonogram."

- **Angiogram.** A procedure to look at blood vessels and the flow of blood. A contrast dye is injected into the blood vessel. As the contrast dye moves through the blood vessel, x-rays are taken to see if there are any blockages.

- **Venous sampling.** A procedure in which a sample of blood is taken from specific veins and checked to measure the amounts of certain substances released into the blood by nearby organs and tissues. If imaging tests do not show which parathyroid gland is overactive, blood samples may be taken from veins near each parathyroid gland to find which one is making too much PTH.

Stages of Parathyroid Cancer

The prognosis and treatment options depend on the following:

- Whether the calcium level in the blood can be controlled

- The stage of the cancer

- Whether the tumor and the capsule around the tumor can be completely removed by surgery

- The patient's general health

Recurrent Parathyroid Cancer

Recurrent parathyroid cancer is cancer that has recurred (come back) after it has been treated. More than half of patients have a recurrence. The parathyroid cancer usually recurs between 2 and 5 years after the first surgery, but can recur up to 20 years later. It usually comes back in the tissues or lymph nodes of the neck. High blood calcium levels that appear after treatment may be the first sign of recurrence.

Treatment of Parathyroid Cancer

Different types of treatment are available for patients with parathyroid cancer. Some treatments are standard (the currently used treatment), and some are being tested in clinical trials. A treatment clinical trial is a research study meant to help improve current treatments or obtain information on new treatments for patients with cancer. When clinical trials show that a new treatment is better than the standard treatment, the new treatment may become the standard treatment. Patients may want to think about taking part in a clinical trial. Some clinical trials are open only to patients who have not started treatment.

Treatment Includes Control of Hypercalcemia in Patients Who Have an Overactive Parathyroid Gland

In order to reduce the amount of parathyroid hormone that is being made and control the level of calcium in the blood, as much of the tumor as possible is removed in surgery. For patients who cannot have surgery, medication may be used.

Four Types of Standard Treatment Are Used
Surgery

Surgery (removing the cancer in an operation) is the most common treatment for parathyroid cancer that is in the parathyroid glands or has spread to other parts of the body. Because parathyroid cancer grows very slowly, cancer that has spread to other parts of the body may be removed by surgery in order to cure the patient or control the effects of the disease for a long time. Before surgery, treatment is given to control hypercalcemia.

The following surgical procedures may be used:

- **En bloc resection.** Surgery to remove the entire parathyroid gland and the capsule around it. Sometimes lymph nodes, half of the thyroid gland on the same side of the body as the cancer, and muscles, tissues, and a nerve in the neck are also removed.

- **Tumor debulking.** A surgical procedure in which as much of the tumor as possible is removed. Some tumors cannot be completely removed.

- **Metastasectomy.** Surgery to remove any cancer that has spread to distant organs such as the lung.

Surgery for parathyroid cancer sometimes damages nerves of the vocal cords. There are treatments to help with speech problems caused by this nerve damage.

Radiation Therapy

Radiation therapy is a cancer treatment that uses high-energy x-rays or other types of radiation to kill cancer cells or keep them from growing. There are two types of radiation therapy:

- **External radiation therapy** uses a machine outside the body to send radiation toward the cancer.

- **Internal radiation therapy** uses a radioactive substance sealed in needles, seeds, wires, or catheters that are placed directly into or near the cancer.

The way the radiation therapy is given depends on the type and stage of the cancer being treated. External radiation therapy is used to treat parathyroid cancer.

Chemotherapy

Chemotherapy is a cancer treatment that uses drugs to stop the growth of cancer cells, either by killing the cells or by stopping them from dividing. When chemotherapy is taken by mouth or injected into a vein or muscle, the drugs enter the bloodstream and can reach cancer cells throughout the body (systemic chemotherapy). When chemotherapy is placed directly into the cerebrospinal fluid (CSF), an organ, or a body cavity such as the abdomen, the drugs mainly affect cancer cells in those areas (regional chemotherapy). The way the chemotherapy is given depends on the type and stage of the cancer being treated.

Supportive Care

Supportive care is given to lessen the problems caused by the disease or its treatment. Supportive care for hypercalcemia caused by parathyroid cancer may include the following:

- Intravenous (IV) fluids
- Drugs that increase how much urine the body makes

- Drugs that stop the body from absorbing calcium from the food we eat

- Drugs that stop the parathyroid gland from making parathyroid hormone

Follow-Up Tests May Be Needed

Some of the tests that were done to diagnose cancer or to find out the stage of the cancer may be repeated. Some tests will be repeated in order to see how well the treatment is working. Decisions about whether to continue, change or stop treatment may be based on the results of these tests.

Some of the tests will continue to be done from time to time after treatment has ended. The results of these tests can show if your condition has changed or if cancer has recurred (come back). These tests are sometimes called "follow-up tests" or "check-ups."

Parathyroid cancer often recurs. Patients should have regular check-ups for the rest of their lives, to find and treat recurrences early.

Part Four

Adrenal Gland Disorders

Chapter 25

About Adrenal Gland Disorders

The adrenal glands, located on the top of each kidney, are responsible for releasing different classes of hormones. These hormones—cortisol, aldosterone, adrenaline, and noradrenaline—control many important functions in the body, including:

- Maintaining metabolic processes, such as managing blood sugar levels and regulating inflammation
- Regulating the balance of salt and water
- Controlling the "fight or flight" response to stress
- Maintaining pregnancy
- Initiating and controlling sexual maturation during childhood and puberty

The adrenal glands are also an important source of sex steroids, such as estrogen and testosterone.

What Are Adrenal Gland Disorders?

The adrenal glands, located on the top of each kidney, are responsible for releasing different hormones. Adrenal gland disorders occur

This chapter includes text excerpted from "About Adrenal Gland Disorders," *Eunice Kennedy Shriver* National Institute of Child Health and Human Development (NICHD), January 31, 2017.

when the adrenal glands do not work properly. They can occur when the adrenal glands produce either too much or too little of these hormones.

Adrenal gland disorders can be classified into disorders that occur when too much hormone is produced or when too little hormone is produced. These disorders can occur if there is a problem with the adrenal gland itself, such as a disease, genetic mutation, tumor, or infection. Or, sometimes the disorder results from a problem in another gland, such as the pituitary gland, which helps to regulate the adrenal gland. In addition, some medications can cause problems with how the adrenal glands function. When the adrenal glands produce too little or too many hormones, or when too many hormones come into the body from an outside source, serious health problems can develop.

Overall, adrenal gland disorders are generally rare. The number of people affected and at risk depends on the specific type of adrenal gland disorder.

What Are Some Types of Adrenal Gland Disorders?

There are several types of adrenal gland disorders, each with its own symptoms and treatments.

- Adrenal gland tumors
- Adrenocortical carcinoma
- Cushing syndrome
- Congenital adrenal hyperplasia (CAH)
- Pituitary tumors
- Pheochromocytoma
- Adrenal gland suppression
- Addison disease
- Hyperaldosteronism

What Causes Adrenal Gland Disorders

Adrenal gland disorders are caused by problems with one or both adrenal glands or by problems with other glands, such as the pituitary gland.

Specific disorders can develop when the adrenal glands produce too few or too many hormones, or when too many hormones are introduced from an outside source.

How Do Healthcare Providers Diagnose Adrenal Gland Disorders?

Methods for diagnosing adrenal gland disorders differ depending on the specific disorder. For example, the severe form of CAH is most commonly identified during newborn screening. But, pheochromocytoma is diagnosed using blood and urine tests.

What Are the Treatments for Adrenal Gland Disorders?

Healthcare providers use a variety of surgical and medical treatments for adrenal gland disorders. These include:

- Surgery to remove tumors in the adrenal gland or, when appropriate, surgery to remove the one or both of the adrenal glands

- Minimally invasive surgery performed through the nostrils to remove tumors in the pituitary gland

- Medication to stop the excess production of hormones

- Hormone replacement

Chapter 26

Adrenal Insufficiency and Addison Disease

What Is Adrenal Insufficiency?

Adrenal insufficiency is a disorder that occurs when the adrenal glands do not make enough of certain hormones. The adrenal glands are located just above the kidneys. Adrenal insufficiency can be primary, secondary, or tertiary. Primary adrenal insufficiency is often called "Addison disease."

Adrenal insufficiency can affect your body's ability to respond to stress and maintain other essential life functions. With treatment, most people with adrenal insufficiency can have a normal, active life.

Addison Disease

Addison disease occurs when the adrenal glands are damaged and cannot make enough of the hormone cortisol and sometimes the hormone aldosterone.

Secondary Adrenal Insufficiency

Secondary adrenal insufficiency starts in the pituitary gland—a pea-sized gland at the base of the brain. The pituitary gland makes

This chapter includes text excerpted from "Adrenal Insufficiency and Addison's Disease," National Institute of Diabetes and Digestive and Kidney Diseases (NIDDK), October 9, 2018.

adrenocorticotropin (ACTH), a hormone that tells the adrenal glands to make cortisol. If the pituitary gland does not make enough ACTH, the adrenal glands do not make enough cortisol. Over time, the adrenal glands can shrink and stop working.

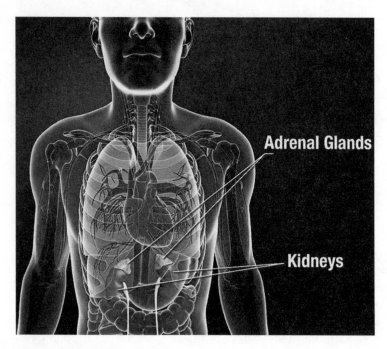

Figure 26.1. *Adrenal Gland*

The adrenal glands, two small glands on top of your kidneys, make hormones that are essential for life.

Tertiary Adrenal Insufficiency

Tertiary adrenal insufficiency starts in the hypothalamus, a small area of the brain near the pituitary gland. The hypothalamus makes corticotropin-releasing hormone (CRH), a hormone that tells the pituitary gland to make ACTH. When the hypothalamus does not make enough CRH, the pituitary gland does not make enough ACTH. In turn, the adrenal glands do not make enough cortisol.

What Do Adrenal Hormones Do?

The adrenal glands make two main types of hormones: cortisol and aldosterone.

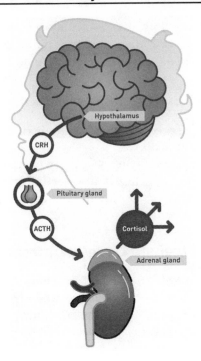

Figure 26.2. *Cortisol Creation*

CRH tells the pituitary gland to make ACTH, which in turn tells the adrenals to make cortisol.

Cortisol

Cortisol is sometimes called the "stress hormone" because it helps your body respond to stress. Cortisol also helps:

- Control blood pressure
- Control blood glucose also called "blood sugar"
- Reduce inflammation
- Control metabolism

Cortisol belongs to a class of hormones called "glucocorticoids."

Aldosterone

Aldosterone helps maintain the balance of the minerals such as sodium and potassium in your blood. Sodium and potassium work together to control the salt and water balance in your body and help keep blood pressure stable. Both help maintain normal nerve and muscle function. Potassium also helps your heartbeat stay regular. Aldosterone belongs to a class of hormones called "mineralocorticoids."

How Common Is Adrenal Insufficiency

Addison disease is rare. In developed countries, it affects about 100 to 140 of every million people.

Secondary adrenal insufficiency is more common, affecting 150 to 280 people per million. Secondary and tertiary adrenal insufficiency are often grouped together, so no numbers for tertiary adrenal insufficiency by itself are available.

Who Is More Likely to Develop Adrenal Insufficiency?

Women are more likely than men to develop Addison disease. This condition occurs most often in people between the ages of 30 and 50, although it can occur at any age, even in children.

Secondary adrenal insufficiency occurs in people with certain conditions that affect the pituitary gland.

People who take glucocorticoid medicines, such as prednisone, for a long time and then stop are most likely to develop tertiary adrenal insufficiency. These medicines are used to treat medical conditions such as asthma, rheumatoid arthritis, lupus, cancer, and inflammation, among others.

What Are the Complications of Adrenal Insufficiency?

The most serious complication of adrenal insufficiency is called "adrenal crisis." If not treated right away, adrenal crisis can cause death. Your body needs much more cortisol than usual during times of physical stress such as illness, serious injury, or surgery. The severe lack of cortisol at these times can cause life-threatening low blood pressure, low blood glucose, low blood sodium, and high blood potassium.

Seek Care Right Away

If you have adrenal insufficiency and have symptoms of adrenal crisis, you need emergency medical treatment. Symptoms include:

- Sudden, severe pain in your lower back, abdomen, or legs

- Vomiting and diarrhea

- Weakness

- Confusion

- Loss of consciousness

An injection, or shot, of corticosteroid—a glucocorticoid medicine—can save your life in an emergency. Make sure you have a corticosteroid injection with you at all times and make sure your friends and family know how and when to give you the injection. Wear a medical alert tag or carry a card with information about your condition in case of an emergency.

Sometimes the lack of aldosterone in Addison disease can cause hyponatremia. This condition occurs when you do not have enough sodium in your blood. Hyponatremia can cause confusion, fatigue, and muscle twitches and seizures. The lack of aldosterone can also cause hyperkalemia, or too much potassium. Mild hyperkalemia may not cause problems, but severe hyperkalemia can cause life-threatening changes in your heart rhythm.

Symptoms of Adrenal Insufficiency

The most common symptoms of adrenal insufficiency are:

- Chronic, or long-lasting, fatigue

- Muscle weakness

- Loss of appetite

- Weight loss

- Abdominal pain

Other symptoms of adrenal insufficiency can include:

- Nausea

- Vomiting

- Diarrhea

- Low blood pressure that drops further when you stand up, causing dizziness or fainting

- Irritability and depression

- Joint pain

- Craving salty foods

- Hypoglycemia, or low blood glucose

- Irregular or no menstrual periods

- Loss of interest in sex

People with Addison disease may also have darkening of their skin. This darkening is most visible on scars; skin folds; pressure points such as the elbows, knees, knuckles, and toes; lips; and mucous membranes such as the lining of the cheek.

Because symptoms of adrenal insufficiency come on slowly over time, they may be overlooked or confused with other illnesses. Sometimes symptoms appear for the first time during an adrenal crisis. If you always feel tired, weak, or are losing weight, ask your healthcare professional if you might have adrenal insufficiency. Early treatment can help avoid an adrenal crisis.

Causes of Adrenal Insufficiency

Different types of adrenal insufficiency have different causes. The most common cause of adrenal insufficiency overall is suddenly stopping corticosteroids after taking them for a long time.

Addison Disease

Damage to the adrenal glands in Addison disease is usually caused by autoimmune disease—when your immune system attacks your body's own cells and organs. In developed countries, the autoimmune disease causes 8 or 9 of every 10 cases of Addison disease.

Certain infections can also cause Addison disease. Tuberculosis (TB) can damage the adrenal glands and used to be the most common cause of Addison disease. As treatment improved over the years, TB became a much less common cause. People with human immunodeficiency virus infection (HIV)/acquired immune deficiency syndrome (AIDS), whose weakened immune systems cannot fight off infections that could cause Addison disease, are also at risk.

Less common causes of Addison disease are:

- Cancer cells in the adrenal glands

- Surgical removal of the adrenal glands to treat other conditions

- Bleeding into the adrenal glands

- Genetic disorders that affect the way the adrenal glands develop or function

- Certain medicines, such as antifungal medicines or etomidate, a type of general anesthesia

Secondary Adrenal Insufficiency

Anything that affects the pituitary gland's ability to make ACTH can cause secondary adrenal insufficiency. The pituitary gland makes many different hormones, so ACTH may not be the only hormone that is lacking.

Causes of secondary adrenal insufficiency include:

- Autoimmune disease

- Pituitary tumors or infection

- Bleeding in the pituitary gland

- Genetic diseases that affect the way the pituitary gland develops or functions

- Surgical removal of the pituitary gland to treat other conditions

- Traumatic brain injury (TBI)

Tertiary Adrenal Insufficiency

The most common cause of tertiary adrenal insufficiency is suddenly stopping corticosteroids after taking them for a long time. Prescription doses of corticosteroids can cause higher levels of cortisol in your blood than your body normally makes. High levels in your blood for a long time cause the hypothalamus to make less CRH. Less CRH means less ACTH, which in turn causes the adrenal glands to stop making cortisol.

Once you stop taking corticosteroids, your adrenal glands may be slow to start working again. To give them time to start making cortisol again, your doctor will gradually reduce your dose over a period of weeks or even months. Even so, your adrenal glands might not begin to work normally for many months. Your doctor should watch you carefully for symptoms of adrenal insufficiency.

Tertiary adrenal insufficiency can also occur after Cushing syndrome is cured. Cushing syndrome is a hormonal disorder caused by high levels of cortisol in the blood for a long time. Sometimes Cushing syndrome is caused by tumors, usually noncancerous, in the pituitary or adrenal glands that make too much ACTH or cortisol. Once the tumors are surgically removed, the source of excess ACTH or cortisol is suddenly gone. Your adrenal glands may be slow to start working again.

How Do Doctors Diagnose Adrenal Insufficiency?

Your doctor will review your symptoms and run tests to confirm that your cortisol levels are low.

Review of Symptoms

In its early stages, adrenal insufficiency can be hard to diagnose since symptoms come on slowly. Your healthcare professional may suspect it after reviewing your medical history and symptoms. The next step is blood testing to see if your cortisol levels are too low and to help find the cause.

Blood Tests
Adrenocorticotropin Stimulation Test

The ACTH stimulation test is the test used most often to diagnose adrenal insufficiency. In this test, a healthcare professional will give you an intravenous (IV) injection of manufactured ACTH, which is just like the ACTH your body makes. Your healthcare professional will take samples of your blood before and 30 minutes or 60 minutes after the injection. The cortisol levels in your blood samples are measured in a lab.

The normal response after an ACTH injection is a rise in blood cortisol levels. People with Addison disease and most people who have had secondary adrenal insufficiency for a long time have little or no increase in cortisol levels. The adrenal glands may be too damaged to respond to ACTH.

The ACTH test may not be accurate in people who have had secondary adrenal insufficiency for a shorter time because their adrenal glands have not yet shrunk and can still respond to ACTH.

Insulin Tolerance Test

If the results of the ACTH stimulation test are not clear or your doctor suspects a problem in the pituitary gland, you may have an insulin tolerance test (ITT). A healthcare professional will give you an IV injection of the hormone insulin, which lowers your levels of blood glucose. The dose is high enough to cause hypoglycemia, which occurs when your blood glucose level drops too low.

Hypoglycemia causes physical stress, which normally triggers the pituitary gland to make more ACTH. A healthcare professional will draw your blood at the beginning of the test and again every half hour during the next two hours. If your cortisol levels are low, your pituitary gland is not making enough ACTH, so your adrenal glands do not make enough cortisol. The ITT is the most reliable test to diagnose secondary adrenal insufficiency.

Very low blood glucose levels can be dangerous, so a healthcare professional must be present at all times during this test to make sure blood glucose levels do not drop too low. The ITT is not safe for people with heart disease, a history of seizures, and other serious illnesses.

Corticotropin-Releasing Hormone Stimulation Test

The CRH stimulation test is another option to help identify secondary insufficiency if the results of the ACTH test are not clear. This test can also tell secondary from tertiary adrenal insufficiency.

A healthcare professional will give you an IV injection of CRH and take samples of your blood before and 30, 60, 90, and 120 minutes after the injection to measure ACTH levels. If the pituitary gland is damaged, it will not make ACTH in response to the CRH injection. This result shows secondary adrenal insufficiency. A slow rise in ACTH levels suggests tertiary adrenal insufficiency.

What Tests Do Doctors Use to Find the Cause of Adrenal Insufficiency?

Once doctors diagnose and identify the type of adrenal insufficiency, they may use blood and imaging tests to find the exact cause.

Addison Disease
Antibody Blood Tests

A blood test can find antibodies that are present in autoimmune Addison disease. Antibodies are proteins made by your immune system to protect your body from bacteria or viruses. In autoimmune Addison disease, the antibodies mistakenly attack the adrenal glands. Most, but not all, people with autoimmune Addison disease have these antibodies. If the test shows antibodies, you do not need further testing.

Computed Tomography Scan

Computed tomography (CT) scans use a combination of x-rays and computer technology to create images of your organs and other internal structures. A CT scan of the abdomen can find changes in your adrenal glands. In autoimmune Addison disease, the glands are small or normal size and do not have other visible abnormalities.

Enlarged adrenal glands or a buildup of calcium in the glands can occur when Addison disease is caused by infection, bleeding in the adrenal glands, or cancer cells in the glands. However, these changes do not always occur in Addison disease caused by TB.

Tuberculosis

Tests to find TB include a chest x-ray, a urine test to look for the bacteria that causes TB, and a TB skin test. In the skin test, a healthcare professional injects a tiny amount of inactive TB bacteria under the skin of your forearm. If you develop a hard, raised bump or swelling on your arm, you have the TB bacteria in your body, even if you do not have active TB.

Secondary and Tertiary Adrenal Insufficiency
Magnetic Resonance Imaging

Magnetic resonance imaging (MRI) machines use radio waves and magnets to create detailed pictures of your internal organs and soft tissues without using x-rays. An MRI can look for changes in your pituitary gland and hypothalamus, such as large, noncancerous pituitary tumors.

How Is Adrenal Insufficiency Treated?

Your doctor will prescribe hormone medicines to replace the hormones that your adrenal glands are not making. You will need higher doses during times of physical stress.

Hormone Replacement

Cortisol is replaced with a corticosteroid, most often hydrocortisone, which you take two or three times a day by mouth. Less often, doctors prescribe prednisone or dexamethasone.

If your adrenal glands are not making aldosterone, you will take a medicine called "fludrocortisone," which helps balance the amount of sodium and fluids in your body. People with secondary adrenal insufficiency usually make enough aldosterone, so they do not need to take this medicine.

Your doctor will adjust the dose of each medicine to meet your body's needs.

Treatment for adrenal crisis includes immediate IV injections of corticosteroids and large amounts of IV saline, a salt solution, with dextrose added. Dextrose is a type of sugar.

Treatment in Special Situations
Surgery

If you are having any type of surgery that uses general anesthesia, you may have treatment with IV corticosteroids and saline. IV treatment begins before surgery and continues until you are fully awake after surgery and can take medicine by mouth. Your doctor will adjust the "stress" dose as you recover until you are back to your presurgery dose.

Illness

Talk with your doctor about how to adjust your dose of corticosteroids during an illness. You will need to increase your dose if you have a high fever. Once you recover, your doctor will adjust your dose back to your regular, preillness level. You will need immediate medical attention if you have a severe infection or diarrhea, or are vomiting and cannot keep your corticosteroid pills down. Without treatment, in an emergency room if necessary, these conditions can lead to an adrenal crisis.

Injury or Other Serious Condition

If you have a severe injury, you may need a higher, "stress" dose of corticosteroids right after the injury and while you recover. The same is true if you have a serious health condition such as suddenly passing out or being in a coma. Often, you must get these stress doses intravenously. Once you recover, your doctor will adjust your dose back to regular, preinjury level.

Pregnancy

If you become pregnant and have adrenal insufficiency, you will take the same dose of medicine as you did before pregnancy. However, if nausea and vomiting in early pregnancy make it hard to take medicine by mouth, your doctor may need to give you corticosteroid shots. During delivery, treatment is similar to that of people needing surgery. Following delivery, your doctor will slowly decrease your dose, and you will be back to your regular dose about 10 days after your baby is born.

Eating, Diet, and Nutrition

Some people with Addison disease who have low aldosterone can benefit from a high-sodium diet. A healthcare professional or a dietitian can recommend the best sodium sources and how much sodium you should have each day.

High doses of corticosteroids are linked to a higher risk of osteoporosis—a condition in which the bones become less dense and more likely to fracture. If you take corticosteroids, you may need to protect your bone health by getting enough dietary calcium and vitamin D. A healthcare professional or a dietitian can tell you how much calcium you should have based on your age. You may also need to take calcium supplements.

Chapter 27

Adrenal-Gland Cancer

What Is Adrenocortical Carcinoma?

Adrenocortical carcinoma is a rare disease in which malignant (cancer) cells form in the outer layer of the adrenal gland. There are two adrenal glands. The adrenal glands are small and shaped like a triangle. One adrenal gland sits on top of each kidney. Each adrenal gland has two parts. The outer layer of the adrenal gland is the adrenal cortex. The center of the adrenal gland is the adrenal medulla.

The adrenal cortex makes important hormones that:

- Balance the water and salt in the body

- Help keep blood pressure normal

- Help control the body's use of protein, fat, and carbohydrates

- Cause the body to have masculine or feminine characteristics

Adrenocortical carcinoma is also called "cancer of the adrenal cortex." A tumor of the adrenal cortex may be functioning (makes more hormones than normal) or nonfunctioning (does not make more hormones than normal). Most adrenocortical tumors are functioning. The hormones made by functioning tumors may cause certain signs or symptoms of disease.

This chapter includes text excerpted from "Adrenocortical Carcinoma Treatment (PDQ®)—Patient Version," National Cancer Institute (NCI), May 21, 2019.

235

The adrenal medulla makes hormones that help the body react to stress. Cancer that forms in the adrenal medulla is called "pheochromocytoma."

Adrenocortical carcinoma and pheochromocytoma can occur in both adults and children. Treatment for children, however, is different than treatment for adults.

Risk Factors of Adrenocortical Carcinoma

Having certain genetic conditions increases the risk of adrenocortical carcinoma. Having a risk factor does not mean that you will get cancer; not having risk factors does not mean that you will not get cancer. Talk with your doctor if you think you may be at risk.

Risk factors for adrenocortical carcinoma include having the following hereditary diseases:

• Li-Fraumeni syndrome

• Beckwith-Wiedemann syndrome

• Carney complex

Symptoms of Adrenocortical Carcinoma

These and other signs and symptoms may be caused by adrenocortical carcinoma:

• A lump in the abdomen

• Pain the abdomen or back

• A feeling of fullness in the abdomen

A nonfunctioning adrenocortical tumor may not cause signs or symptoms in the early stages.

A functioning adrenocortical tumor makes too much of one of the following hormones:

• Cortisol

• Aldosterone

• Testosterone

• Estrogen

Too much cortisol may cause:

• Weight gain in the face, neck, and trunk of the body and thin arms and legs

- Growth of fine hair on the face, upper back, or arms
- A round, red, full face
- A lump of fat on the back of the neck
- A deepening of the voice and swelling of the sex organs or breasts in both males and females
- Muscle weakness
- High blood sugar
- High blood pressure
- Too much aldosterone may cause:
- High blood pressure
- Muscle weakness or cramps
- Frequent urination
- Feeling thirsty

Too much testosterone (in women) may cause:

- Growth of fine hair on the face, upper back, or arms
- Acne
- Balding
- A deepening of the voice
- No menstrual periods

Men who make too much testosterone do not usually have signs or symptoms.

Too much estrogen (in women) may cause:

- Irregular menstrual periods in women who have not gone through menopause
- Vaginal bleeding in women who have gone through menopause
- Weight gain

Too much estrogen (in men) may cause:

- Growth of breast tissue
- Lower sex drive
- Impotence

These and other signs and symptoms may be caused by adrenocortical carcinoma or by other conditions. Check with your doctor if you have any of these problems.

Diagnosis of Adrenocortical Carcinoma

Imaging studies and tests that examine the blood and urine are used to detect (find) and diagnose adrenocortical carcinoma.

The tests and procedures used to diagnose adrenocortical carcinoma depend on the patient's signs and symptoms. The following tests and procedures may be used:

- **Physical examination and history.** An examination of the body to check general signs of health, including checking for signs of disease, such as lumps or anything else that seems unusual. A history of the patient's health habits and past illnesses and treatments will also be taken.

- **Twenty-four-hour urine test.** A test in which urine is collected for 24 hours to measure the amounts of cortisol or 17-ketosteroids. A higher than normal amount of these in the urine may be a sign of disease in the adrenal cortex.

- **Low-dose dexamethasone suppression test.** A test in which one or more small doses of dexamethasone are given. The level of cortisol is checked from a sample of blood or from urine that is collected for three days. This test is done to check if the adrenal gland is making too much cortisol.

- **High-dose dexamethasone suppression test.** A test in which one or more high doses of dexamethasone are given. The level of cortisol is checked from a sample of blood or from urine that is collected for three days. This test is done to check if the adrenal gland is making too much cortisol or if the pituitary gland is telling the adrenal glands to make too much cortisol.

- **Blood chemistry study.** A procedure in which a blood sample is checked to measure the amounts of certain substances, such as potassium or sodium, released into the blood by organs and tissues in the body. An unusual (higher or lower than normal) amount of a substance can be a sign of disease.

- **Computed tomography (CT) scan.** A procedure that makes a series of detailed pictures of areas inside the body, taken from different angles. The pictures are made by a computer linked to an x-ray machine. A dye may be injected into a vein or swallowed to help the organs or tissues show up more clearly. This procedure is also called "computed tomography," "computerized tomography," or "computerized axial tomography."

- **Magnetic resonance imaging (MRI).** A procedure that uses a magnet, radio waves, and a computer to make a series of detailed pictures of areas inside the body. This procedure is also called "nuclear magnetic resonance imaging" (NMRI). An MRI of the abdomen is done to diagnose adrenocortical carcinoma.

- **Adrenal angiography.** A procedure to look at the arteries and the flow of blood near the adrenal glands. A contrast dye is injected into the adrenal arteries. As the dye moves through the arteries, a series of x-rays are taken to see if any arteries are blocked.

- **Adrenal venography.** A procedure to look at the adrenal veins and the flow of blood near the adrenal glands. A contrast dye is injected into an adrenal vein. As the contrast dye moves through the veins, a series of x-rays are taken to see if any veins are blocked. A catheter (very thin tube) may be inserted into the vein to take a blood sample, which is checked for abnormal hormone levels.

- **Positron emission tomography (PET) scan.** A procedure to find malignant tumor cells in the body. A small amount of radioactive glucose (sugar) is injected into a vein. The PET scanner rotates around the body and makes a picture of where glucose is being used in the body. Malignant tumor cells show up brighter in the picture because they are more active and take up more glucose than normal cells do.

- **Metaiodobenzylguanidine (MIBG) scan.** A very small amount of radioactive material called "MIBG" is injected into a vein and travels through the bloodstream. Adrenal gland cells take up the radioactive material and are detected by a device that measures radiation. This scan is done to tell the difference between adrenocortical carcinoma and pheochromocytoma.

- **Biopsy.** The removal of cells or tissues so they can be viewed under a microscope by a pathologist to check for signs of cancer. The sample may be taken using a thin needle, called a "fine-needle aspiration (FNA) biopsy" or a wider needle, called a "core biopsy."

Factors That Affect Prognosis and Treatment Options

The prognosis and treatment options depend on the following:

- The stage of the cancer (the size of the tumor and whether it is in the adrenal gland only or has spread to other places in the body)

- Whether the tumor can be completely removed in surgery

- Whether the cancer has been treated in the past

- The patient's general health

- The grade of tumor cells (how different they look from normal cells under a microscope)

Adrenocortical carcinoma may be cured if treated at an early stage.

Stages of Adrenocortical Carcinoma

The process used to find out if cancer has spread within the adrenal gland or to other parts of the body is called "staging." The information gathered from the staging process determines the stage of the disease. It is important to know the stage in order to plan treatment. The following tests and procedures may be used in the staging process:

- **Computed tomography.** A procedure that makes a series of detailed pictures of areas inside the body, such as the abdomen or chest, taken from different angles. The pictures are made by a computer linked to an x-ray machine. A dye may be injected into a vein or swallowed to help the organs or tissues show up more clearly. This procedure is also called "computed tomography," "computerized tomography," or "computerized axial tomography."

- **Magnetic resonance imaging with gadolinium.** A procedure that uses a magnet, radio waves, and a computer to make a series of detailed pictures of areas inside the body, such as the abdomen. A substance called "gadolinium" may be injected into a vein. The gadolinium collects around the cancer cells so they show up brighter in the picture. This procedure is also called "nuclear magnetic resonance imaging" (NMRI).

- **Positron emission tomography (PET) scan.** A procedure to find malignant tumor cells in the body. A small amount of radioactive glucose (sugar) is injected into a vein. The PET scanner rotates around the body and makes a picture of where glucose is being used in the body. Malignant tumor cells show up brighter in the picture because they are more active and take up more glucose than normal cells do.

- **Ultrasound exam.** A procedure in which high-energy sound waves (ultrasound) are bounced off internal tissues or organs, such as the vena cava, and make echoes. The echoes form a picture of body tissues called a "sonogram."

- **Adrenalectomy.** A procedure to remove the affected adrenal gland. A tissue sample is viewed under a microscope by a pathologist to check for signs of cancer.

Cancer May Spread from Where It Began to Other Parts of the Body

When cancer spreads to another part of the body, it is called "metastasis." Cancer cells break away from where they began (the primary tumor) and travel through the lymph system or blood.

- **Lymph system.** The cancer gets into the lymph system, travels through the lymph vessels, and forms a tumor (metastatic tumor) in another part of the body.

- **Blood.** The cancer gets into the blood, travels through the blood vessels, and forms a tumor (metastatic tumor) in another part of the body.

The metastatic tumor is the same type of cancer as the primary tumor. For example, if adrenocortical carcinoma spreads to the lung, the cancer cells in the lung are actually adrenocortical carcinoma cells. The disease is metastatic adrenocortical carcinoma, not lung cancer.

Stages Used for Adrenocortical Carcinoma
Stage I

In stage I, the tumor is five centimeters or smaller and is found in the adrenal gland only.

Stage II

In stage II, the tumor is larger than five centimeters and is found in the adrenal gland only.

Stage III

In stage III, the tumor is any size and has spread:

- To nearby lymph nodes

- To nearby tissues or organs (kidney, diaphragm, pancreas, spleen, or liver) or to large blood vessels (renal vein or vena cava) and may have spread to nearby lymph nodes

Stage IV

In stage IV, the tumor is any size, may have spread to nearby lymph nodes, and has spread to other parts of the body, such as the lung, bone, or peritoneum.

Recurrent Adrenocortical Carcinoma

Recurrent adrenocortical carcinoma is cancer that has recurred (come back) after it has been treated. The cancer may come back in the adrenal cortex or in other parts of the body.

Treatment Options for Adrenocortical Carcinoma
Types of Treatment for Adrenocortical Carcinoma Patients

Different types of treatments are available for patients with adrenocortical carcinoma. Some treatments are standard (the currently used treatment), and some are being tested in clinical trials. A treatment clinical trial is a research study meant to help improve current treatments or obtain information on new treatments for patients with cancer. When clinical trials show that a new treatment is better than the standard treatment, the new treatment may become the standard treatment. Patients may want to think about taking part in a clinical trial. Some clinical trials are open only to patients who have not started treatment.

Types of Standard Treatment
Surgery

Surgery to remove the adrenal gland (adrenalectomy) is often used to treat adrenocortical carcinoma. Sometimes surgery is done to remove the nearby lymph nodes and other tissue where the cancer has spread.

Radiation Therapy

Radiation therapy is a cancer treatment that uses high-energy x-rays or other types of radiation to kill cancer cells or keep them from growing. There are two types of radiation therapy:

- **External radiation therapy** uses a machine outside the body to send radiation toward the cancer.

- **Internal radiation therapy** uses a radioactive substance sealed in needles, seeds, wires, or catheters that are placed directly into or near the cancer.

The way the radiation therapy is given depends on the type and stage of the cancer being treated. External radiation therapy is used to treat adrenocortical carcinoma.

Chemotherapy

Chemotherapy is a cancer treatment that uses drugs to stop the growth of cancer cells, either by killing the cells or by stopping them from dividing. When chemotherapy is taken by mouth or injected into a vein or muscle, the drugs enter the bloodstream and can reach cancer cells throughout the body (systemic chemotherapy). When chemotherapy is placed directly into the cerebrospinal fluid (CBF), an organ, or a body cavity such as the abdomen, the drugs mainly affect cancer cells in those areas (regional chemotherapy). Combination chemotherapy is treatment using more than one anticancer drug. The way the chemotherapy is given depends on the type and stage of the cancer being treated.

New Types of Treatment Are Being Tested in Clinical Trials

This section describes treatments that are being studied in clinical trials.

Biologic Therapy

Biologic therapy is a treatment that uses the patient's immune system to fight cancer. Substances made by the body or made in a laboratory are used to boost, direct, or restore the body's natural defenses against cancer. This type of cancer treatment is also called "biotherapy" or "immunotherapy."

Targeted Therapy

Targeted therapy is a type of treatment that uses drugs or other substances to identify and attack specific cancer cells without harming normal cells.

Follow-Up Tests May Be Needed

Some of the tests that were done to diagnose the cancer or to find out the stage of the cancer may be repeated. Some tests will be repeated in order to see how well the treatment is working. Decisions about whether to continue, change, or stop treatment may be based on the results of these tests.

Some of the tests will continue to be done from time to time after treatment has ended. The results of these tests can show if your condition has changed or if the cancer has recurred. These tests are sometimes called "follow-up tests" or "check-ups."

Chapter 28

Congenital Adrenal Hyperplasia

What Is Congenital Adrenal Hyperplasia?

Congenital adrenal hyperplasia (CAH) refers to a group of genetic disorders that affect the adrenal glands. These glands sit on top of the kidneys and release hormones the body needs to function. CAH is caused by three disturbances:

- **Too little cortisol.** The adrenal glands of infants born with CAH cannot make enough of the hormone cortisol. This hormone affects energy levels, blood sugar levels, blood pressure, and the body's response to stress, illness, and injury.

- **Too little aldosterone.** In about three-fourths of cases, infants born with CAH cannot make enough of the hormone aldosterone, which helps the body maintain the proper level of sodium (salt) and water and helps maintain blood pressure.

- **Too much androgens.** In certain cases, infants born with CAH produce too much of male hormones, androgens. Proper levels of these hormones are needed for normal growth and development in both boys and girls.

This chapter includes text excerpted from "Congenital Adrenal Hyperplasia (CAH): Condition Information," *Eunice Kennedy Shriver* National Institute of Child Health and Human Development (NICHD), December 1, 2016. Reviewed September 2019.

Congenital adrenal hyperplasia can also cause imbalances in the hormone adrenaline, which affects blood sugar levels, blood pressure, and the body's response to stress.

The hormone imbalance most often seen in CAH cases is too little of a substance called "21-hydroxylase." The adrenal glands need 21-hydroxylase to make proper amounts of hormones. This type of CAH is sometimes referred to as 21-hydroxylase deficiency. In CAH due to 21-hydroxylase deficiency, the adrenal glands cannot make enough cortisol or aldosterone. In addition, the glands make too much androgen. People with 21-hydroxylase deficiency also may not produce enough adrenaline.

A small number of cases of CAH are caused by a deficiency in a substance similar to 21-hydroxylase, called "11-hydroxylase." This type of CAH is sometimes referred to as 11-hydroxylase deficiency. In CAH due to 11-hydroxylase deficiency, the adrenal glands make too little cortisol and too many androgens. This type of CAH does not result in aldosterone deficiency.

Other very rare types of CAH include 3-beta-hydroxysteroid dehydrogenase deficiency, lipoid CAH, and 17-hydroxylase deficiency. They are not discussed here.

Congenital adrenal hyperplasia can be categorized as classic or nonclassic types based on severity:

- **Classic congenital adrenal hyperplasia** is more severe than the nonclassic form. It can be life-threatening in newborns if it is not diagnosed. Classic CAH can be caused by either 21-hydroxylase or 11-hydroxylase deficiency.

- **Nonclassic congenital adrenal hyperplasia** is sometimes called "late-onset CAH." It is a milder form of the disorder that is usually diagnosed in late childhood or early adolescence. Sometimes, people have nonclassic CAH and never know it. This form of CAH is almost always caused by 21-hydroxylase deficiency.

What Causes Congenital Adrenal Hyperplasia

Congenital adrenal hyperplasia is caused by changes (mutations) in one of several genes. These changes lead to deficiencies in 21-hydroxylase or, less commonly, 11-hydroxylase. Both of these are chemicals called "enzymes." The adrenal glands need these enzymes to make proper amounts of the hormones: cortisol, aldosterone, androgens, and adrenaline.

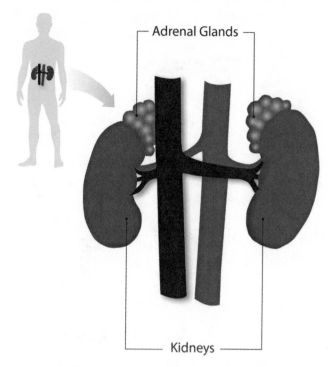

Figure 28.1. *Position of the Adrenal Glands and Kidneys in the Human Body*

How Is Congenital Adrenal Hyperplasia Inherited?

The genes for CAH are passed down from parents to their children. In general, people have two copies of every gene in their bodies. They receive one copy from each parent. For an infant to have CAH, both copies must have an error that affects an adrenal-gland enzyme.

Congenital adrenal hyperplasia is an example of an autosomal recessive disorder:

- "Autosomal" means the gene is not on the X chromosome or the Y chromosome.

- "Recessive" means that both copies of the gene must have the error for the disease or disorder to occur.

If both parents have CAH, all of their children will also have it. If each parent carries one affected gene and one normal gene (called a "carrier"), there is a one-in-four chance of their child having CAH.

247

Autosomal recessive

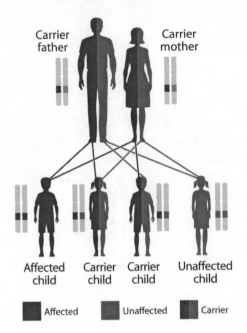

Figure 28.2. *Inheritance of an Autosomal Recessive Disorder from Carrier Parents*

What Are the Symptoms of Congenital Adrenal Hyperplasia?

Classic Congenital Adrenal Hyperplasia

Symptoms of classic CAH due to 21-hydroxylase deficiency (the most common type of CAH) can be grouped into two types according to their severity: salt wasting and simple virilizing (also called "nonsalt wasting").

Symptoms of classic CAH due to 11-hydroxylase deficiency are similar to those of simple virilizing CAH. About two-thirds of people with classic 11-hydroxylase deficiency also have high blood pressure (hypertension).

Salt-Wasting Congenital Adrenal Hyperplasia

Salt-wasting CAH is the severe form of classic 21-hydroxylase deficiency. In this type of CAH, the adrenal glands make too little aldosterone, causing the body to be unable to retain enough sodium (salt). Too much sodium is lost in urine (thus the name, "salt-wasting"). If undiagnosed, symptoms of classic salt-wasting CAH appear within days or weeks of birth and, in some cases, death occurs.

Symptoms may include:

- Dehydration

- Poor feeding

- Diarrhea

- Vomiting

- Heart rhythm problems (arrhythmias)

- Low blood pressure

- Very low blood sodium levels

- Low blood glucose

- Too much acid in the blood, called "metabolic acidosis"

- Weight loss

- Shock, a condition where not enough blood gets to the brain and other organs. Shock in infants with salt-wasting is called "adrenal crisis." Signs include confusion, irritability, rapid heart rate, and/or coma.

Even when carefully treated, children with salt-wasting CAH are still at risk for adrenal crises when they become ill or are under physical stress. The body needs more than the usual amount of adrenal hormones during illness, injury, or physical stress. This means a child with CAH must be given more medication during these times to prevent an adrenal crisis.

Salt-wasting CAH also involves symptoms caused by low cortisol and high androgens. These symptoms may include:

- In female newborns, external genitalia can be ambiguous, i.e., not typical female appearing, with normal internal reproductive organs (ovaries, uterus, and fallopian tubes)

- Enlarged genitalia in male newborns

- Development of certain qualities called "virilization" in boys or girls before the normal age of puberty, sometimes as early as age two or three. This is a condition characterized by:

  - Rapid growth

- Appearance of pubic and armpit hair
- Deep voice
- Failure to menstruate, or abnormal or irregular menstrual periods (females)
- Well-developed muscles
- Enlarged penis (males)
- Unusually tall height as children, but being shorter than normal as adults
- Possible difficulties getting pregnant (females)
- Excess facial hair (females)
- Early beard (males)
- Severe acne
- Benign testicular tumors and infertility (males)

Simple Virilizing (Nonsalt Wasting) Congenital Adrenal Hyperplasia

Simple virilizing CAH is the moderate form of classic 21-hydroxylase deficiency. This type of CAH involves less severe aldosterone deficiency. Therefore, there are no severe or life-threatening sodium-deficiency symptoms in newborns. Like salt-wasting CAH, simple virilizing CAH involves too little cortisol and too much androgen. Female newborns have ambiguous genitalia and young children display virilization.

Nonclassic Congenital Adrenal Hyperplasia

Almost all cases of nonclassic CAH are caused by a mild 21-hydroxylase deficiency. Most symptoms of nonclassic CAH are related to increased androgens. Symptoms can show up in childhood, adolescence, or early adulthood.

Symptoms of nonclassic CAH can include:

- Rapid growth in childhood and early teens but shorter height than both parents
- Early signs of puberty
- Acne
- Irregular menstrual periods (females)

- Fertility problems (in about 10 to 15% of women)

- Excess facial or body hair in women

- Male-pattern baldness (hair loss near the temples)

- Enlarged penis (males)

- Small testicles (males)

Some people have nonclassic CAH and never know it because the symptoms are so mild.

How Do Healthcare Providers Diagnose Congenital Adrenal Hyperplasia?
During Pregnancy

If a woman already has a child with CAH and becomes pregnant with the same partner, her fetus has a one in four chance of having CAH. For this reason, prenatal testing can be done for some forms of CAH. A healthcare provider checks for the disorder by using techniques called "amniocentesis" or "chorionic villus sampling" (CVS).

- **Amniocentesis.** This involves inserting a needle into the womb, through the abdomen, to withdraw a small amount of fluid from the sac that surrounds the fetus. The procedure is usually done between the 15th and 20th week of pregnancy.

- **Chorionic villus sampling.** This is similar to amniocentesis. A healthcare provider inserts a needle into the womb, either through the abdomen or the cervix, and extracts a small piece of tissue from the chorionic villi (the tissue that will later become the placenta). This procedure is usually done between the 10th and 12th week of pregnancy.

After a healthcare provider takes a sample using one of these techniques, she or he will perform a genetic test on the sample. This test will reveal whether the fetus has a gene change that causes CAH.

Parents may also choose to wait until birth to have the newborn tested. Talking to their healthcare providers may help parents identify the option that is right for them.

At Birth

All states in the U.S. have neonatal screening for CAH. Infants who test positive need to have follow-up testing done to confirm the diagnosis. If for some reason, the neonatal screening is negative but there is a high suspicion for CAH (such as ambiguous genitalia), further evaluation is also indicated.

Later in Life

Newborns do not show symptoms of nonclassic CAH, and the test done on newborns does not detect nonclassic CAH. Nonclassic CAH is diagnosed in childhood or adulthood, when symptoms appear. To diagnose nonclassic CAH, a healthcare provider may:

- Ask whether family members have CAH

- Do a physical exam

- Take blood and urine to measure hormone levels

- Do a genetic test to determine if the patient has the gene change that causes CAH

An x-ray can help to diagnose CAH in children. Because some children with CAH grow too quickly, their bones will be more developed than normal for their age.

What Are the Treatments for Congenital Adrenal Hyperplasia?

Treatments for CAH include medication and surgery as well as psychological support.

Medication
Classic Congenital Adrenal Hyperplasia

Newborns with classic CAH should start treatment very soon after birth to reduce the effects of CAH. Classic CAH is treated with steroids that replace the low hormones.

- Infants and children usually take a form of cortisol called "hydrocortisone."

- Adults take hydrocortisone, prednisone, or dexamethasone, which also replace cortisol.

- Patients with classic CAH also take another medicine, fludrocortisone, to replace aldosterone.

- Eating salty foods or taking salt pills may also help salt-wasters retain salt.

The body needs more cortisol when it is under physical stress. Adults and children with classic CAH need close medical attention and may need to take more of their medication during these times. They may also need more medication if they:

- Have an illness with a high fever

- Undergo surgery

- Sustain a major injury

People who have classic CAH need to wear a medical-alert identification bracelet or necklace. To alert medical professionals in case of an emergency, the bracelet or necklace should read: "adrenal insufficiency, requires hydrocortisone." Adults or parents also need to learn how to give an injection of hydrocortisone if there is an emergency.

Patients with classic CAH need to take medication daily for their entire lives. If a patient stops taking her or his medication, symptoms will return.

The body makes different amounts of cortisol at different times in life, so sometimes a patient's dose of medication may be too high or too low. Taking too much medication to replace cortisol can cause symptoms of Cushing syndrome. These include:

- Weight gain

- Slowed growth

- Stretch marks on the skin

- Rounded face

- High blood pressure

- Bone loss

- High blood sugar

It is important to alert the healthcare provider if these symptoms appear so that she or he can adjust the medication dose.

Nonclassic Congenital Adrenal Hyperplasia

People with nonclassic CAH may not need treatment if they do not have symptoms. Individuals with symptoms are given low doses of the same cortisol replacing medication taken by people with classic CAH.

Symptoms of nonclassic CAH that signal that the patient may need treatment are:

253

- Early puberty

- Excess body hair

- Irregular menstrual periods (females)

- Infertility

It may be possible for patients with nonclassic CAH to stop medication as adults if their symptoms go away.

Surgery
Classic Congenital Adrenal Hyperplasia

Girls who are born with ambiguous external genitalia may need surgery. For example, surgery is necessary if changes to the genitals have affected urine flow.

Surgery for treatment of classic CAH should be done by an experienced surgeon who has expertise with this specific type of surgery. Parents may want to consider surgery for their child during infancy, or they may want to delay until later in childhood. Parents should work with their child's healthcare providers to determine the best timing of treatments.

The Endocrine Society provides care recommendations on classic CAH, and can help parents find a healthcare provider who specializes in CAH. The American Association of Clinical Endocrinologists (AACE) also offers a way to find an endocrinologist. The Congenital Adrenal Hyperplasia Research, Education, and Support (CARES) Foundation also provides information about classic CAH, including considering surgical treatment and how to find a knowledgeable surgeon.

Parents may also want to find a psychologist, social worker, or other mental-health professional to support them in their decision making. It is important to find an experienced mental-health provider whose expertise includes working with children who have CAH and their special needs.

Nonclassic Congenital Adrenal Hyperplasia

Congenital adrenal hyperplasia girls with nonclassic CAH have normal genitals, so they do not need surgery.

Congenital Adrenal Hyperplasia: Other FAQs
If My Children Have Congenital Adrenal Hyperplasia Can They Go to Day care and School?

Yes, children with CAH can attend day care and school. Before enrolling children in day care, parents should explain that the child has adrenal insufficiency, which might require the administration of emergency medication. Parents should discuss the day-care provider's policy on giving medications to children. They should also provide a set of written instructions, as well as a list of emergency contact names and numbers.

Before a child starts school, parents should consider meeting with the teacher, principal, and school nurse to explain the child's condition. Parents can also discuss precautions to take if the child becomes ill.

The Congenital Adrenal Hyperplasia Research Education and Support (CARES) Foundation provides a list of suggestions to help parents and children get ready to attend school.

I Have Congenital Adrenal Hyperplasia and Want to Start a Family. What Should I Be Thinking About?

Anyone with CAH, or from a family in which CAH has been diagnosed, should consider genetic counseling. Genetic counselors discuss all options for having a child. They explain the risks and benefits of each option.

The genes for CAH are passed down from parents to their children. In general, people have two copies of every gene in their bodies. They receive one copy from each parent. For an infant to have CAH, both copies must have an error that affects an adrenal-gland enzyme.

Congenital adrenal hyperplasia is an example of an autosomal recessive disorder:

- Autosomal means the gene is not on the X chromosome or the Y chromosome.

- Recessive means that both copies of the gene must have the error for the disease or disorder to occur.

If both parents have CAH, all of their children will also have it. If each parent carries one affected gene and one normal gene, there is a one in four chance of a child having CAH.

For Women

Women with CAH can get pregnant. In some of the women, high levels of androgens disrupt the regular release of the egg from the ovary, a process known as "ovulation." Some women also have irregular menstrual cycles. These problems can make it more difficult to get pregnant. These women often can be helped with medicines. Women with CAH who want to become pregnant can meet with a reproductive endocrinologist. This is a healthcare provider who specializes in fertility issues.

Women with CAH who become pregnant should continue taking their medications.

For Men

Men with CAH can father children. The main challenges for these men are low testosterone (a hormone important for male fertility and sexual function), and growths in the testicles called "adrenal rest tissue." These problems can cause reduced sperm production. These issues tend to occur when hormone imbalances are not well controlled with medicines. Men who wish to father children should take all medicines as directed. A healthcare provider may recommend that males with CAH who have gone through puberty get an ultrasound of the testicles. The ultrasound provides a picture of the inside of the testicle and can help a healthcare provider detect abnormal growths. Future ultrasounds can be compared with the original to quickly identify any problems.

Chapter 29

X-Linked Adrenal Hypoplasia Congenita

What Is X-Linked Adrenal Hypoplasia Congenita?

X-linked adrenal hypoplasia congenita is an inherited disorder that mainly affects males. It involves many hormone-producing (endocrine) tissues in the body, particularly a pair of small glands on top of each kidney called the "adrenal glands." These glands produce a variety of hormones that regulate many essential functions in the body. Congenital adrenal hypoplasia is characterized by adrenal insufficiency, which may be life-threatening, and hypogonadotropic hypogonadism. Congenital adrenal hypoplasia (CAH) is caused by mutations in the *NR0B1* gene. It is inherited in an X-linked recessive pattern.

Symptoms of X-Linked Adrenal Hypoplasia Congenita

X-linked adrenal hypoplasia congenita is a disorder that mainly affects males. One of the main signs of this disorder is adrenal insufficiency, which occurs when the adrenal glands do not produce enough hormones. Adrenal insufficiency typically begins in infancy or

This chapter includes text excerpted from "X-Linked Adrenal Hypoplasia Congenita," Genetic and Rare Diseases Information Center (GARD), National Center for Advancing Translational Sciences (NCATS), August 15, 2012. Reviewed September 2019.

childhood and can cause vomiting, difficulty with feeding, dehydration, extremely low blood sugar (hypoglycemia), and shock. If untreated, these complications may be life-threatening.

Affected males may also have a shortage of male sex hormones, which leads to underdeveloped reproductive tissues, undescended testicles, delayed puberty, and an inability to father children. Together, these characteristics are known as "hypogonadotropic hypogonadism."

The onset and severity of these signs and symptoms can vary, even among affected members of the same family.

Causes of X-Linked Adrenal Hypoplasia Congenita

X-linked adrenal hypoplasia congenita is caused by mutations in the *NR0B1* gene. The *NR0B1* gene provides instructions to make a protein called "DAX1." This protein plays an important role in the development and function of several hormone-producing tissues including the adrenal glands, two hormone-secreting glands in the brain (the hypothalamus and pituitary), and the gonads (ovaries in females and testes in males). The hormones produced by these glands control many important body functions.

Some *NR0B1* mutations result in the production of an inactive version of the DAX1 protein, while other mutations delete the entire gene. The resulting shortage of DAX1 disrupts the normal development and function of hormone-producing tissues in the body. The signs and symptoms of adrenal insufficiency and hypogonadotropic hypogonadism occur when endocrine glands do not produce the right amounts of certain hormones.

Inheritance of X-Linked Adrenal Hypoplasia Congenita

X-linked adrenal hypoplasia congenita is inherited in an X-linked recessive pattern. A condition is considered X-linked if the mutated gene that causes the disorder is located on the X chromosome, one of the two sex chromosomes. In males (who have only one X chromosome), one altered copy of the gene in each cell is sufficient to cause the condition. In females (who have two X chromosomes), a mutation must be present in both copies of the gene to cause the disorder. Males are affected by X-linked recessive disorders much more frequently than females. A characteristic of X-linked inheritance is that fathers cannot pass X-linked traits to their sons.

In X-linked recessive inheritance, a female with one mutated copy of the gene in each cell is called a "carrier." She can pass on the altered gene but usually does not experience signs and symptoms of the disorder. In rare cases, however, females who carry an *NR0B1* mutation may experience adrenal insufficiency or signs of hypogonadotropic hypogonadism, such as underdeveloped reproductive tissues, delayed puberty, and an absence of menstruation.

Chapter 30

Cushing Syndrome

What Is Cushing Syndrome?

Cushing syndrome is a hormonal disorder caused by prolonged exposure of the body's tissues to high levels of the hormone cortisol. Sometimes called "hypercortisolism," Cushing syndrome is relatively rare and most commonly affects adults aged 20 to 50. People who are obese and have type 2 diabetes, along with poorly controlled blood glucose—also called "blood sugar"—and high blood pressure, have an increased risk of developing the disorder.

What Are the Signs and Symptoms of Cushing Syndrome?

Signs and symptoms of Cushing syndrome vary, but most people with the disorder have upper body obesity, a rounded face, increased fat around the neck, and relatively slender arms and legs. Children tend to be obese with slowed growth rates.

Other signs appear in the skin, which becomes fragile and thin, bruises easily, and heals poorly. Purple or pink stretch marks may appear on the abdomen, thighs, buttocks, arms, and breasts. The bones are weakened, and routine activities such as bending, lifting, or rising from a chair may lead to backaches and rib or spinal column fractures.

This chapter includes text excerpted from "Cushing's Syndrome," National Institutes of Health (NIH), July 2008. Reviewed September 2019.

Women with Cushing syndrome usually have excess hair growth on their face, neck, chest, abdomen, and thighs. Their menstrual periods may become irregular or stop. Men may have decreased fertility with diminished or absent desire for sex and, sometimes, erectile dysfunction.

Other common signs and symptoms include:

- Severe fatigue

- Weak muscles

- High blood pressure

- High blood glucose

- Increased thirst and urination

- Irritability, anxiety, or depression

- A fatty hump between the shoulders

Sometimes other conditions have many of the same signs as Cushing syndrome, even though people with these disorders do not have abnormally elevated cortisol levels. For example, polycystic ovary syndrome (POS) can cause menstrual disturbances, weight gain beginning in adolescence, excess hair growth, and impaired insulin action and diabetes. Metabolic syndrome—a combination of problems that includes excess weight around the waist, high blood pressure, abnormal levels of cholesterol and triglycerides in the blood, and insulin resistance—also mimics the symptoms of Cushing syndrome.

What Causes Cushing Syndrome

Cushing syndrome occurs when the body's tissues are exposed to high levels of cortisol for too long. Many people develop Cushing syndrome because they take glucocorticoids—steroid hormones that are chemically similar to naturally produced cortisol—such as prednisone for asthma, rheumatoid arthritis (RA), lupus, and other inflammatory diseases. Glucocorticoids are also used to suppress the immune system after transplantation to keep the body from rejecting the new organ or tissue.

Other people develop Cushing syndrome because their bodies produce too much cortisol. Normally, the production of cortisol follows a precise chain of events. First, the hypothalamus, a part of the brain about the size of a small sugar cube, sends corticotropin-releasing hormone (CRH) to the pituitary gland. CRH causes the pituitary gland to secrete adrenocorticotropic hormone (ACTH), which stimulates the adrenal glands. When the adrenals, which are located just above the kidneys, receive the ACTH, they respond by releasing cortisol into the bloodstream. Cortisol performs vital tasks in the body including:

- Helping maintain blood pressure and cardiovascular function

- Reducing the immune system's inflammatory response

- Balancing the effects of insulin, which breaks down glucose for energy

- Regulating the metabolism of proteins, carbohydrates, and fats

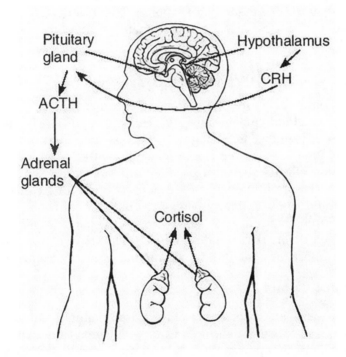

Figure 30.1. *How Cortisol Is Released into the Bloodstream*

The hypothalamus sends CRH to the pituitary gland, which responds by secreting ACTH. ACTH then causes the adrenals to release cortisol into the bloodstream.

One of cortisol's most important jobs is to help the body respond to stress. For this reason, women in their last three months of pregnancy and highly trained athletes normally have high levels of the hormone. People suffering from depression, alcoholism, malnutrition, or panic disorders also have increased cortisol levels.

When the amount of cortisol in the blood is adequate, the hypothalamus and pituitary gland release less CRH and ACTH. This process ensures the amount of cortisol released by the adrenal glands is precisely balanced to meet the body's daily needs. However, if something goes wrong with the adrenals, or regulating switches in the pituitary gland or hypothalamus, cortisol production can go awry.

Pituitary Adenomas

Pituitary adenomas cause 70 percent of Cushing syndrome cases, excluding those caused by glucocorticoid use. These benign, or noncancerous, tumors of the pituitary gland secrete extra ACTH. Most people with the disorder have a single adenoma. This form of the syndrome, known as "Cushing disease," affects women five times more often than men.

Ectopic Adrenocorticotropic Hormone Syndrome

Some benign or, more often, cancerous tumors that arise outside the pituitary gland can produce ACTH. This condition is known as "ectopic ACTH syndrome." Lung tumors cause more than half of these cases, and men are affected three times more often than women. The most common forms of ACTH-producing tumors are small cell lung cancer, which accounts for about 13 percent of all lung cancer cases, and carcinoid tumors—small, slow-growing tumors that arise from hormone-producing cells in various parts of the body. Other less common types of tumors that can produce ACTH are thymomas, pancreatic islet cell tumors, and medullary carcinomas of the thyroid.

Adrenal Tumors

In rare cases, an abnormality of the adrenal glands, most often an adrenal tumor, causes Cushing syndrome. Adrenal tumors are four to five times more common in women than men, and the average age of onset is about 40. Most of these cases involve noncancerous tumors of adrenal tissue called "adrenal adenomas," which releases excess cortisol into the blood. Adrenocortical carcinomas—adrenal cancers—are the least common cause of Cushing syndrome. With adrenocortical carcinomas, cancer cells secrete excess levels of several adrenocortical hormones, including cortisol and adrenal androgens, a type of male hormone. Adrenocortical carcinomas usually cause very high hormone levels and rapid development of symptoms.

Familial Cushing Syndrome

Most cases of Cushing syndrome are not inherited. Rarely, however, Cushing syndrome results from an inherited tendency to develop tumors of one or more endocrine glands. Endocrine glands release hormones into the bloodstream. With primary pigmented micronodular adrenal disease (PPNAD), children or young adults develop small cortisol-producing tumors of the adrenal glands. With multiple endocrine neoplasia type 1 (MEN1), hormone-secreting tumors of the parathyroid glands, pancreas, and pituitary gland develop; Cushing syndrome in MEN1 may be due to pituitary, ectopic, or adrenal tumors.

How Is Cushing Syndrome Diagnosed?

Diagnosis is based on a review of a person's medical history, a physical examination, and laboratory tests. X-rays of the adrenal or pituitary glands can be useful in locating tumors.

Tests to Diagnose Cushing Syndrome

No single lab test is perfect and usually several are needed. The three most common tests used to diagnose Cushing syndrome are the 24-hour urinary free cortisol test, measurement of midnight plasma cortisol or late-night salivary cortisol, and the low-dose dexamethasone suppression test. Another test, the dexamethasone-corticotropin-releasing hormone test, may be needed to distinguish Cushing syndrome from other causes of excess cortisol.

- **A 24-hour urinary free cortisol level.** In this test, a person's urine is collected several times over a 24-hour period and tested for cortisol. Levels higher than 50 to 100 micrograms a day for an adult suggest Cushing syndrome. The normal upper limit varies in different laboratories, depending on which measurement technique is used.

- **Midnight plasma cortisol and late-night salivary cortisol measurements.** The midnight plasma cortisol test measures cortisol concentrations in the blood. Cortisol production is normally suppressed at night, but in Cushing syndrome, this suppression does not occur. If the cortisol level is more than 50 nanomoles per liter (nmol/L), Cushing syndrome is suspected.

The test generally requires a 48-hour hospital stay to avoid falsely elevated cortisol levels due to stress.

However, a late-night or bedtime saliva sample can be obtained at home, then tested to determine the cortisol level. Diagnostic ranges vary, depending on the measurement technique used.

- **Low-dose dexamethasone suppression test (LDDST).** In the LDDST, a person is given a low dose of dexamethasone, a synthetic glucocorticoid, by mouth every six hours for two days. Urine is collected before dexamethasone is administered and several times on each day of the test. A modified LDDST uses a one-time overnight dose.

Cortisol and other glucocorticoids signal the pituitary gland to release less ACTH, so the normal response after taking dexamethasone is a drop in blood and urine cortisol levels. If cortisol levels do not drop, Cushing syndrome is suspected.

The LDDST may not show a drop in cortisol levels in people with depression, alcoholism, high estrogen levels, acute illness, or stress, falsely indicating Cushing syndrome. On the other hand, drugs such as phenytoin and phenobarbital may cause cortisol levels to drop, falsely indicating that Cushing is not present in people who actually have the syndrome. For this reason, physicians usually advise their patients to stop taking these drugs at least one week before the test.

- **Dexamethasone-corticotropin-releasing hormone (CRH) test.** Some people have high cortisol levels but do not develop the progressive effects of Cushing syndrome, such as muscle weakness, fractures, and thinning of the skin. These people may have pseudo-Cushing syndrome, a condition sometimes found in people who have depression or anxiety disorders, drink excess alcohol, have poorly controlled diabetes, or are severely obese. Pseudo-Cushing does not have the same long-term effects on health as Cushing syndrome and does not require treatment directed at the endocrine glands.

The dexamethasone-CRH test rapidly distinguishes pseudo-Cushing from mild cases of Cushing. This test combines the LDDST and a CRH stimulation test. In the CRH stimulation test, an injection of CRH causes the pituitary gland to secrete ACTH. Pretreatment with dexamethasone prevents CRH from causing an increase in cortisol in people with pseudo-Cushing. Elevations of cortisol during this test suggest Cushing syndrome.

Tests to Find the Cause of Cushing Syndrome

Once Cushing syndrome has been diagnosed, other tests are used to find the exact location of the abnormality that leads to excess cortisol production. The choice of test depends, in part, on the preference of the endocrinologist or the center where the test is performed.

- **Corticotropin-releasing hormone stimulation test.** The CRH test, without pretreatment with dexamethasone, helps separate people with pituitary adenomas from those with ectopic ACTH syndrome or adrenal tumors. As a result of the CRH injection, people with pituitary adenomas usually experience a rise in blood levels of ACTH and cortisol because CRH acts directly on the pituitary gland. This response is rarely seen in people with ectopic ACTH syndrome and practically never in those with adrenal tumors.

- **High-dose dexamethasone suppression test (HDDST).** The HDDST is the same as the LDDST, except it uses higher doses of dexamethasone. This test helps separate people with excess production of ACTH due to pituitary adenomas from those with ectopic ACTH-producing tumors. High doses of dexamethasone usually suppress cortisol levels in people with pituitary adenomas but not in those with ectopic ACTH-producing tumors.

- **Radiologic imaging: Direct visualization of the endocrine glands.** Imaging tests reveal the size and shape of the pituitary and adrenal glands and help determine if a tumor is present. The most common imaging tests are the computerized tomography (CT) scan and magnetic resonance imaging (MRI). A CT scan produces a series of x-ray pictures giving a cross-sectional image of a body part. MRI also produces images of internal organs but without exposing patients to ionizing radiation.

Imaging procedures are used to find a tumor after a diagnosis has been made. Imaging is not used to make the diagnosis of Cushing syndrome because benign tumors are commonly found in the pituitary and adrenal glands. These tumors, sometimes called "incidentalomas," do not produce hormones in quantities that are harmful. They are not removed unless blood tests show they are a cause of symptoms or they are unusually large. Conversely, pituitary tumors may not be detectable by imaging in almost half of the people who ultimately need pituitary gland surgery for Cushing syndrome.

- **Petrosal sinus sampling.** This test is not always required, but in many cases, it is the best way to distinguish pituitary from ectopic causes of Cushing syndrome. Samples of blood are drawn from the petrosal sinuses—veins that drain the pituitary gland—by inserting tiny tubes through a vein in the upper thigh or groin region. A local anesthetic and mild sedation are given, and x-rays are taken to confirm the correct position of the tubes. Often CRH, the hormone that causes the pituitary gland to release ACTH, is given during this test to improve diagnostic accuracy. Levels of ACTH in the petrosal sinuses are measured and compared with ACTH levels in a forearm vein. Higher levels of ACTH in the sinuses than in the forearm vein indicate a pituitary adenoma. Similar levels of ACTH in the petrosal sinuses and the forearm suggest ectopic ACTH syndrome.

How Is Cushing Syndrome Treated?

Treatment depends on the specific reason for excess cortisol and may include surgery, radiation, chemotherapy, or the use of cortisol-inhibiting drugs. If the cause is long-term use of glucocorticoid hormones to treat another disorder, the doctor will gradually reduce the dosage to the lowest dose adequate for control of that disorder. Once control is established, the daily dose of glucocorticoid hormones may be doubled and given on alternate days to lessen side effects. In some cases, noncorticosteroid drugs can be prescribed.

Pituitary Adenomas

Several therapies are available to treat the ACTH-secreting pituitary adenomas of Cushing disease. The most widely used treatment is surgical removal of the tumor, known as "transsphenoidal adenomectomy." Using a special microscope and fine instruments, the surgeon approaches the pituitary gland through a nostril or an opening made below the upper lip. Because this procedure is extremely delicate, patients are often referred to centers specializing in this type of surgery. The success, or cure, rate of this procedure is more than 80 percent when performed by a surgeon with extensive experience. If surgery fails or only produces a temporary cure, surgery can be repeated, often with good results.

After a curative pituitary gland surgery, the production of ACTH drops two levels below normal. This drop is natural and temporary, and patients are given a synthetic form of cortisol such as hydrocortisone or prednisone to compensate. Most people can stop this replacement therapy in less than 1 or 2 years, but some must be on it for life. If transsphenoidal surgery fails or a patient is not a suitable candidate for surgery, radiation therapy is another possible treatment. Radiation to the pituitary gland is given over a 6-week period, with improvement occurring in 40 to 50 percent of adults and up to 85 percent of children. Another technique, called "stereotactic radiosurgery" (SRS) or "gamma knife radiation," can be given in a single high-dose treatment. It may take several months or years before people feel better from radiation treatment alone. Combining radiation with cortisol-inhibiting drugs can help speed recovery.

Drugs used alone or in combination to control the production of excess cortisol are ketoconazole, mitotane, aminoglutethimide, and metyrapone. Each drug has its own side effects that doctors consider when prescribing medical therapy for individual patients.

Ectopic Adrenocorticotropic Hormone Syndrome

To cure the overproduction of cortisol caused by ectopic ACTH syndrome, all of the cancerous tissue that is secreting ACTH must be eliminated. The choice of cancer treatment—surgery, radiation, chemotherapy, immunotherapy, or a combination of these treatments—depends on the type of cancer and how far it has spread. Because ACTH-secreting tumors may be small or widespread at the time of diagnosis, making them difficult to locate and treat directly, cortisol-inhibiting drugs are an important part of treatment. In some cases, if other treatments fail, surgical removal of the adrenal glands, called "bilateral adrenalectomy," may replace drug therapy.

Adrenal Tumors

Surgery is the mainstay of treatment for benign and cancerous tumors of the adrenal glands. Primary pigmented micronodular adrenal disease and the inherited Carney complex (CNC)—primary tumors of the heart that can lead to endocrine overactivity and Cushing syndrome—require surgical removal of the adrenal glands.

Chapter 31

Primary Hyperaldosteronism and Familial Hyperaldosteronism

What Is Primary Hyperaldosteronism?

Primary hyperaldosteronism is a disorder caused by excess production of the hormone aldosterone by the adrenal glands.

Symptoms

The main symptom of primary hyperaldosteronism is high blood pressure (hypertension), but other symptoms may include headaches, weakness, swelling (edema), and muscle spasms (tetany).

This chapter contains text excerpted from the following sources: Text under the heading "What Is Primary Hyperaldosteronism?" is excerpted from "Primary Hyperaldosteronism," Genetic and Rare Diseases Information Center (GARD), National Center for Advancing Translational Sciences (NCATS), July 26, 2016. Reviewed September 2019; Text beginning with the heading "What Is Familial Hyperaldosteronism?" is excerpted from "Familial Hyperaldosteronism," Genetics Home Reference (GHR), National Institutes of Health (NIH), April 2014. Reviewed September 2019.

Causes

The cause of primary hyperaldosteronism can vary. One cause may be an adenoma, or benign tumor, on the adrenal glands, which causes them to produce too much aldosterone. If primary hyperaldosteronism is caused by an adenoma, it is known as "Conn syndrome." The condition may also be caused by enlarged adrenal glands without adenomas (adrenal hyperplasia). In some cases, primary hyperaldosteronism is inherited in an autosomal dominant manner, but in most cases, the exact cause of the disease is unknown (idiopathic).

Diagnosis

A diagnosis is made by testing the blood for high levels of aldosterone.

Treatment

Treatment for Conn syndrome includes surgical removal of adenomas. Medication is used to treat primary hyperaldosteronism if it is caused by adrenal hyperplasia.

What Is Familial Hyperaldosteronism?

Familial hyperaldosteronism is a group of inherited conditions in which the adrenal glands, which are small glands located on top of each kidney, produce too much of the hormone aldosterone. Aldosterone helps control the amount of salt retained by the kidneys. Excess aldosterone causes the kidneys to retain more salt than normal, which in turn increases the body's fluid levels and blood pressure. People with familial hyperaldosteronism may develop severe high blood pressure (hypertension), often early in life. Without treatment, hypertension increases the risk of strokes, heart attacks, and kidney failure.

Familial hyperaldosteronism is categorized into three types, distinguished by their clinical features and genetic causes. In familial hyperaldosteronism type I, hypertension generally appears in childhood to early adulthood and can range from mild to severe. This type can be treated with steroid medications called "glucocorticoids," so it is also known as "glucocorticoid-remediable aldosteronism" (GRA). In familial hyperaldosteronism type II, hypertension usually appears in early to middle adulthood and does not improve with glucocorticoid treatment. In most individuals with familial hyperaldosteronism type III, the adrenal glands are enlarged up to six times their normal size. These affected individuals have severe hypertension that starts in childhood. The hypertension is difficult to treat and often results in damage to organs, such as the heart and kidneys. Rarely, individuals with type III have milder symptoms with treatable hypertension and no adrenal gland enlargement.

There are other forms of hyperaldosteronism that are not familial. These conditions are caused by various problems in the adrenal glands or kidneys. In some cases, a cause for the increase in aldosterone levels cannot be found.

Frequency

The prevalence of familial hyperaldosteronism is unknown. Familial hyperaldosteronism type II appears to be the most common variety. All types of familial hyperaldosteronism combined account for fewer than 1 out of 10 cases of hyperaldosteronism.

Causes

The various types of familial hyperaldosteronism have different genetic causes. Familial hyperaldosteronism type I is caused by the abnormal joining together (fusion) of two similar genes called "*CYP11B1*" and "*CYP11B2*," which are located close together on chromosome 8. These genes provide instructions for making two enzymes that are found in the adrenal glands.

The *CYP11B1* gene provides instructions for making an enzyme called "11-beta-hydroxylase." This enzyme helps produce hormones called "cortisol" and "corticosterone." The *CYP11B2* gene provides instructions for making another enzyme called "aldosterone synthase," which helps produce aldosterone. When *CYP11B1* and *CYP11B2* are abnormally fused together, too much aldosterone synthase is produced. This overproduction causes the adrenal glands to make excess aldosterone, which leads to the signs and symptoms of familial hyperaldosteronism type I.

Familial hyperaldosteronism type III is caused by mutations in the *KCNJ5* gene. The *KCNJ5* gene provides instructions for making a protein that functions as a potassium channel, which means that it transports positively charged atoms (ions) of potassium into and out of cells. In the adrenal glands, the flow of ions through potassium channels produced from the *KCNJ5* gene is thought to help regulate the production of aldosterone. Mutations in the *KCNJ5* gene likely result in the production of potassium channels that are less selective, allowing other ions (predominantly sodium) to pass as well. The abnormal ion flow results in the activation of biochemical processes (pathways) that lead to increased aldosterone production, causing hypertension associated with familial hyperaldosteronism type III.

The genetic cause of familial hyperaldosteronism type II is unknown.

Inheritance Pattern

This condition is inherited in an autosomal dominant pattern, which means one copy of the altered gene in each cell is sufficient to cause the disorder.

Chapter 32

Pheochromocytoma and Paraganglioma

Pheochromocytoma and paraganglioma are rare tumors that come from the same type of tissue.

Paragangliomas form in nerve tissue in the adrenal glands and near certain blood vessels and nerves. Paragangliomas that form in the adrenal glands are called "pheochromocytomas." Paragangliomas that form outside the adrenal glands are called "extra-adrenal paragangliomas." In this chapter, extra-adrenal paragangliomas are called "paragangliomas."

Pheochromocytomas and paragangliomas may be benign (noncancerous) or malignant (cancerous).

Pheochromocytoma

Pheochromocytoma forms in the adrenal glands. There are two adrenal glands, one on top of each kidney in the back of the upper abdomen. Each adrenal gland has two parts. The outer layer of the adrenal gland is the adrenal cortex. The center of the adrenal gland is the adrenal medulla.

Pheochromocytoma is a rare tumor of the adrenal medulla. Usually, pheochromocytoma affects one adrenal gland, but it may affect

This chapter includes text excerpted from "Pheochromocytoma and Paraganglioma Treatment (PDQ®)—Patient Version," National Cancer Institute (NCI), May 24, 2019.

275

both adrenal glands. Sometimes there is more than one tumor in one adrenal gland.

The adrenal glands make important hormones called "catechol-amines." Adrenaline (epinephrine) and noradrenaline (norepineph-rine) are two types of catecholamines that help control heart rate, blood pressure, blood sugar, and the way the body reacts to stress. Sometimes a pheochromocytoma will release extra adrenaline and noradrenaline into the blood and cause signs or symptoms of the disease.

Paraganglioma

Paragangliomas form outside the adrenal gland and are rare tumors that form near the carotid artery, along nerve pathways in the head and neck, and in other parts of the body. Some paragangliomas make extra catecholamines called "adrenaline" and "noradrenaline." The release of these extra catecholamines into the blood may cause signs or symptoms of the disease.

Risk Factors of Pheochromocytoma or Paraganglioma

Certain inherited disorders and changes in certain genes increase the risk of pheochromocytoma or paraganglioma. Anything that increases your chance of getting a disease is called a "risk factor." Having a risk factor does not mean that you will get cancer; not having risk factors does not mean that you will not get cancer. Talk to your doctor if you think you may be at risk.

The following inherited syndromes or gene changes increase the risk of pheochromocytoma or paraganglioma:

- Multiple endocrine neoplasia 2 syndrome, types A and B (MEN2A and MEN2B)

- von Hippel-Lindau (VHL) syndrome

- Neurofibromatosis type 1 (NF1)

- Hereditary paraganglioma syndrome

- Carney-Stratakis dyad (paraganglioma and gastrointestinal stromal tumor (GIST))

- Carney triad (paraganglioma, GIST, and pulmonary chondroma)

Signs and Symptoms of Pheochromocytoma and Paraganglioma

Signs and symptoms of pheochromocytoma and paraganglioma include high blood pressure and headache. Some tumors do not make extra adrenaline or noradrenaline and do not cause signs and symptoms. These tumors are sometimes found when a lump form in the neck or when a test or procedure is done for another reason. Signs and symptoms of pheochromocytoma and paraganglioma occur when too much adrenaline or noradrenaline is released into the blood. These and other signs and symptoms may be caused by pheochromocytoma and paraganglioma or by other conditions. Check with your doctor if you have any of the following:

- High blood pressure

- Headache

- Heavy sweating for no known reason

- A strong, fast, or irregular heartbeat

- Being shaky

- Being extremely pale

The most common sign is high blood pressure. It may be hard to control. Very high blood pressure can cause serious health problems, such as irregular heartbeat, heart attack, stroke, or death.

Diagnosis of Pheochromocytoma and Paraganglioma

Tests that examine the blood and urine are used to detect and diagnose pheochromocytoma and paraganglioma. The following tests and procedures may be used:

- **Physical exam and history.** An exam of the body to check general signs of health, including checking for signs of disease, such as high blood pressure or anything else that seems unusual. A history of the patient's health habits and past illnesses and treatments will also be taken.

- **Twenty-four-hour urine test.** A test in which urine is collected for 24 hours to measure the amounts of catecholamines in the urine. Substances caused by the breakdown of these catecholamines are also measured. An unusual (higher or lower than normal) amount of a substance can be a sign of disease in the organ or tissue that makes it. Higher-than-normal amounts of certain catecholamines may be a sign of pheochromocytoma.

- **Blood catecholamine studies.** A procedure in which a blood sample is checked to measure the amount of certain catecholamines released into the blood. Substances caused by the breakdown of these catecholamines are also measured. An unusual (higher than or lower than normal) amount of a substance can be a sign of disease in the organ or tissue that makes it. Higher-than-normal amounts of certain catecholamines may be a sign of pheochromocytoma.

- **Computed tomography (CT) scan.** A procedure that makes a series of detailed pictures of areas inside the body, such as the neck, chest, abdomen, and pelvis, taken from different angles. The pictures are made by a computer linked to an x-ray machine. A dye may be injected into a vein or swallowed to help the organs or tissues show up more clearly. This procedure is also called "computed tomography," "computerized tomography," or "computerized axial tomography."

- **Magnetic resonance imaging (MRI).** A procedure that uses a magnet, radio waves, and a computer to make a series of detailed pictures of areas inside the body, such as the neck, chest, abdomen, and pelvis. This procedure is also called "nuclear magnetic resonance imaging" (NMRI).

Treatment Plan of Pheochromocytoma or Paraganglioma

Genetic counseling is part of the treatment plan for patients with pheochromocytoma or paraganglioma. All patients who are diagnosed with pheochromocytoma or paraganglioma should have genetic counseling to find out their risk for having an inherited syndrome and other related cancers.

Genetic testing may be recommended by a genetic counselor for patients who:

- Have a personal or family history of traits linked with inherited pheochromocytoma or paraganglioma syndrome

- Have tumors in both adrenal glands

- Have more than one tumor in one adrenal gland

- Have signs or symptoms of extra catecholamines being released into the blood or malignant paraganglioma

- Are diagnosed before the age of 40

Genetic testing is sometimes recommended for patients with pheochromocytoma who:

- Are aged 40 to 50 years

- Have a tumor in one adrenal gland

- Do not have a personal or family history of an inherited syndrome

When certain gene changes are found during genetic testing, the testing is usually offered to family members who are at risk but do not have signs or symptoms.

Genetic testing is not recommended for patients older than 50 years.

Certain Factors Affect Prognosis and Treatment Options

The prognosis (chance of recovery) and treatment options depend on the following:

- Whether the tumor is benign or malignant

- Whether the tumor is in one area only or has spread to other places in the body

- Whether there are signs or symptoms caused by a higher-than-normal amount of catecholamines

- Whether the tumor has just been diagnosed or has recurred

Chapter 33

Laparoscopic Adrenal Gland Removal

Adrenal glands are triangular-shaped organs located at the top of each kidney. They are classified as endocrine glands because they produce hormones, such as aldosterone, cortisol, epinephrine, and norepinephrine, as well as a small amount of estrogen and androgen. These hormones control many bodily functions, including metabolism, blood chemistry, immune system regulation, blood pressure, electrolytes, glucose usage and the ability to react quickly in times of stress (the "fight or flight" response).

When the adrenal glands produce more or less of these hormones than the body needs, a variety of illnesses can develop. For example, overproduction of aldosterone can result in hyperaldosteronism, which causes low blood pressure and low potassium levels, whereas too little aldosterone may have the opposite effect, hypoaldosteronism. Similarly, if the adrenal glands produce too much cortisol, Cushing syndrome could be the result, while underproduction is associated with Addison disease. And either under- or overproduction of some hormones can lead to several types of tumors, some benign and some cancerous.

Disorders of the adrenal glands can be treated in a number of ways, including medication and hormone replacement, but when removal becomes necessary, there are at least five ways the surgery, called "adrenalectomy," may be performed. Four of them come under the heading of the "open" approach, in which a six-to-twelve-inch incision is made in the abdomen, flank, or back to give the surgeon access to the adrenal gland and surrounding area. The alternative is laparoscopic surgery, a procedure in which three to five holes of just one-quarter to one-half inch are required.

The Laparoscopic Adrenalectomy Procedure

Removal of the adrenal gland may be recommended for patients with functioning adrenal-gland disorders, in which the organ is producing excess hormones, or nonfunctioning disorders, a condition in which the gland does not produce any hormones. Either may be caused by a benign or malignant tumor.

Preparation for Surgery

• When an adrenal tumor is suspected, the doctor will typically order urine and blood tests to determine the level of various hormones in the body.

• A computerized tomography (CT) scan or magnetic resonance imaging (MRI) might then be used to confirm the presence of the tumor and pinpoint its location.

• Depending on the patient's age and condition, a chest x-ray and an electrocardiogram (EKG) might be administered.

• Prior to the operation, some patients may need to take medication to control the symptoms of the adrenal disorder. Others might need to discontinue certain drugs.

• The surgeon will review the procedure in detail, explaining the benefits and potential risks of the operation, and ask the patient to sign a consent form.

• The patient will be advised not to eat or drink after midnight on the day of the surgery.

How Laparoscopic Adrenalectomy Is Performed

• The procedure will take place in a hospital with the patient under general anesthesia, so she or he is asleep during the surgery.

- The patient will be positioned on her or his back or side, depending on how the adrenal gland will be removed.

- One or more IV lines will be inserted in order to administer fluids during the procedure.

- The surgeon will make three to five small incisions and insert tubes into them through which various instruments will be introduced.

- One such instrument, called a "laparoscope," connects to a camera that is attached to a television screen and gives the surgeon a magnified view of the internal organs.

- Other instruments, such as forceps and scissors, inserted through the rest of the tubes allow the doctor to separate the adrenal gland from the kidney.

- Once the gland is detached it is placed in a small bag, also introduced through a tube, which makes it easier to remove from the body.

- Finally, the instruments and tubes are withdrawn, the surgeon closes the incisions, and dressings are applied.

After Surgery

- When the adrenalectomy is completed, the patient is moved to a recovery room where she or he will rest for several hours and be monitored closely by hospital staff.

- Assuming no complications, the patient will then be moved to a regular hospital room for one to three days.

- Although laparoscopic surgery is much less invasive than an open procedure, some discomfort at the incision sites is to be expected, so during their hospital stay patient are usually given pain medication.

- No special home care is generally required. Patients can engage in light activities almost immediately, resume showering as long as the incision sites are kept dry, and change dressings as needed.

- The doctor may prescribe pain pills and will let the patient know when she or he can begin taking regular medicines again.

- Within about a week, most patients are able to resume normal activities, including work, climbing stairs, driving, and light lifting.

- The surgeon will schedule a follow-up visit about two weeks after the surgery to be sure that recovery is proceeding satisfactorily and discuss any of the patient's concerns.

Advantages of Laparoscopic Adrenal Gland Removal

In some cases, such as when a tumor is very large, open surgery must be used, but laparoscopic adrenalectomy is now commonly performed whenever possible. Some of the advantages of this technique include:

- Less time in surgery
- Smaller incisions
- Shorter hospital stays
- Less postoperative pain
- Fewer complications
- Faster recovery time
- Less scarring
- Very high success rate

Risks and Complications

Although laparoscopic adrenal gland removal is considerably less invasive and generally safer than open surgery, any surgical procedure carries risks, and postoperative complications, though rare and usually not serious, can occur. Some of these include:

- Excessive bleeding during surgery
- Injury to other internal organs during the procedure
- Adverse reaction to general anesthesia
- High blood pressure
- Excessive postoperative pain
- Infection at the wound site
- Drainage and bleeding from the wound
- Swelling and redness
- Nausea

- Dizziness

- Fluid retention

- Sudden weight gain

Life after Adrenal Gland Removal

The long-term effects of adrenalectomy vary from individual to individual, but one major determining factor is whether one or both glands have been removed. In general, a single adrenal gland can produce enough hormones to meet the body's needs. A lot depends on the type of tumor or disorder that necessitated the surgery in the first place, but most patients are able to function normally with one adrenal gland without the need for hormone replacement. The doctor will monitor the function of the remaining organ to be sure it is working properly and recommend medication if necessary.

If both adrenal glands have been removed, or if the remaining gland is not functioning properly, the patient may need to take steroids, such as hydrocortisone or fludrocortisone to replace the hormones that had been produced by these organs. These substances may be necessary to support life, so it is critical that their use be continued unless instructed otherwise by a doctor. It is also wise for the patient to inform all of her or his healthcare providers of the operation and get a medical alert bracelet stating that an adrenalectomy has been performed and that in an emergency special life-saving medication may be required.

References

1. "Adrenal Gland Removal," DoveMed.com, October 18, 2015.

2. "Adrenal Gland Removal," George Washington University Medical Faculty Associates, n.d.

3. "Laparoscopic Adrenal Gland Removal," Society of American Gastrointestinal and Endoscopic Surgeons (SAGES), n.d.

4. Norman, James MD, FACS, FACE. "Surgical Approaches to the Adrenal Gland," EndocrineWeb.com, April 18, 2016.

Part Five

Pancreatic and Diabetic Disorders

Chapter 34

About Pancreatic and Diabetic Disorders

How much you eat alters more than your waistline. It also affects your body's organs, starting with your pancreas. With each bite, your pancreas must release enough digestive juices and hormones for you to benefit from the food you eat. Putting too much stress on your pancreas—by too much eating, drinking, or smoking—can cause serious health issues.

The pancreas lies behind your stomach. It is surrounded by the intestines, liver, and gallbladder. These neighboring organs work together to help you digest your food.

"The pancreas produces a variety of enzymes to help break down the carbohydrates, proteins, and fats in your diet into smaller elements that are more easily used for energy," says Dr. Dana Andersen, a pancreatic specialist at the National Institutes of Health (NIH). "It also produces specialized hormones that travel through the blood and help regulate a variety of body functions."

The best-known hormone produced by the pancreas is insulin. Insulin controls how much sugar, or glucose, is taken up by your body's cells. If the insulin-producing cells in the pancreas are damaged, diabetes may arise. Type 2 diabetes occurs when the pancreas cannot

---

This chapter includes text excerpted from "The Power of Your Pancreas," *NIH News in Health*, National Institutes of Health (NIH), February 2017.

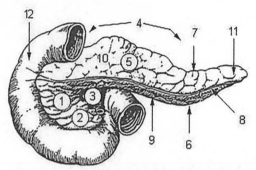

1. Head of pancreas	7. Superior margin
2. Uncinate process	8. Anterior margin
3. Pancreatic notch	9. Inferior margin
4. Body of pancreas	10. Omental tuber
5. Anterior surface	11. Tail of pancreas
6. Inferior surface	12. Duodenum

Figure 34.1. *Anatomy of Pancreas* (Source: "Anatomy of the Pancreas and Duodenum," Surveillance, Epidemiology, and End Results Program (SEER), National Cancer Institute (NCI).)

produce enough insulin to handle the sugar in your blood. Obesity worsens type 2 diabetes.

"Obesity can make your body less sensitive to insulin, so it takes more insulin to achieve the same metabolic work. That puts more stress on the pancreas," Andersen says. "Just losing 5 or 10 pounds can help the pancreas to work more efficiently."

High levels of fat in the blood can also lead to inflammation of the pancreas, or pancreatitis, which can be chronic or acute. With chronic pancreatitis, the inflammation does not heal and gets worse over time. Eventually, it can lead to permanent damage.

Acute pancreatitis occurs suddenly and is very painful. It usually resolves in a few days with treatment. In severe cases, bleeding and permanent tissue damage may occur. The most common causes of acute pancreatitis are gallstones and heavy alcohol use. Gallstones are small, pebble-like substances made of hardened bile (a liquid produced by the liver to digest fat). Other causes of acute pancreatitis include abdominal trauma, medications, and infections.

Genetic disorders of the pancreas and certain autoimmune disorders can also lead to pancreatitis. But in nearly half of cases, the cause is unknown—a condition known as "idiopathic pancreatitis."

Tracking your family's medical history can help you learn if you are at risk for pancreatic problems. "It's always a good idea to tell your doctor if there's been a family history of pancreatic disease," Andersen says. "That may not sound like much, but to a doctor it's very important information."

Knowledge of family health history is especially important for possible early detection of pancreatic cancer, which usually has no symptoms in its early stages. When caught early, pancreatic cancer may be curable with surgery. But most patients with pancreatic cancer are not diagnosed until more advanced stages, when the chances for survival are low.

Researchers at the NIH are looking for new ways to detect pancreatic diseases early and predict who is most at risk. Eating a healthy diet and limiting your exposure to harmful substances, such as tobacco and alcohol, can help keep your pancreas and your entire digestive system working properly.

Chapter 35

Pancreatitis

What Is Pancreatitis?

Pancreatitis is an inflammation of the pancreas. The pancreas is a large gland behind the stomach, close to the first part of the small intestine, called "duodenum." The pancreas has two main functions—to make insulin and to make digestive juices, or enzymes, to help you digest food. These enzymes digest food in the intestine. Pancreatitis occurs when the enzymes damage the pancreas, which causes inflammation. Pancreatitis can be acute or chronic. Either form is serious and can lead to complications.

Acute Pancreatitis

Acute pancreatitis occurs suddenly and is a short-term condition. Most people with acute pancreatitis get better, and it goes away in several days with treatment. Some people can have a more severe form of acute pancreatitis, which requires a lengthy hospital stay.

Chronic Pancreatitis

Chronic pancreatitis is a long-lasting condition. The pancreas does not heal or improve. Instead, it gets worse over time, which can lead to lasting damage to your pancreas.

This chapter includes text excerpted from "Pancreatitis," National Institute of Diabetes and Digestive and Kidney Diseases (NIDDK), November 15, 2017.

How Common Is Pancreatitis?

Acute pancreatitis has become more common, for reasons that are not clear. Each year, about 275,000 hospital stays for acute pancreatitis occur in the United States. Although pancreatitis is rare in children, the number of children with acute pancreatitis has grown.

Chronic pancreatitis is less common, with about 86,000 hospital stays per year.

Who Is More Likely to Get Pancreatitis?

Certain groups of people are more likely to get acute or chronic pancreatitis than others:

- Men are more likely to get pancreatitis than women
- African Americans have a higher risk of getting pancreatitis
- People with a family history of pancreatitis have a higher risk
- People with a personal or family history of gallstones also have a higher risk

People with Certain Health Conditions

You are more likely to get pancreatitis if you have one of the following health conditions:

- Diabetes
- Gallstones
- High triglycerides
- Genetic disorders of the pancreas
- Certain autoimmune conditions
- Cystic fibrosis (CF)

People with Other Health Concerns

You are also more likely to get pancreatitis if you:

- Have obesity
- Are a heavy alcohol user
- Are a smoker

What Are the Complications of Pancreatitis?

Both acute and chronic pancreatitis can lead to complications that include:

- Narrowing or blockage in a bile or pancreatic duct
- Leakage from the pancreatic duct
- Pancreatic pseudocysts
- Damage to your pancreas
- Heart, lung, or kidney failure
- Death

Acute Pancreatitis

Repeat episodes of acute pancreatitis may lead to chronic pancreatitis. Other complications of acute pancreatitis include:

- Dehydration
- Bleeding
- Infection

Chronic Pancreatitis

Complications of chronic pancreatitis include:

- Chronic pain in your abdomen
- Maldigestion, when you cannot digest food properly
- Malnutrition and malabsorption
- Problems with how well your pancreas works
- Scars in your pancreas
- Diabetes
- Pancreatic cancer, which is more likely in people with both diabetes and pancreatitis
- Osteopenia, osteoporosis, and bone fractures

Symptoms of Pancreatitis

The main symptom of acute and chronic pancreatitis is:

- Pain in your upper abdomen that may spread to your back

People with acute or chronic pancreatitis may feel the pain in different ways.

Acute Pancreatitis

Acute pancreatitis usually starts with pain that:

- Begins slowly or suddenly in your upper abdomen
- Sometimes spreads to your back
- Can be mild or severe
- May last for several days

Other symptoms may include:

- Fever
- Nausea and vomiting
- Fast heartbeat
- Swollen or tender abdomen

People with acute pancreatitis usually look and feel seriously ill and need to see a doctor right away.

Chronic Pancreatitis

Most people with chronic pancreatitis:

- Feel pain in the upper abdomen, although some people have no pain at all.

The pain may:

- Spread to your back
- Become constant and severe
- Become worse after eating
- Go away as your condition gets worse

People with chronic pancreatitis may not have symptoms until they have complications.
Other symptoms may include:

- Diarrhea
- Nausea

- Greasy, foul-smelling stools
- Vomiting
- Weight loss

Seek Care Right Away for Pancreatitis

Seek care right away for the following symptoms of severe pancreatitis:

- Pain or tenderness in the abdomen that is severe or becomes worse
- Nausea and vomiting
- Fever or chills
- Fast heartbeat
- Shortness of breath
- Yellowish color of the skin or whites of the eyes, called "jaundice"

These symptoms may be a sign of:

- Serious infection
- Inflammation
- Blockage of the pancreas, gallbladder, or a bile and pancreatic duct

Left untreated, these problems can be fatal.

Causes of Pancreatitis

The most common causes of both acute and chronic pancreatitis are:

- Gallstones
- Heavy alcohol use
- Genetic disorders of your pancreas
- Some medicines

Other causes include:

- Infections, such as viruses or parasites
- Injury to your abdomen

- Pancreatic cancer
- Having a procedure called "endoscopic retrograde cholangiopancreatography" (ERCP) to treat another condition
- Pancreas divisum

Acute Pancreatitis

The most common cause of acute pancreatitis is having gallstones. Gallstones cause inflammation of your pancreas as stones pass through and get stuck in a bile or pancreatic duct. This condition is called "gallstone pancreatitis."

Chronic Pancreatitis

The most common causes of chronic pancreatitis are:

- Heavy alcohol use
- Genetic disorders of your pancreas

Other causes include:

- Blockage in your pancreatic duct
- High levels of blood fats, called "lipids"
- High level of calcium in your blood

In many cases, doctors cannot find the cause of pancreatitis. This is called "idiopathic pancreatitis."

Diagnosis and Tests of Pancreatitis
How Do Doctors Diagnose Pancreatitis?

To diagnose pancreatitis and find its causes, doctors use:

- Your medical history
- A physical exam
- Lab and imaging tests

A healthcare professional will ask:

- About your symptoms
- If you have a history of health conditions or concerns that make you more likely to get pancreatitis—including medicines you are taking

- If you have a personal or family medical history of pancreatitis or gallstones

During a physical exam, the healthcare professional will:

- Examine your body

- Check your abdomen for pain, swelling, or tenderness

What Tests Do Healthcare Professionals Use to Diagnose Pancreatitis?

Healthcare professionals may use lab or imaging tests to diagnose pancreatitis and find its causes. Diagnosing chronic pancreatitis can be hard in the early stages. Your doctor will also test for other conditions that have similar symptoms, such as peptic ulcers or pancreatic cancer.

Lab Tests

Lab tests to help diagnose pancreatitis include the following:

Blood tests. A healthcare professional may take a blood sample from you and send the sample to a lab to test for:

- High amylase and lipase levels—digestive enzymes made in your pancreas

- High blood glucose, also called "blood sugar"

- High levels of blood fats, called "lipids"

- Signs of infection or inflammation of the bile ducts, pancreas, gallbladder, or liver

- Pancreatic cancer

Stool tests. Your doctor may test a stool sample to find out if a person has fat malabsorption.

Imaging Tests

Healthcare professionals also use imaging tests to diagnose pancreatitis. A technician performs most tests in an outpatient center, a hospital, or a doctor's office. You do not need anesthesia, a medicine to keep you calm, for most of these tests.

Ultrasound. Ultrasound uses a device called a "transducer," which bounces safe, painless sound waves off your organs to create a picture of their structure. Ultrasound can find gallstones.

Computed tomography (CT) scan. CT scans create pictures of your pancreas, gallbladder, and bile ducts. CT scans can show pancreatitis or pancreatic cancer.

Magnetic resonance cholangiopancreatography (MRCP). MRCP uses a magnetic resonance imaging (MRI) machine, which creates pictures of your organs and soft tissues without x-rays. Your doctor or a specialist may use MRCP to look at your pancreas, gallbladder, and bile ducts for causes of pancreatitis.

Endoscopic ultrasound (EUS). Your doctor inserts an endoscope—a thin, flexible tube—down your throat, through your stomach, and into your small intestine. The doctor turns on an ultrasound attachment to create pictures of your pancreas and bile ducts. Your doctor may send you to a gastroenterologist to perform this test.

Pancreatic function test (PFT). Your doctor may use this test to measure how your pancreas responds to secretin, a hormone made by the small intestine. This test is done only at some centers in the United States.

Treatment, Management, and Prevention of Pancreatitis
How Do Healthcare Professionals Treat Pancreatitis?

Treatment for acute or chronic pancreatitis may include:

- A hospital stay to treat dehydration with intravenous (IV) fluids and if you can swallow them, fluids by mouth

- Pain medicine, and antibiotics by mouth or through an IV if you have an infection in your pancreas

- A low-fat diet, or nutrition by feeding tube or IV if you cannot eat

Your doctor may send you to a gastroenterologist or surgeon for one of the following treatments, depending on the type of pancreatitis that you have.

Acute Pancreatitis

Mild acute pancreatitis usually goes away in a few days with rest and treatment. If your pancreatitis is more severe, your treatment may also include:

Surgery. Your doctor may recommend surgery to remove the gallbladder, called "cholecystectomy," if gallstones cause your pancreatitis. Having surgery within a few days after you are admitted to the hospital lowers the chance of complications. If you have severe pancreatitis, your doctor may advise delaying surgery to first treat complications.

Procedures. Your doctor or specialist will drain fluid in your abdomen if you have an abscess or infected pseudocyst, or a large pseudocyst causing pain or bleeding. Your doctor may remove damaged tissue from your pancreas.

Endoscopic cholangiopancreatography (ERCP). Doctors use ERCP to treat both acute and chronic pancreatitis. ERCP combines upper gastrointestinal endoscopy and x-rays to treat narrowing or blockage of a bile or pancreatic duct. Your gastroenterologist may use ERCP to remove gallstones blocking the bile or pancreatic ducts.

Chronic pancreatitis

Treatment for chronic pancreatitis may help relieve pain, improve how well the pancreas works, and manage complications.

Your doctor may prescribe or provide the following:

Medicines and vitamins. Your doctor may give you enzyme pills to help with digestion, or vitamins A, D, E, and K if you have malabsorption. She or he may also give you vitamin B_{12} shots if you need them.

Treatment for diabetes. Chronic pancreatitis may cause diabetes. If you get diabetes, your doctor and healthcare team will work with you to create an eating plan and a routine of medicine, blood glucose monitoring, and regular checkups.

Surgery. Your doctor may recommend surgery to relieve pressure or blockage in your pancreatic duct, or to remove a damaged or infected part of your pancreas. Surgery is done in a hospital, where you may have to stay a few days.

In patients who do not get better with other treatments, surgeons may perform surgery to remove your whole pancreas, followed by islet auto-transplantation. Islets are groups of cells in your pancreas that make hormones, including insulin. After removing your pancreas, doctors will take islets from your pancreas and transplant them into your liver. The islets will begin to make hormones and release them into your bloodstream.

Procedures. Your doctor may suggest a nerve block, which is a shot of numbing medicine through your skin and directly into nerves that carry the pain message from your pancreas. If you have stones blocking your pancreatic duct, your doctor may use a procedure to break up and remove the stones.

How Can I Help Manage My Pancreatitis?
Stop Drinking Alcohol

Healthcare professionals strongly advise people with pancreatitis to stop drinking alcohol, even if your pancreatitis is mild or in the early stages. Continuing to drink alcohol when you have acute pancreatitis can lead to:

- More episodes of acute pancreatitis
- Chronic pancreatitis

When people with chronic pancreatitis caused by alcohol use continue to drink alcohol, the condition is more likely to lead to severe complications and even death.

Talk with your healthcare professional if you need help to stop drinking alcohol.

Stop Smoking

Healthcare professionals strongly advise people with pancreatitis to stop smoking, even if your pancreatitis is mild or in the early stages. Smoking with acute pancreatitis, especially if it is caused by alcohol use, greatly raises the chances that your pancreatitis will become chronic. Smoking with pancreatitis also may raise your risk of pancreatic cancer.

Talk with your healthcare professional if you need help to stop smoking.

How Can I Help Prevent Pancreatitis?

You cannot prevent pancreatitis, but you can take steps to help you stay healthy.

Maintain a Healthy Weight or Lose Weight Safely

Maintaining a healthy lifestyle and a healthy weight—or losing weight if needed—can help to:

- Make your pancreas work better
- Lower your chance of getting gallstones, a leading cause of pancreatitis
- Prevent obesity—a risk factor for pancreatitis
- Prevent diabetes—a risk factor for pancreatitis

Avoid Alcohol Use

Alcohol use can cause acute and chronic pancreatitis. Talk with your healthcare professional if you need help to stop drinking alcohol.

Avoid Smoking

Smoking is a common risk factor for pancreatitis—and the chances of getting pancreatitis are even higher in people who smoke and drink alcohol. Talk with your healthcare professional if you need help to stop smoking.

Eating, Diet, and Nutrition for Pancreatitis

During pancreatitis treatment, your doctor may tell you not to eat or drink for a while. Instead, your doctor may use a feeding tube to give you nutrition. Once you may start eating again, she or he will prescribe a healthy, low-fat eating plan that includes small, frequent meals.

If you have pancreatitis, drink plenty of fluids and limit caffeine. Healthcare professionals strongly advise people with pancreatitis not to drink any alcohol, even if your pancreatitis is mild.

Having an eating plan high in fat and calories can lead to high levels of fat in your blood, which raises your risk of pancreatitis. You can lower your chances of getting pancreatitis by sticking with a low-fat, healthy eating plan.

Chapter 36

Insulin Resistance and Prediabetes

What Is Insulin?

Insulin is a hormone made by the pancreas that helps glucose in your blood enter cells in your muscle, fat, and liver, where it's used for energy. Glucose comes from the food you eat. The liver also makes glucose in times of need, such as when you are fasting. When blood glucose, also called "blood sugar," levels rise after you eat, your pancreas releases insulin into the blood. Insulin then lowers blood glucose to keep it in the normal range.

What Is Insulin Resistance?

Insulin resistance is when cells in your muscles, fat, and liver do not respond well to insulin and cannot easily take up glucose from your blood. As a result, your pancreas makes more insulin to help glucose enter your cells. As long as your pancreas can make enough insulin to overcome your cells' weak response to insulin, your blood glucose levels will stay in the healthy range.

This chapter includes text excerpted from "Insulin Resistance and Prediabetes," National Institute of Diabetes and Digestive and Kidney Diseases (NIDDK), May 2018.

What Is Prediabetes?

Prediabetes means your blood glucose levels are higher than normal but not high enough to be diagnosed as diabetes. Prediabetes usually occurs in people who already have some insulin resistance or whose beta cells in the pancreas are not making enough insulin to keep blood glucose in the normal range. Without enough insulin, extra glucose stays in your bloodstream rather than entering your cells. Over time, you could develop type 2 diabetes.

How Common Is Prediabetes?

More than 84 million people ages 18 and older have prediabetes in the United States. That is about 1 out of every 3 adults.

Who Is More Likely to Develop Insulin Resistance or Prediabetes?

People who have genetic or lifestyle risk factors are more likely to develop insulin resistance or prediabetes. Risk factors include:

- Overweight or obesity
- Age 45 or older
- A parent, brother, or sister with diabetes
- African American, Alaska Native, American Indian, Asian American, Hispanic/Latinx, Native Hawaiian, or Pacific Islander American ethnicity
- Physical inactivity
- Health conditions such as high blood pressure and abnormal cholesterol levels
- A history of gestational diabetes
- A history of heart disease or stroke
- Polycystic ovary syndrome (PCOS)

People who have metabolic syndrome—a combination of high blood pressure, abnormal cholesterol levels, and large waist size—are more likely to have prediabetes.

Along with these risk factors, other things that may contribute to insulin resistance include:

- Certain medicines, such as glucocorticoids, some antipsychotics, and some medicines for human immunodeficiency virus (HIV)

- Hormonal disorders, such as Cushing syndrome and acromegaly

- Sleep problems, especially sleep apnea

Although you cannot change risk factors such as family history, age, or ethnicity, you can change lifestyle risk factors around eating, physical activity, and weight. These lifestyle changes can lower your chances of developing insulin resistance or prediabetes.

What Causes Insulin Resistance and Prediabetes

Researchers do not fully understand what causes insulin resistance and prediabetes, but they think excess weight and lack of physical activity are major factors.

Excess Weight

Experts believe obesity, especially too much fat in the abdomen and around the organs, called "visceral fat," is a main cause of insulin resistance. A waist measurement of 40 inches or more for men and 35 inches or more for women is linked to insulin resistance. This is true even if your body mass index (BMI) falls within the normal range. However, research has shown that Asian Americans may have an increased risk for insulin resistance even without a high BMI.

Researchers used to think that fat tissue was only for energy storage. However, studies have shown that belly fat makes hormones and other substances that can contribute to chronic, or long-lasting, inflammation in the body. Inflammation may play a role in insulin resistance, type 2 diabetes, and cardiovascular disease.

Excess weight may lead to insulin resistance, which in turn may play a part in the development of fatty liver disease.

Physical Inactivity

Not getting enough physical activity is linked to insulin resistance and prediabetes. Regular physical activity causes changes in your body that make it better able to keep your blood glucose levels in balance.

What Are the Symptoms of Insulin Resistance and Prediabetes?

Insulin resistance and prediabetes usually have no symptoms. Some people with prediabetes may have darkened skin in the armpit or on the back and sides of the neck, a condition called "acanthosis nigricans." Many small skin growths called "skin tags" often appear in these same areas.

Even though blood glucose levels are not high enough to cause symptoms for most people, a few research studies have shown that some people with prediabetes may already have early changes in their eyes that can lead to retinopathy. This problem more often occurs in people with diabetes.

How Do Doctors Diagnose Insulin Resistance and Prediabetes?

Doctors use blood tests to find out if someone has prediabetes, but they do not usually test for insulin resistance. The most accurate test for insulin resistance is complicated and used mostly for research.

Doctors most often use the fasting plasma glucose (FPG) test or the A1C test to diagnose prediabetes. Less often, doctors use the oral glucose tolerance test (OGTT), which is more expensive and not as easy to give.

The A1C test reflects your average blood glucose over the past three months. The FPG and OGTT show your blood glucose level at the time of the test. The A1C test is not as sensitive as the other tests. In some people, it may miss prediabetes that the OGTT could catch. The OGTT can identify how your body handles glucose after a meal—often before your fasting blood glucose level becomes abnormal. Often doctors use the OGTT to check for gestational diabetes, a type of diabetes that develops during pregnancy.

People with prediabetes have up to a 50 percent chance of developing diabetes over the next 5 to 10 years. You can take steps to manage your prediabetes and prevent type 2 diabetes.

The following test results show prediabetes:

- A1C—5.7 to 6.4 percent
- FPG—100 to 125 mg/dL (milligrams per deciliter)
- OGTT—140 to 199 mg/dL

You should be tested for prediabetes if you are overweight or have obesity and have one or more other risk factors for diabetes, or if your parents, siblings, or children have type 2 diabetes. Even if you do not have risk factors, you should start getting tested once you reach age 45.

If the results are normal but you have other risk factors for diabetes, you should be retested at least every three years.

How Can You Prevent or Reverse Insulin Resistance and Prediabetes?

Physical activity and losing weight if you need to may help your body respond better to insulin. Taking small steps, such as eating healthier foods and moving more to lose weight, can help reverse insulin resistance and prevent or delay type 2 diabetes in people with prediabetes.

The National Institutes of Health (NIH)-funded research study, the Diabetes Prevention Program (DPP), showed that for people at high risk of developing diabetes, losing 5 to 7 percent of their starting weight helped reduce their chance of developing the disease. That is 10 to 14 pounds for someone who weighs 200 pounds. People in the study lost weight by changing their diet and being more physically active.

The DPP also showed that taking metformin, a medicine used to treat diabetes, could delay diabetes. Metformin worked best for women with a history of gestational diabetes, younger adults, and people with obesity. Ask your doctor if metformin might be right for you.

Making a plan, tracking your progress, and getting support from your healthcare professional, family, and friends can help you make lifestyle changes that may prevent or reverse insulin resistance and prediabetes. You may be able to take part in a lifestyle change program as part of the National Diabetes Prevention Program (NDPP).

Chapter 37

Diabetes Mellitus

Diabetes is a disease that occurs when your blood glucose, also called "blood sugar," is too high. Blood glucose is your main source of energy and comes from the food you eat. Insulin, a hormone made by the pancreas, helps glucose from food get into your cells to be used for energy. Sometimes your body does not make enough—or any—insulin or does not use insulin well. Glucose then stays in your blood and does not reach your cells.

Over time, having too much glucose in your blood can cause health problems. Although diabetes has no cure, you can take steps to manage your diabetes and stay healthy.

Sometimes people call diabetes "a touch of sugar" or "borderline diabetes." These terms suggest that someone does not really have diabetes or has a less serious case, but every case of diabetes is serious.

What Are the Different Types of Diabetes?

The most common types of diabetes are type 1, type 2, and gestational diabetes.

Type 1 Diabetes

If you have type 1 diabetes, your body does not make insulin. Your immune system attacks and destroys the cells in your pancreas that

This chapter includes text excerpted from "Diabetes Overview," National Institute of Diabetes and Digestive and Kidney Diseases (NIDDK), December 21, 2016. Reviewed September 2019.

make insulin. Type 1 diabetes is usually diagnosed in children and young adults, although it can appear at any age. People with type 1 diabetes need to take insulin every day to stay alive.

Type 2 Diabetes

If you have type 2 diabetes, your body does not make or use insulin well. You can develop type 2 diabetes at any age, even during childhood. However, this type of diabetes occurs most often in middle-aged and older people. Type 2 is the most common type of diabetes.

Gestational Diabetes

Gestational diabetes develops in some women when they are pregnant. Most of the time, this type of diabetes goes away after the baby is born. However, if you have had gestational diabetes, you have a greater chance of developing type 2 diabetes later in life. Sometimes diabetes diagnosed during pregnancy is actually type 2 diabetes.

Other Types of Diabetes

Less common types include monogenic diabetes, which is an inherited form of diabetes, and cystic fibrosis (CF)-related diabetes.

How Common Is Diabetes

As of 2015, 30.3 million people in the United States, or 9.4 percent of the population, had diabetes. More than 1 in 4 of them did not know they had the disease. Diabetes affects 1 in 4 people over the age of 65. About 90 to 95 percent of cases in adults are type 2 diabetes.

Who Is More Likely to Develop Type 2 Diabetes?

You are more likely to develop type 2 diabetes if you are age 45 or older, have a family history of diabetes, or are overweight. Physical inactivity, race, and certain health problems such as high blood pressure also affect your chance of developing type 2 diabetes. You are also more likely to develop type 2 diabetes if you have prediabetes or had gestational diabetes when you were pregnant.

What Health Problems Can People with Diabetes Develop?

Over time, high blood glucose leads to problems such as:

- Heart disease
- Stroke
- Kidney disease
- Eye problems
- Dental disease
- Nerve damage
- Foot problems

You can take steps to lower your chances of developing these diabetes-related health problems.

Symptoms and Causes of Diabetes
Symptoms of Diabetes

Symptoms of diabetes include:

- Increased thirst and urination
- Increased hunger
- Fatigue
- Blurred vision
- Numbness or tingling in the feet or hands
- Sores that do not heal
- Unexplained weight loss

Symptoms of type 1 diabetes can start quickly, in a matter of weeks. Symptoms of type 2 diabetes often develop slowly—over the course of several years—and can be so mild that you might not even notice them. Many people with type 2 diabetes have no symptoms. Some people do not find out they have the disease until they have diabetes-related health problems, such as blurred vision or heart trouble.

What Causes Type 1 Diabetes

Type 1 diabetes occurs when your immune system, the body's system for fighting infection, attacks and destroys the insulin-producing beta cells of the pancreas. Scientists think type 1 diabetes is caused by genes and environmental factors, such as viruses, that might trigger the disease.

What Causes Type 2 Diabetes

Type 2 diabetes—the most common form of diabetes—is caused by several factors, including lifestyle factors and genes.

Overweight, Obesity, and Physical Inactivity

You are more likely to develop type 2 diabetes if you are not physically active and are overweight or obese. Extra weight causes insulin resistance and is common in people with type 2 diabetes. The location of body fat also makes a difference. Extra belly fat is linked to insulin resistance, type 2 diabetes, and heart and blood vessel disease.

Insulin Resistance

Type 2 diabetes usually begins with insulin resistance, a condition in which muscle, liver, and fat cells do not use insulin well. As a result, the body needs more insulin to help glucose enter cells. At first, the pancreas makes more insulin to keep up with the added demand. Over time, the pancreas cannot make enough insulin, and blood glucose levels rise.

Genes and Family History

As in type 1 diabetes, certain genes may make you more likely to develop type 2 diabetes. The disease tends to run in families and occurs more often in these racial or ethnic groups:

- African Americans
- Alaska Natives
- American Indians
- Asian Americans
- Hispanics or Latinos
- Native Hawaiians
- Pacific Islanders

Genes also can increase the risk of type 2 diabetes by increasing a person's tendency to become overweight or obese.

What Causes Gestational Diabetes

Scientists believe gestational diabetes, a type of diabetes that develops during pregnancy, is caused by the hormonal changes of pregnancy along with genetic and lifestyle factors.

Insulin Resistance

Hormones produced by the placenta contribute to insulin resistance, which occurs in all women during late pregnancy. Most pregnant women can produce enough insulin to overcome insulin resistance, but some cannot. Gestational diabetes occurs when the pancreas cannot make enough insulin.

As with type 2 diabetes, extra weight is linked to gestational diabetes. Women who are overweight or obese may already have insulin resistance when they become pregnant. Gaining too much weight during pregnancy may also be a factor.

Genes and Family History

Having a family history of diabetes makes it more likely that a woman will develop gestational diabetes, which suggests that genes play a role. Genes may also explain why the disorder occurs more often in African Americans, American Indians, Asians, and Hispanics or Latinxs.

What Else Can Cause Diabetes

Genetic mutations, other diseases, damage to the pancreas, and certain medicines may also cause diabetes.

Risk Factors of Type 2 Diabetes

Your chances of developing type 2 diabetes depend on a combination of risk factors such as your genes and lifestyle. Although you cannot change risk factors such as family history, age, or ethnicity, you can change lifestyle risk factors around eating, physical activity, and weight. These lifestyle changes can affect your chances of developing type 2 diabetes.

Read about risk factors for type 2 diabetes below and see which ones apply to you. Taking action on the factors you can change can help you delay or prevent type 2 diabetes.

You are more likely to develop type 2 diabetes if you:

- Are overweight or obese

- Are age 45 or older

- Have a family history of diabetes

- Are African American, Alaska Native, American Indian, Asian American, Hispanic or Latino, Native Hawaiian, or Pacific Islander

- Have high blood pressure

- Have a low level of HDL ("good") cholesterol, or a high level of triglycerides

Table 37.1. Body Mass Index Chart

If You Are Not Asian American or Pacific Islander		If You Are Asian American		If You Are Pacific Islander	
At-risk BMI≥ 25		At-risk BMI≥ 23		At-risk BMI≥ 26	
Height	Weight	Height	Weight	Height	Weight
4'10"	119	4'10"	110	4'10"	124
4'11"	124	4'11"	114	4'11"	128
5'0"	128	5'0"	118	5'0"	133
5'1"	132	5'1"	122	5'1"	137
5'2"	136	5'2"	126	5'2"	142
5'3"	141	5'3"	130	5'3"	146
5'4"	145	5'4"	134	5'4"	151
5'5"	150	5'5"	138	5'5"	156
5'6"	155	5'6"	142	5'6"	161
5'7"	159	5'7"	146	5'7"	166
5'8"	164	5'8"	151	5'8"	171
5'9"	169	5'9"	155	5'9"	176
5'10"	174	5'10"	160	5'10"	181
5'11"	179	5'11"	165	5'11"	186
6'0"	184	6'0"	169	6'0"	191
6'1"	189	6'1"	174	6'1"	197
6'2"	194	6'2"	179	6'2"	202
6'3"	200	6'3"	184	6'3"	208
6'4"	205	6'4"	189	6'4"	213

- Have a history of gestational diabetes or gave birth to a baby weighing nine pounds or more
- Are not physically active
- Have a history of heart disease or stroke
- Have depression
- Have polycystic ovary syndrome, also called "PCOS"
- Have acanthosis nigricans—dark, thick, and velvety skin around your neck or armpits

To see if your weight puts you at risk for type 2 diabetes, find your height in the Table 37.1 (BMI) charts above. If your weight is equal to or more than the weight listed, you have a greater chance of developing the disease.

Preventing Type 2 Diabetes

Diabetes can cause serious health problems, such as heart disease, stroke, and eye and foot problems. Prediabetes also can cause health problems. The good news is that type 2 diabetes can be delayed or even prevented. The longer you have diabetes, the more likely you are to develop health problems, so delaying diabetes by even a few years will benefit your health. You can help prevent or delay type 2 diabetes by losing a modest amount of weight by following a reduced-calorie eating plan and being physically active most days of the week. Ask your doctor if you should take the diabetes drug metformin to help prevent or delay type 2 diabetes.

You can take steps to help prevent or delay type 2 diabetes by losing weight if you are overweight, eating fewer calories, and being more physically active. Talk with your healthcare professional about any of the health conditions listed above that may require medical treatment. Managing these health problems may help reduce your chances of developing type 2 diabetes. Also, ask your healthcare professional about any medicines you take that might increase your risk.

Research such as the Diabetes Prevention Program (DPP) shows that you can do a lot to reduce your chances of developing type 2 diabetes. Here are some things you can change to lower your risk:

- **Lose weight and keep it off.** You may be able to prevent or delay diabetes by losing 5 to 7 percent of your starting weight. For instance, if you weigh 200 pounds, your goal would be to lose about 10 to 14 pounds.

- **Move more.** Get at least 30 minutes of physical activity 5 days a week. If you have not been active, talk with your healthcare professional about which activities are best. Start slowly to build up to your goal.

- **Eat healthy foods most of the time.** Eat smaller portions to reduce the amount of calories you eat each day and help you lose weight. Choosing foods with less fat is another way to reduce calories. Drink water instead of sweetened beverages.

Ask your healthcare professional about what other changes you can make to prevent or delay type 2 diabetes.

Steps to Take If You Have Prediabetes

Prediabetes is when your blood glucose, also called "blood sugar," levels are higher than normal, but not high enough to be called "diabetes." Having prediabetes is serious because it raises your chance of developing type 2 diabetes. Many of the same factors that raise your chance of developing type 2 diabetes put you at risk for prediabetes.

Other names for prediabetes include impaired fasting glucose or impaired glucose tolerance. Some people call prediabetes "borderline diabetes."

About one in three Americans has prediabetes, according to diabetes statistics from the Centers for Disease Control and Prevention (CDC). You will not know if you have prediabetes unless you are tested.

If you have prediabetes, you can lower your chance of developing type 2 diabetes. Lose weight if you need to, become more physically active, and follow a reduced-calorie eating plan.

Steps to Lower Your Chances of Developing Type 2 Diabetes If You Had Gestational Diabetes

Gestational diabetes is a type of diabetes that develops during pregnancy. Most of the time, gestational diabetes goes away after your baby is born. Even if your gestational diabetes goes away, you still have a greater chance of developing type 2 diabetes within 5 to 10 years. Your child may also be more likely to become obese and develop type 2 diabetes later in life. Making healthy choices helps the whole family and may protect your child from becoming obese or developing diabetes.

Here are the steps you should take for yourself and your child if you had gestational diabetes:

- Get tested for diabetes 6 to 12 weeks after your baby is born. If your blood glucose is still high, you may have type 2 diabetes. If your blood glucose is normal, you should get tested every 3 years to see if you have developed type 2 diabetes.

- Be more active and make healthy food choices to get back to a healthy weight.

- Breastfeed your baby. Breastfeeding gives your baby the right balance of nutrients and helps you burn calories.

- Ask your doctor if you should take the diabetes drug metformin to help prevent type 2 diabetes.

Tests and Diagnosis of Diabetes

Your healthcare professional can diagnose diabetes, prediabetes, and gestational diabetes through blood tests. The blood tests show if your blood glucose, also called "blood sugar," is too high.

Do not try to diagnose yourself if you think you might have diabetes. Testing equipment that you can buy over the counter, such as a blood glucose meter, cannot diagnose diabetes.

Who Should Be Tested for Diabetes?

Anyone who has symptoms of diabetes should be tested for the disease. Some people will not have any symptoms but may have risk factors for diabetes and need to be tested. Testing allows healthcare professionals to find diabetes sooner and work with their patients to manage diabetes and prevent complications.

Testing also allows healthcare professionals to find prediabetes. Making lifestyle changes to lose a modest amount of weight if you are overweight may help you delay or prevent type 2 diabetes.

Type 1 Diabetes

Most often, testing for type 1 diabetes occurs in people with diabetes symptoms. Doctors usually diagnose type 1 diabetes in children and young adults.

Type 2 Diabetes

Experts recommend routine testing for type 2 diabetes if you:

- Are age 45 or older

- Are between the ages of 19 and 44, are overweight or obese, and have one or more other diabetes risk factors

- Are a woman who had gestational diabetes

Medicare covers the cost of diabetes tests for people with certain risk factors for diabetes. If you have Medicare, find out if you qualify for coverage. If you have different insurance, ask your insurance company if it covers diabetes tests.

Though type 2 diabetes most often develops in adults, children can also develop type 2 diabetes. Experts recommend testing children between the ages of 10 and 18 who are overweight or obese and have at least two other risk factors for developing diabetes.

- Low birthweight

- A mother who had diabetes while pregnant with them

Gestational Diabetes

All pregnant women who do not have a prior diabetes diagnosis should be tested for gestational diabetes. If you are pregnant, you will take a glucose challenge test between 24 and 28 weeks of pregnancy.

What Tests Are Used to Diagnose Diabetes and Prediabetes?

Healthcare professionals most often use the fasting plasma glucose (FPG) test or the A1C test to diagnose diabetes. In some cases, they may use a random plasma glucose (RPG) test.

Fasting Plasma Glucose Test

The FPG blood test measures your blood glucose level at a single point in time. For the most reliable results, it is best to have this test in the morning, after you fast for at least 8 hours. Fasting means having nothing to eat or drink except sips of water.

A1C Test

The A1C test is a blood test that provides your average levels of blood glucose over the past three months. Other names for the A1C test are hemoglobin A1C, HbA1C, glycated hemoglobin, and glycosylated hemoglobin test. You can eat and drink before this test. When it comes to using the A1C to diagnose diabetes, your doctor will consider factors such as your age and whether you have anemia or another problem with your blood. The A1C test is not accurate in people with anemia.

If you are of African, Mediterranean, or Southeast Asian descent, your A1C test results may be falsely high or low. Your healthcare professional may need to order a different type of A1C test.

Your healthcare professional will report your A1C test result as a percentage, such as an A1C of seven percent. The higher the percentage, the higher your average blood glucose levels.

People with diabetes also use information from the A1C test to help manage their diabetes.

Random Plasma Glucose Test

Sometimes healthcare professionals use the RPG test to diagnose diabetes when diabetes symptoms are present and they do not want to wait until you have fasted. You do not need to fast overnight for the RPG test. You may have this blood test at any time.

What Tests Are Used to Diagnose Gestational Diabetes?

Pregnant women may have the glucose challenge test, the oral glucose tolerance test, or both. These tests show how well your body handles glucose.

Glucose Challenge Test

If you are pregnant and a healthcare professional is checking you for gestational diabetes, you may first receive the glucose challenge test. Another name for this test is the glucose screening test. In this test, a healthcare professional will draw your blood one hour after you drink a sweet liquid containing glucose. You do not need to fast for this test. If your blood glucose is too high—135 to 140 or more—you may need to return for an oral glucose tolerance test while fasting.

Oral Glucose Tolerance Test

The oral glucose tolerance test (OGTT) measures blood glucose after you fast for at least eight hours. First, a healthcare professional will draw your blood. Then you will drink the liquid containing glucose. For diagnosing gestational diabetes, you will need your blood drawn every hour for two to three hours.

High blood glucose levels at any two or more blood test times during the OGTT—fasting, one hour, two hours, or three hours—mean you have gestational diabetes. Your healthcare team will explain what your OGTT results mean.

Healthcare professionals also can use the OGTT to diagnose type 2 diabetes and prediabetes in people who are not pregnant. The OGTT helps healthcare professionals detect type 2 diabetes and prediabetes better than the FPG test. However, the OGTT is a more expensive test and is not as easy to give. To diagnose type 2 diabetes and pre-diabetes, a healthcare professional will need to draw your blood one hour after you drink the liquid containing glucose and again after two hours.

Which Tests Help My Healthcare Professional Know What Kind of Diabetes I Have?

Even though the tests described here can confirm that you have diabetes, they cannot identify what type you have. Sometimes health-care professionals are unsure if diabetes is type 1 or type 2. A rare type of diabetes that can occur in babies, called "monogenic diabetes," can also be mistaken for type 1 diabetes. Treatment depends on the type of diabetes, so knowing which type you have is important.

To find out if your diabetes is type 1, your healthcare professional may look for certain autoantibodies. Autoantibodies are antibodies that mistakenly attack your healthy tissues and cells. The presence of one or more of several types of autoantibodies specific to diabetes is common in type 1 diabetes, but not in type 2 or monogenic diabetes. A healthcare professional will have to draw your blood for this test.

If you had diabetes while you were pregnant, you should get tested no later than 12 weeks after your baby is born to see if you have type 2 diabetes.

Diabetes Management

You can manage your diabetes and live a long and healthy life by taking care of yourself each day.

Diabetes can affect almost every part of your body. Therefore, you will need to manage your blood glucose levels, also called "blood sugar." Managing your blood glucose, as well as your blood pressure and cholesterol, can help prevent the health problems that can occur when you have diabetes.

How Can I Manage My Diabetes?

With the help of your healthcare team, you can create a diabetes self-care plan to manage your diabetes. Your self-care plan may include these steps:

- Manage your diabetes ABCs.
- Follow your diabetes meal plan.
- Make physical activity part of your routine.
- Take your medicine.
- Check your blood glucose levels.
- Work with your healthcare team.
- Cope with your diabetes in healthy ways.

Manage Your Diabetes ABCs

Knowing your diabetes ABCs will help you manage your blood glucose, blood pressure, and cholesterol. Stopping smoking if you smoke will also help you manage your diabetes. Working toward your ABC goals can help lower your chances of having a heart attack, stroke, or other diabetes problems.

A for the A1C Test

The A1C test shows your average blood glucose level over the past three months. The A1C goal for many people with diabetes is below seven percent. Ask your healthcare team what your goal should be.

B for Blood Pressure

The blood pressure goal for most people with diabetes is below 140/90 mm Hg. Ask what your goal should be.

C for Cholesterol

You have two kinds of cholesterol in your blood: LDL and HDL. LDL or "bad" cholesterol can build up and clog your blood vessels. Too much bad cholesterol can cause a heart attack or stroke. HDL or "good" cholesterol helps remove the "bad" cholesterol from your blood vessels.

Ask your healthcare team what your cholesterol numbers should be. If you are over 40 years of age, you may need to take a statin drug for heart health.

S for Stop Smoking

Not smoking is especially important for people with diabetes because both smoking and diabetes narrow blood vessels. Blood vessel narrowing makes your heart work harder. E-cigarettes are not a safe option either.

If you quit smoking:

- You will lower your risk for heart attack, stroke, nerve disease, kidney disease, diabetic eye disease, and amputation

- Your cholesterol and blood pressure levels may improve

- Your blood circulation will improve

- You may have an easier time being physically active

If you smoke or use other tobacco products, stop. Ask for help so you do not have to do it alone. You can start by calling the national quitline at 800-QUITNOW or 800-784-8669. For keeping your A1C, blood pressure, and cholesterol levels close to your goals and stopping smoking may help prevent the long-term harmful effects of diabetes. These health problems include heart disease, stroke, kidney disease, nerve damage, and eye disease.

Follow Your Diabetes Meal Plan

Make a diabetes meal plan with help from your healthcare team. Following a meal plan will help you manage your blood glucose, blood pressure, and cholesterol.

Choose fruits and vegetables, beans, whole grains, chicken or turkey without the skin, fish, lean meats, and nonfat or low-fat milk and cheese. Drink water instead of sugar-sweetened beverages. Choose foods that are lower in calories, saturated fat, trans fat, sugar, and salt.

Make Physical Activity Part of Your Daily Routine

Set a goal to be more physically active. Try to work up to 30 minutes or more of physical activity on most days of the week.

Brisk walking and swimming are good ways to move more. If you are not active, ask your healthcare team about the types and amounts of physical activity that are right for you. Following your meal plan and being more active can help you stay at or get to a healthy weight. If you are overweight or obese, work with your healthcare team to create a weight-loss plan that is right for you.

Take Your Medicine

Take your medicines for diabetes and any other health problems, even when you feel good or have reached your blood glucose, blood pressure, and cholesterol goals. These medicines help you manage your ABCs. Ask your doctor if you need to take aspirin to prevent a heart attack or stroke. Tell your healthcare professional if you cannot afford your medicines or if you have any side effects from your medicine.

Check Your Blood Glucose Levels

For many people with diabetes, checking their blood glucose level each day is an important way to manage their diabetes. Monitoring your blood glucose level is most important if you take insulin. The results of blood glucose monitoring can help you make decisions about food, physical activity, and medicines.

The most common way to check your blood glucose level at home is with a blood glucose meter. You get a drop of blood by pricking the side of your fingertip with a lancet. Then you apply the blood to a test strip. The meter will show you how much glucose is in your blood at the moment.

Ask your healthcare team how often you should check your blood glucose levels. Make sure to keep a record of your blood glucose self-checks.

Work with Your Healthcare Team

Most people with diabetes get healthcare from a primary care professional. Primary care professionals include internists, family physicians, and pediatricians. Sometimes physician assistants and nurses with extra training, called "nurse practitioners," provide primary care. You also will need to see other care professionals from time to time. A team of healthcare professionals can help you improve your diabetes self-care. Remember, you are the most important member of your healthcare team.

Besides a primary care professional, your healthcare team may include:

- An endocrinologist for more specialized diabetes care

- A registered dietitian, also called a "nutritionist"

- A nurse

- A certified diabetes educator

- A pharmacist

- A dentist

- An eye doctor

- A podiatrist, or foot doctor, for foot care

- A social worker, who can help you find financial aid for treatment and community resources

- A counselor or other mental-healthcare professional

When you see members of your healthcare team, ask questions. Write a list of questions you have before your visit so you do not forget what you want to ask. Watch a video to help you get ready for your diabetes care visit.

You should see your healthcare team at least twice a year, and more often if you are having problems or are having trouble reaching your blood glucose, blood pressure, or cholesterol goals. At each visit, be sure you have a blood pressure check, foot check, and weight check; and review your self-care plan. Talk with your healthcare team about your medicines and whether you need to adjust them. Routine healthcare will help you find and treat any health problems early, or may be able to help prevent them.

Talk with your doctor about what vaccines you should get to keep from getting sick, such as a flu shot and pneumonia shot. Preventing illness is an important part of taking care of your diabetes. Your blood glucose levels are more likely to go up when you are sick or have an infection.

Cope with Your Diabetes in Healthy Ways

Feeling stressed, sad, or angry is common when you live with diabetes. Stress can raise your blood glucose levels, but you can learn ways to lower your stress. Try deep breathing, gardening, taking a walk, doing yoga, meditating, doing a hobby, or listening to your favorite music. Consider taking part in a diabetes education program or support group that teaches you techniques for managing stress. Depression is common among people with a chronic, or long-term, illness. Depression can get in the way of your efforts to manage your diabetes. Ask for help if you feel down. A mental-health counselor, support group, clergy member, friend, or family member who will listen to your feelings may help you feel better.

Try to get seven to eight hours of sleep each night. Getting enough sleep can help improve your mood and energy level. You can take steps to improve your sleep habits. If you often feel sleepy during the day, you may have obstructive sleep apnea, a condition in which your breathing briefly stops many times during the night. Sleep apnea is common in people who have diabetes. Talk with your healthcare team if you think you have a sleep problem. Remember, managing diabetes is not easy, but it is worth it.

Chapter 38

Hypoglycemia

What Is Hypoglycemia?

Hypoglycemia, also called "low blood glucose" or "low blood sugar," occurs when blood glucose drops below normal levels. Glucose, an important source of energy for the body, comes from food. Carbohydrates are the main dietary source of glucose. Rice, potatoes, bread, tortillas, cereal, milk, fruits, and sweets are all carbohydrate-rich foods.

After a meal, glucose is absorbed into the bloodstream and carried to the body's cells. Insulin, a hormone made by the pancreas, helps the cells use glucose for energy. If a person takes in more glucose than the body needs at the time, the body stores the extra glucose in the liver and muscles in a form called "glycogen." The body can use glycogen for energy between meals. Extra glucose can also be changed to fat and stored in fat cells. Fat can also be used for energy.

When blood glucose begins to fall, glucagon—another hormone made by the pancreas—signals the liver to break down glycogen and release glucose into the bloodstream. Blood glucose will then rise toward a normal level. In some people with diabetes, this glucagon response to hypoglycemia is impaired and other hormones such as epinephrine also called "adrenaline," may raise the blood glucose level. But, with diabetes treated with insulin or pills that increase insulin production, glucose levels cannot easily return to the normal range.

This chapter includes text excerpted from "Hypoglycemia," National Institute of Diabetes and Digestive and Kidney Diseases (NIDDK), October 2008. Reviewed September 2019.

Hypoglycemia can happen suddenly. It is usually mild and can be treated quickly and easily by eating or drinking a small amount of glucose-rich food. If left untreated, hypoglycemia can get worse and cause confusion, clumsiness, or fainting. Severe hypoglycemia can lead to seizures, coma, and even death.

In adults and children older than 10 years, hypoglycemia is uncommon except as a side effect of diabetes treatment. Hypoglycemia can also result, however, from other medications or diseases, hormone or enzyme deficiencies, or tumors.

What Are the Symptoms of Hypoglycemia?

Hypoglycemia causes symptoms such as:

- Hunger
- Shakiness
- Nervousness
- Sweating
- Dizziness or light-headedness
- Sleepiness
- Confusion
- Difficulty speaking
- Anxiety
- Weakness

Hypoglycemia can also happen during sleep. Some signs of hypoglycemia during sleep include:

- Crying out or having nightmares
- Finding pajamas or sheets damp from perspiration
- Feeling tired, irritable, or confused after waking up

What Causes Hypoglycemia in People with Diabetes
Diabetes Medications

Hypoglycemia can occur as a side effect of some diabetes medications, including insulin and oral diabetes medications—pills—that increase insulin production, such as:

- Chlorpropamide (Diabinese®)
- Glimepiride (Amaryl®)
- Glipizide (Glucotrol®, Glucotrol XL®)
- Glyburide (DiaBeta®, Glynase®, Micronase®)
- Nateglinide (Starlix®)
- Repaglinide (Prandin®)
- Sitagliptin (Januvia®)
- Tolazamide
- Tolbutamide

Certain combination pills can also cause hypoglycemia, including:

- Glipizide + metformin (Metaglip™)
- Glyburide + metformin (Glucovance®)
- Pioglitazone + glimepiride (Duetact)
- Rosiglitazone + glimepiride (Avandaryl®)
- Sitagliptin + metformin (Janumet®)

Other types of diabetes pills, when taken alone, do not cause hypoglycemia. Examples of these medications are:

- Acarbose (Precose®)
- Metformin (Glucophage®)
- Miglitol (Glyset®)
- Pioglitazone (Actos®)
- Rosiglitazone (Avandia®)

However, taking these pills along with other diabetes medications—insulin, pills that increase insulin production, or both—increases the risk of hypoglycemia.

In addition, the use of the following injectable medications can cause hypoglycemia:

- Pramlintide (Symlin®), which is used along with insulin
- Exenatide (Byetta®), which can cause hypoglycemia when used in combination with chlorpropamide, glimepiride, glipizide, glyburide, tolazamide, and tolbutamide

Other Causes of Hypoglycemia

In people on insulin or pills that increase insulin production, low blood glucose can be due to:

- Meals or snacks that are too small, delayed, or skipped

- Increased physical activity

- Alcoholic beverages

How Can Hypoglycemia Be Prevented?

Diabetes treatment plans are designed to match the dose and timing of medication to a person's usual schedule of meals and activities. Mismatches could result in hypoglycemia. For example, taking a dose of insulin—or other medication that increases insulin levels—but then skipping a meal could result in hypoglycemia.

To help prevent hypoglycemia, people with diabetes should always consider their:

- **Diabetes medications.** A healthcare provider can explain which diabetes medications can cause hypoglycemia and explain how and when to take medications. For good diabetes management, people with diabetes should take diabetes medications in the recommended doses at the recommended times. In some cases, healthcare providers may suggest that patients learn how to adjust medications to match changes in their schedule or routine.

- **Meal plan.** A registered dietitian can help design a meal plan that fits one's personal preferences and lifestyle. Following one's meal plan is important for managing diabetes. People with diabetes should eat regular meals, have enough food at each meal, and try not to skip meals or snacks. Snacks are particularly important for some people before going to sleep or exercising. Some snacks may be more effective than others in preventing hypoglycemia overnight. The dietitian can make recommendations for snacks.

- **Daily activity.** To help prevent hypoglycemia caused by physical activity, healthcare providers may advise:

  - Checking blood glucose before sports, exercise, or other physical activity and having a snack if the level is below 100 milligrams per deciliter (mg/dL)

- Adjusting medication before physical activity

- Checking blood glucose at regular intervals during extended periods of physical activity and having snacks as needed

- Checking blood glucose periodically after physical activity

- **Use of alcoholic beverages.** Drinking alcoholic beverages, especially on an empty stomach, can cause hypoglycemia, even a day or two later. Heavy drinking can be particularly dangerous for people taking insulin or medications that increase insulin production. Alcoholic beverages should always be consumed with a snack or meal at the same time. A healthcare provider can suggest how to safely include alcohol in a meal plan.

- **Diabetes management plan.** Intensive diabetes management—keeping blood glucose as close to the normal range as possible to prevent long-term complications—can increase the risk of hypoglycemia. Those whose goal is tight control should talk with a healthcare provider about ways to prevent hypoglycemia and how best to treat it if it occurs.

What to Ask the Doctor about Diabetes Medications

People who take diabetes medications should ask their doctor or healthcare provider:

- Whether their diabetes medications could cause hypoglycemia

- When they should take their diabetes medications

- How much medication they should take

- Whether they should keep taking their diabetes medications when they are sick

- Whether they should adjust their medications before physical activity

- Whether they should adjust their medications if they skip a meal

How Is Hypoglycemia Treated?

Signs and symptoms of hypoglycemia vary from person to person. People with diabetes should get to know their signs and symptoms and describe them to their friends and family so they can help if needed. School staff should be told how to recognize a child's signs and symptoms of hypoglycemia and how to treat it.

People who experience hypoglycemia several times a week should call their healthcare provider. They may need a change in their treatment plan: less medication or a different medication, a new schedule for insulin or medication, a different meal plan, or a new physical activity plan.

Prompt Treatment for Hypoglycemia

When people think their blood glucose is too low, they should check the blood glucose level of a blood sample using a meter. If the level is below 70 mg/dL, one of these quick-fix foods should be consumed right away to raise blood glucose:

- 3 or 4 glucose tablets

- 1 serving of glucose gel—an amount equal to 15 grams of carbohydrate

- ½ cup, or 4 ounces, of any fruit juice

- ½ cup, or 4 ounces, of a regular—not diet—soft drink

- 1 cup, or 8 ounces, of milk

- 5 or 6 pieces of hard candy

- 1 tablespoon of sugar or honey

Recommended amounts may be less for small children. The child's doctor can advise about the right amount to give a child.

The next step is to recheck blood glucose in 15 minutes to make sure it is 70 mg/dL or above. If it is still too low, another serving of a quick-fix food should be eaten. These steps should be repeated until the blood glucose level is 70 mg/dL or above. If the next meal is an hour or more away, a snack should be eaten once the quick-fix foods have raised the blood glucose level to 70 mg/dL or above.

Hypoglycemia When Driving

Hypoglycemia is particularly dangerous if it happens to someone who is driving. People with hypoglycemia may have trouble concentrating or seeing clearly behind the wheel and may not be able to react quickly to road hazards or to the actions of other drivers.

To prevent problems, people at risk for hypoglycemia should check their blood glucose level before driving. During longer trips, they should check their blood glucose level frequently and eat snacks as needed to keep the level at 70 mg/dL or above. If necessary, they should stop for treatment and then make sure their blood glucose level is 70 mg/dL or above before starting to drive again.

Hypoglycemia Unawareness

Some people with diabetes do not have early warning signs of low blood glucose, a condition called "hypoglycemia unawareness." This condition occurs most often in people with type 1 diabetes, but it can also occur in people with type 2 diabetes. People with hypoglycemia unawareness may need to check their blood glucose level more often so they know when hypoglycemia is about to occur. They also may need a change in their medications, meal plan, or physical activity routine.

Hypoglycemia unawareness develops when frequent episodes of hypoglycemia lead to changes in how the body reacts to low blood glucose levels. The body stops releasing the hormone epinephrine and other stress hormones when blood glucose drops too low. The loss of the body's ability to release stress hormones after repeated episodes of hypoglycemia is called "hypoglycemia-associated autonomic failure," or "HAAF."

Epinephrine causes early warning symptoms of hypoglycemia such as shakiness, sweating, anxiety, and hunger. Without the release of epinephrine and the symptoms it causes, a person may not realize that hypoglycemia is occurring and may not take action to treat it. A vicious cycle can occur in which frequent hypoglycemia leads to hypoglycemia unawareness and HAAF, which in turn leads to even more severe and dangerous hypoglycemia. Studies have shown that preventing hypoglycemia for a period as short as several weeks can sometimes break this cycle and restore awareness of symptoms. Healthcare providers may, therefore, advise people who have had severe hypoglycemia to aim for higher-than-usual blood glucose targets for short-term periods.

Being Prepared for Hypoglycemia

People who use insulin or take an oral diabetes medication that can cause low blood glucose should always be prepared to prevent and treat low blood glucose by:

- Learning what can trigger low blood glucose levels
- Having their blood glucose meter available to test glucose levels; frequent testing may be critical for those with hypoglycemia

unawareness, particularly before driving a car or engaging in any hazardous activity

- Always having several servings of quick-fix foods or drinks handy

- Wearing a medical identification bracelet or necklace

- Planning what to do if they develop severe hypoglycemia

- Telling their family, friends, and coworkers about the symptoms of hypoglycemia and how they can help if needed

Help from Others for Severe Hypoglycemia

Severe hypoglycemia—very low blood glucose—can cause a person to pass out and can be life-threatening. Severe hypoglycemia is more likely to occur in people with type 1 diabetes. People should ask a healthcare provider what to do about severe hypoglycemia. Another person can help someone who has passed out by giving an injection of glucagon. Glucagon will rapidly bring the blood glucose level back to normal and help the person regain consciousness. A healthcare provider can prescribe a glucagon emergency kit. Family, friends, or coworkers—the people who will be around the person at risk of hypoglycemia—can learn how to give a glucagon injection and when to call 911 or get medical help.

Chapter 39

Pancreatic Cancer

About Pancreatic Cancer

The pancreas is a gland about six inches long that is shaped like a thin pear lying on its side. The wider end of the pancreas is called the "head," the middle section is called the "body," and the narrow end is called the "tail." The pancreas lies between the stomach and the spine.

The pancreas has two main jobs in the body:

- To make juices that help digest (break down) food.

- To make hormones, such as insulin and glucagon, that help control blood sugar levels. Both of these hormones help the body use and store the energy it gets from food.

The digestive juices are made by exocrine pancreas cells and the hormones are made by endocrine pancreas cells. About 95 percent of pancreatic cancers begin in exocrine cells.

Risk Factors of Pancreatic Cancer

Anything that increases your risk of getting a disease is called a "risk factor." Having a risk factor does not mean that you will get cancer; not having risk factors does not mean that you will not get cancer. Talk with your doctor if you think you may be at risk.

This chapter includes text excerpted from "Pancreatic Cancer Treatment (PDQ®)—Patient Version," National Cancer Institute (NCI), May 23, 2018.

Risk factors for pancreatic cancer include the following:

- Smoking

- Being very overweight

- Having a personal history of diabetes or chronic pancreatitis

- Having a family history of pancreatic cancer or pancreatitis

- Having certain hereditary conditions, such as:

  - Multiple endocrine neoplasia type 1 (MEN1) syndrome

  - Hereditary nonpolyposis colon cancer (HNPCC; Lynch syndrome)

  - von Hippel-Lindau syndrome

  - Peutz-Jeghers syndrome

  - Hereditary breast and ovarian cancer syndrome

  - Familial atypical multiple mole melanoma (FAMMM) syndrome

Signs and Symptoms of Pancreatic Cancer

Pancreatic cancer may not cause early signs or symptoms. Signs and symptoms may be caused by pancreatic cancer or by other conditions. Check with your doctor if you have any of the following:

- Jaundice (yellowing of the skin and whites of the eyes)

- Light-colored stools

- Dark urine

- Pain in the upper or middle abdomen and back

- Weight-loss for no known reason

- Loss of appetite

- Feeling very tired

Difficulty in Detecting and Diagnosing Pancreatic Cancer

Pancreatic cancer is difficult to detect and diagnose for the following reasons:

- There are not any noticeable signs or symptoms in the early stages of pancreatic cancer.

- The signs and symptoms of pancreatic cancer, when present, are similar to the signs and symptoms of many other illnesses.

- The pancreas is hidden behind other organs such as the stomach, small intestine, liver, gallbladder, spleen, and bile ducts.

Diagnostic Tests of Pancreatic Cancer

Pancreatic cancer is usually diagnosed with tests and procedures that make pictures of the pancreas and the area around it. The process used to find out if cancer cells have spread within and around the pancreas is called "staging." Tests and procedures to detect, diagnose, and stage pancreatic cancer are usually done at the same time. In order to plan treatment, it is important to know the stage of the disease and whether or not the pancreatic cancer can be removed by surgery.

The following tests and procedures may be used:

- **Physical exam and history.** An exam of the body to check general signs of health, including checking for signs of disease, such as lumps or anything else that seems unusual. A history of the patient's health habits and past illnesses and treatments will also be taken.

- **Blood chemistry studies.** A procedure in which a blood sample is checked to measure the amounts of certain substances, such as bilirubin, released into the blood by organs and tissues in the body. An unusual (higher or lower than normal) amount of a substance can be a sign of disease.

- **Tumor marker test.** A procedure in which a sample of blood, urine, or tissue is checked to measure the amounts of certain substances, such as CA 19-9, and carcinoembryonic antigen (CEA), made by organs, tissues, or tumor cells in the body. Certain substances are linked to specific types of cancer when found in increased levels in the body. These are called "tumor markers."

- **Magnetic resonance imaging (MRI).** A procedure that uses a magnet, radio waves, and a computer to make a series of detailed pictures of areas inside the body. This procedure is also called "nuclear magnetic resonance imaging" (NMRI).

- **Computerized tomography (CT) scan.** A procedure that makes a series of detailed pictures of areas inside the body, taken from different angles. The pictures are made by a computer linked to an x-ray machine. A dye may be injected into a vein or swallowed to help the organs or tissues show up more clearly. This procedure is also called "computed tomography," "computerized tomography," or "computerized axial tomography." A spiral or helical CT scan makes a series of very detailed pictures of areas inside the body using an x-ray machine that scans the body in a spiral path.

- **Positron emission tomography (PET) scan.** A procedure to find malignant tumor cells in the body. A small amount of radioactive glucose (sugar) is injected into a vein. The PET scanner rotates around the body and makes a picture of where glucose is being used in the body. Malignant tumor cells show up brighter in the picture because they are more active and take up more glucose than normal cells do. A PET scan and CT scan may be done at the same time. This is called a "PET-CT."

- **Abdominal ultrasound.** An ultrasound examination is used to make pictures of the inside of the abdomen. The ultrasound transducer is pressed against the skin of the abdomen and directs high-energy sound waves (ultrasound) into the abdomen. The sound waves bounce off the internal tissues and organs and make echoes. The transducer receives the echoes and sends them to a computer, which uses the echoes to make pictures called "sonograms." The picture can be printed to be looked at later.

- **Endoscopic ultrasound (EUS).** A procedure in which an endoscope is inserted into the body, usually through the mouth or rectum. An endoscope is a thin, tube-like instrument with a light and a lens for viewing. A probe at the end of the endoscope is used to bounce high-energy sound waves (ultrasound) off internal tissues or organs and make echoes. The echoes form a picture of body tissues called "sonogram." This procedure is also called "endosonography."

- **Endoscopic retrograde cholangiopancreatography (ERCP).** A procedure used to x-ray the ducts (tubes) that carry bile from the liver to the gallbladder and from the gallbladder to the small intestine. Sometimes pancreatic cancer causes these ducts to narrow and block or slow the flow of bile, causing jaundice. An endoscope (a thin, lighted tube) is passed through the mouth, esophagus, and stomach into the first part of the small intestine. A catheter (a smaller tube) is then inserted through the endoscope into the pancreatic ducts. A dye is injected through the catheter into the ducts and an x-ray is taken. If the ducts are blocked by a tumor, a fine tube may be inserted into the duct to unblock it. This tube (or stent) may be left in place to keep the duct open. Tissue samples may also be taken.

- **Percutaneous transhepatic cholangiography (PTC).** A procedure used to x-ray the liver and bile ducts. A thin needle is inserted through the skin below the ribs and into the liver. A dye is injected into the liver or bile ducts and an x-ray is taken. If a blockage is found, a thin, flexible tube called a "stent" is sometimes left in the liver to drain bile into the small intestine or a collection bag outside the body. This test is done only if ERCP cannot be done.

- **Laparoscopy.** A surgical procedure to look at the organs inside the abdomen to check for signs of disease. Small incisions (cuts) are made in the wall of the abdomen and a laparoscope (a thin, lighted tube) is inserted into one of the incisions. The laparoscope may have an ultrasound probe at the end in order to bounce high-energy sound waves off internal organs, such as the pancreas. This is called "laparoscopic ultrasound." Other instruments may be inserted through the same or other incisions to perform procedures such as taking tissue samples from the pancreas or a sample of fluid from the abdomen to check for cancer.

- **Biopsy.** The removal of cells or tissues so they can be viewed under a microscope by a pathologist to check for signs of cancer. There are several ways to do a biopsy for pancreatic cancer. A fine needle or a core needle may be inserted into the pancreas during an x-ray or ultrasound to remove cells. Tissue may also be removed during a laparoscopy or surgery to remove the tumor.

Factors Affecting Prognosis and Treatment Options of Pancreatic Cancer

The prognosis and treatment options depend on the following:

- Whether or not the tumor can be removed by surgery.

- The stage of the cancer (the size of the tumor and whether the cancer has spread outside the pancreas to nearby tissues or lymph nodes or to other places in the body).

- The patient's general health.

- Whether the cancer has just been diagnosed or has recurred.

Pancreatic cancer can be controlled only if it is found before it has spread, when it can be completely removed by surgery. If the cancer has spread, palliative treatment can improve the patient's quality of life by controlling the symptoms and complications of this disease.

Chapter 40

Islet Cell Cancer

Pancreatic Neuroendocrine Tumors

Pancreatic neuroendocrine tumors (pancreatic NETs) form in hormone-making cells (islet cells) of the pancreas.

The pancreas is a gland about six inches long that is shaped like a thin pear lying on its side. The wider end of the pancreas is called the "head," the middle section is called the "body," and the narrow end is called the "tail." The pancreas lies behind the stomach and in front of the spine.

There are two kinds of cells in the pancreas:

- **Endocrine pancreas cells** make several kinds of hormones (chemicals that control the actions of certain cells or organs in the body), such as insulin to control blood sugar. They cluster together in many small groups (islets) throughout the pancreas. Endocrine pancreas cells are also called "islet cells" or "islets of Langerhans." Tumors that form in islet cells are called "islet cell tumors," "pancreatic endocrine tumors," or "pancreatic neuroendocrine tumors."

- **Exocrine pancreas cells** make enzymes that are released into the small intestine to help the body digest food. Most of

This chapter includes text excerpted from "Pancreatic Neuroendocrine Tumors (Islet Cell Tumors) Treatment (PDQ®)—Patient Version," National Cancer Institute (NCI), April 19, 2019.

the pancreas is made of ducts with small sacs at the end of the ducts, which are lined with exocrine cells.

Pancreatic NETs may be benign (not cancer) or malignant (cancer). When pancreatic NETs are malignant, they are called "pancreatic endocrine cancer" or "islet cell carcinoma."

Pancreatic NETs are much less common than pancreatic exocrine tumors and have a better prognosis.

Pancreatic NETs May or May Not Cause Signs or Symptoms

Pancreatic NETs may be functional or nonfunctional:

- **Functional tumors** make extra amounts of hormones, such as gastrin, insulin, and glucagon, that cause signs and symptoms.

- **Nonfunctional tumors** do not make extra amounts of hormones. Signs and symptoms are caused by the tumor as it spreads and grows. Most nonfunctional tumors are malignant (cancer).

Most pancreatic NETs are functional tumors.

Different Kinds of Functional Pancreatic NETs

Pancreatic NETs make different kinds of hormones such as gastrin, insulin, and glucagon. Functional pancreatic NETs include the following:

- **Gastrinoma.** A tumor that forms in cells that make gastrin. Gastrin is a hormone that causes the stomach to release an acid that helps digest food. Both gastrin and stomach acid are increased by gastrinomas. When increased stomach acid, stomach ulcers, and diarrhea are caused by a tumor that makes gastrin, it is called "Zollinger-Ellison syndrome." A gastrinoma usually forms in the head of the pancreas and sometimes forms in the small intestine. Most gastrinomas are malignant (cancer).

- **Insulinoma.** A tumor that forms in cells that make insulin. Insulin is a hormone that controls the amount of glucose (sugar) in the blood. It moves glucose into the cells, where it can be used by the body for energy. Insulinomas are usually slow-growing tumors that rarely spread. An insulinoma forms in the head, body, or tail of the pancreas. Insulinomas are usually benign (not cancer).

- **Glucagonoma.** A tumor that forms in cells that make glucagon. Glucagon is a hormone that increases the amount of glucose in the blood. It causes the liver to break down glycogen. Too much glucagon causes hyperglycemia (high blood sugar). A glucagonoma usually forms in the tail of the pancreas. Most glucagonomas are malignant.

- **Other types of tumors.** There are other rare types of functional pancreatic NETs that make hormones, including hormones that control the balance of sugar, salt, and water in the body. These tumors include:

  - VIPomas, which make vasoactive intestinal peptide. VIPoma may also be called "Verner-Morrison syndrome."

  - Somatostatinomas, which make somatostatin

These other types of tumors are grouped together because they are treated in much the same way.

Risk of Pancreatic NETs

Having certain syndromes can increase the risk of pancreatic NETs. Talk with your doctor if you think you may be at risk. Multiple endocrine neoplasia type 1 (MEN1) syndrome is a risk factor for pancreatic NETs.

Signs and Symptoms of Pancreatic NETs

Different types of pancreatic NETs have different signs and symptoms.

Signs or symptoms can be caused by the growth of the tumor and/ or by hormones the tumor makes or by other conditions. Some tumors may not cause signs or symptoms. Check with your doctor if you have any of these problems.

Signs and Symptoms of a Nonfunctional Pancreatic NET

A nonfunctional pancreatic NET may grow for a long time without showing signs or symptoms. It may grow large or spread to other parts of the body before it shows signs or symptoms, such as:

- Diarrhea
- Indigestion
- A lump in the abdomen
- Pain in the abdomen or back
- Yellowing of the skin and whites of the eyes

Signs and Symptoms of a Functional Pancreatic NET

The signs and symptoms of a functional pancreatic NET depend on the type of hormone being made.

Too much gastrin may cause:

- Stomach ulcers that keep coming back
- Pain in the abdomen, which may spread to the back. The pain may come and go and it may go away after taking an antacid.
- The flow of stomach contents back into the esophagus (gastroesophageal reflux)
- Diarrhea

Too much insulin may cause:

- **Low blood sugar.** This can cause blurred vision, headache, and feeling lightheaded, tired, weak, shaky, nervous, irritable, sweaty, confused, or hungry.
- Fast heartbeat

Too much glucagon may cause:

- Skin rash on the face, stomach, or legs
- **High blood sugar.** This can cause headaches, frequent urination, dry skin and mouth, or feeling hungry, thirsty, tired, or weak.
- **Blood clots.** Blood clots in the lung can cause shortness of breath, cough, or pain in the chest. Blood clots in the arm or leg can cause pain, swelling, warmth, or redness of the arm or leg.

- Diarrhea

- Weight loss for no known reason

- Sore tongue or sores at the corners of the mouth

Too much vasoactive intestinal peptide (VIP) may cause:

- Very large amounts of watery diarrhea

- **Dehydration.** This can cause feeling thirsty, making less urine, dry skin and mouth, headaches, dizziness, or feeling tired.

- **Low potassium level in the blood.** This can cause muscle weakness, aching, or cramps, numbness and tingling, frequent urination, fast heartbeat, and feeling confused or thirsty.

- Cramps or pain in the abdomen

- Weight loss for no known reason

Too much somatostatin may cause:

- **High blood sugar.** This can cause headaches, frequent urination, dry skin and mouth, or feeling hungry, thirsty, tired, or weak.

- Diarrhea

- Steatorrhea (very foul-smelling stool that floats)

- Gallstones

- Yellowing of the skin and whites of the eyes

- Weight loss for no known reason

A pancreatic NET may also make too much adrenocorticotropic hormone (ACTH) and cause Cushing syndrome. Signs and symptoms of Cushing syndrome include the following:

- Headache

- Some loss of vision

- Weight gain in the face, neck, and trunk of the body, and thin arms and legs

- A lump of fat on the back of the neck

- Thin skin that may have purple or pink stretch marks on the chest or abdomen

- Easy bruising

- Growth of fine hair on the face, upper back, or arms

- Bones that break easily

- Sores or cuts that heal slowly

- Anxiety, irritability, and depression

Lab Tests and Imaging Tests

Lab tests and imaging tests are used to detect (find) and diagnose pancreatic NETs.

The following tests and procedures may be used:

- **Physical exam and history.** An exam of the body to check general signs of health, including checking for signs of disease, such as lumps or anything else that seems unusual. A history of the patient's health habits and past illnesses and treatments will also be taken.

- **Blood chemistry studies.** A procedure in which a blood sample is checked to measure the amounts of certain substances, such as glucose (sugar), released into the blood by organs and tissues in the body. An unusual (higher or lower than normal) amount of a substance can be a sign of disease.

- **Chromogranin A test.** A test in which a blood sample is checked to measure the amount of chromogranin A in the blood. A higher than normal amount of chromogranin A and normal amounts of hormones such as gastrin, insulin, and glucagon can be a sign of a nonfunctional pancreatic NET.

- **Abdominal computed tomography (CT/CAT) scan.** A procedure that makes a series of detailed pictures of the abdomen, taken from different angles. The pictures are made by a computer linked to an x-ray machine. A dye may be injected into a vein or swallowed to help the organs or tissues show up more clearly. This procedure is also called "computed tomography," "computerized tomography," or "computerized axial tomography."

- **Magnetic resonance imaging (MRI).** A procedure that uses a magnet, radio waves, and a computer to make a series of detailed pictures of areas inside the body. This procedure is also called "nuclear magnetic resonance imaging" (NMRI).

- **Somatostatin receptor scintigraphy (SRS).** A type of radionuclide scan that may be used to find small pancreatic NETs. A small amount of radioactive octreotide (a hormone that attaches to tumors) is injected into a vein and travels through the blood. The radioactive octreotide attaches to the tumor and a special camera that detects radioactivity is used to show where the tumors are in the body. This procedure is also called "octreotide scan" and "SRS."

- **Endoscopic ultrasound (EUS).** A procedure in which an endoscope is inserted into the body, usually through the mouth or rectum. An endoscope is a thin, tube-like instrument with a light and a lens for viewing. A probe at the end of the endoscope is used to bounce high-energy sound waves (ultrasound) off internal tissues or organs and make echoes. The echoes form a picture of body tissues called a "sonogram." This procedure is also called "endosonography."

- **Endoscopic retrograde cholangiopancreatography (ERCP).** A procedure used to x-ray the ducts (tubes) that carry bile from the liver to the gallbladder and from the gallbladder to the small intestine. Sometimes pancreatic cancer causes these ducts to narrow and block or slow the flow of bile, causing jaundice. An endoscope is passed through the mouth, esophagus, and stomach into the first part of the small intestine. An endoscope is a thin, tube-like instrument with a light and a lens for viewing. A catheter (a smaller tube) is then inserted through the endoscope into the pancreatic ducts. A dye is injected through the catheter into the ducts and an x-ray is taken. If the ducts are blocked by a tumor, a fine tube may be inserted into the duct to unblock it. This tube (or stent) may be left in place to keep the duct open. Tissue samples may also be taken and checked under a microscope for signs of cancer.

- **Angiogram.** A procedure to look at blood vessels and the flow of blood. A contrast dye is injected into the blood vessel. As the contrast dye moves through the blood vessel, x-rays are taken to see if there are any blockages.

- **Laparotomy.** A surgical procedure in which an incision (cut) is made in the wall of the abdomen to check the inside of the abdomen for signs of disease. The size of the incision depends on the reason the laparotomy is being done. Sometimes organs are removed or tissue samples are taken and checked under a microscope for signs of disease.

- **Intraoperative ultrasound.** A procedure that uses high-energy sound waves (ultrasound) to create images of internal organs or tissues during surgery. A transducer placed directly on the organ or tissue is used to make the sound waves, which create echoes. The transducer receives the echoes and sends them to a computer, which uses the echoes to make pictures called "sonograms."

- **Biopsy.** The removal of cells or tissues so they can be viewed under a microscope by a pathologist to check for signs of cancer. There are several ways to do a biopsy for pancreatic NETs. Cells may be removed using a fine or wide needle inserted into the pancreas during an x-ray or ultrasound. Tissue may also be removed during a laparoscopy (a surgical incision made in the wall of the abdomen).

- **Bone scan.** A procedure to check if there are rapidly dividing cells, such as cancer cells, in the bone. A very small amount of radioactive material is injected into a vein and travels through the bloodstream. The radioactive material collects in bones with cancer and is detected by a scanner.

Factors That Affect Prognosis and Treatment Options

Certain factors affect prognosis and treatment options.

Pancreatic NETs can often be cured. The prognosis and treatment options depend on the following:

- The type of cancer cell
- Where the tumor is found in the pancreas
- Whether the tumor has spread to more than one place in the pancreas or to other parts of the body
- Whether the patient has MEN1 syndrome
- The patient's age and general health
- Whether the cancer has just been diagnosed or has recurred (come back)

Treatments of Pancreatic NETs

Different types of treatments are available for patients with pancreatic NETs. Some treatments are standard (the currently used treatment), and some are being tested in clinical trials. A treatment clinical trial is a research study meant to help improve current treatments or obtain information on new treatments for patients with cancer. When clinical trials show that a new treatment is better than the standard treatment, the new treatment may become the standard treatment. Patients may want to think about taking part in a clinical trial. Some clinical trials are open only to patients who have not started treatment.

Surgery

An operation may be done to remove the tumor. One of the following types of surgery may be used:

- **Enucleation:** Surgery to remove the tumor only. This may be done when cancer occurs in one place in the pancreas.

- **Pancreatoduodenectomy:** A surgical procedure in which the head of the pancreas, gallbladder, nearby lymph nodes and part of the stomach, small intestine, and bile duct are removed. Enough of the pancreas is left to make digestive juices and insulin. The organs removed during this procedure depend on the patient's condition. This is also called the "Whipple procedure."

- **Distal pancreatectomy:** Surgery to remove the body and tail of the pancreas. The spleen may also be removed if cancer has spread to the spleen.

- **Total gastrectomy:** Surgery to remove the whole stomach.

- **Parietal cell vagotomy:** Surgery to cut the nerve that causes stomach cells to make acid.

- **Liver resection:** Surgery to remove part or all of the liver.

- **Radiofrequency ablation:** The use of a special probe with tiny electrodes that kill cancer cells. Sometimes the probe is inserted directly through the skin and only local anesthesia is needed. In other cases, the probe is inserted through an incision in the abdomen. This is done in the hospital with general anesthesia.

351

- **Cryosurgical ablation:** A procedure in which tissue is frozen to destroy abnormal cells. This is usually done with a special instrument that contains liquid nitrogen or liquid carbon dioxide. The instrument may be used during surgery or laparoscopy or inserted through the skin. This procedure is also called "cryoablation."

Chemotherapy

Chemotherapy is a cancer treatment that uses drugs to stop the growth of cancer cells, either by killing the cells or by stopping them from dividing. When chemotherapy is taken by mouth or injected into a vein or muscle, the drugs enter the bloodstream and can reach cancer cells throughout the body (systemic chemotherapy). When chemotherapy is placed directly into the cerebrospinal fluid, an organ, or a body cavity such as the abdomen, the drugs mainly affect cancer cells in those areas (regional chemotherapy). Combination chemotherapy is the use of more than one anticancer drug. The way the chemotherapy is given depends on the type of cancer being treated.

Hormone Therapy

Hormone therapy is a cancer treatment that removes hormones or blocks their action and stops cancer cells from growing. Hormones are substances made by glands in the body and circulated in the bloodstream. Some hormones can cause certain cancers to grow. If tests show that the cancer cells have places where hormones can attach (receptors), drugs, surgery, or radiation therapy is used to reduce the production of hormones or block them from working.

Hepatic Arterial Occlusion or Chemoembolization

Hepatic arterial occlusion uses drugs, small particles, or other agents to block or reduce the flow of blood to the liver through the hepatic artery (the major blood vessel that carries blood to the liver). This is done to kill cancer cells growing in the liver. The tumor is prevented from getting the oxygen and nutrients it needs to grow. The liver continues to receive blood from the hepatic portal vein, which carries blood from the stomach and intestine.

Chemotherapy delivered during hepatic arterial occlusion is called "chemoembolization." The anticancer drug is injected into the hepatic artery through a catheter (thin tube). The drug is mixed with a substance that blocks the artery and cuts off blood flow to the tumor. Most of the anticancer drug is trapped near the tumor and only a small amount of the drug reaches other parts of the body.

The blockage may be temporary or permanent, depending on the substance used to block the artery.

Targeted Therapy

Targeted therapy is a type of treatment that uses drugs or other substances to identify and attack specific cancer cells without harming normal cells. Certain types of targeted therapies are being studied in the treatment of pancreatic NETs.

Supportive Care

Supportive care is given to lessen the problems caused by the disease or its treatment. Supportive care for pancreatic NETs may include treatment for the following:

- **Stomach ulcers** may be treated with drug therapy such as:
  - Proton pump inhibitor drugs such as omeprazole, lansoprazole, or pantoprazole
  - Histamine blocking drugs such as cimetidine, ranitidine, or famotidine
  - Somatostatin-type drugs such as octreotide
- **Diarrhea** may be treated with:
  - Intravenous (IV) fluids with electrolytes such as potassium or chloride
  - Somatostatin-type drugs such as octreotide
- **Low blood sugar** may be treated by having small, frequent meals or with drug therapy to maintain a normal blood sugar level.
- **High blood sugar** may be treated with drugs taken by mouth or insulin by injection.

Chapter 41

Zollinger-Ellison Syndrome

What Is Zollinger-Ellison Syndrome?

Zollinger-Ellison syndrome (ZES) is a rare disorder that occurs when one or more tumors form in the pancreas and duodenum. The tumors, called "gastrinomas," release large amounts of gastrin that causes the stomach to produce large amounts of acid. Normally, the body releases small amounts of gastrin after eating, which triggers the stomach to make gastric acid that helps break down food and liquid in the stomach. The extra acid causes peptic ulcers to form in the duodenum and elsewhere in the upper intestine.

The tumors seen with ZES are sometimes cancerous and may spread to other areas of the body.

What Are the Stomach, Duodenum, and Pancreas?

The stomach, duodenum, and pancreas are digestive organs that break down food and liquid.

This chapter includes text excerpted from "Zollinger-Ellison Syndrome," National Institute of Diabetes and Digestive and Kidney Diseases (NIDDK), December 15, 2013. Reviewed September 2019.

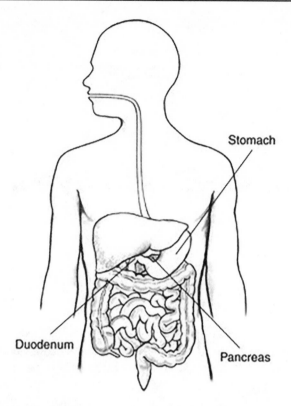

Figure 41.1. *Position of Stomach, Duodenum, and Pancreas*

These are digestive organs that break down food and liquid.

- The stomach stores swallowed food and liquid. The muscle action of the lower part of the stomach mixes the food and liquid with digestive juice. Partially digested food and liquid slowly move into the duodenum and are further broken down.

- The duodenum is the first part of the small intestine—the tube-shaped organ between the stomach and the large intestine—where digestion of the food and liquid continues.

- The pancreas is an organ that makes the hormone insulin and enzymes for digestion. A hormone is a natural chemical produced in one part of the body and released into the blood to trigger or regulate particular functions of the body. Insulin helps cells throughout the body to remove glucose, also called "sugar," from the blood and use it for energy. The pancreas is located behind the stomach and close to the duodenum.

What Causes Zollinger-Ellison Syndrome

Experts do not know the exact cause of ZES. About 25 to 30 percent of gastrinomas are caused by an inherited genetic disorder called "multiple endocrine neoplasia type 1" (MEN1). MEN1 causes hormone-releasing tumors in the endocrine glands and the duodenum. Symptoms of MEN1 include increased hormone levels in the blood, kidney stones, diabetes, muscle weakness, weakened bones, and fractures.

How Common Is Zollinger-Ellison Syndrome

Zollinger-Ellison syndrome is rare and only occurs in about one in every 1 million people. Although anyone can get ZES, the disease is more common among men 30 to 50 years old. A child who has a parent with MEN1 is also at increased risk for ZES.

What Are the Signs and Symptoms of Zollinger-Ellison Syndrome?

Zollinger-Ellison syndrome signs and symptoms are similar to those of peptic ulcers. A dull or burning pain felt anywhere between the navel and midchest is the most common symptom of a peptic ulcer. This discomfort usually:

- Occurs when the stomach is empty—between meals or during the night—and maybe briefly relieved by eating food
- Lasts for minutes to hours
- Comes and goes for several days, weeks, or months

Other symptoms include:
- Diarrhea
- Bloating
- Burping
- Nausea
- Vomiting
- Weight loss
- Poor appetite

Some people with ZES have only diarrhea, with no other symptoms. Others develop gastroesophageal reflux (GER), which occurs when stomach contents flow back up into the esophagus—a muscular tube that carries food and liquids to the stomach. In addition to nausea and vomiting, reflux symptoms include a painful, burning feeling in the midchest.

Seek Help for Emergency Symptoms

A person who has any of the following emergency symptoms should call or see a healthcare provider right away:

- Chest pain
- Sharp, sudden, persistent, and severe stomach pain
- Red blood in stool or black stools
- Red blood in vomit or vomit that looks like coffee grounds

These symptoms could be signs of a serious problem, such as:

- **Internal bleeding**—when gastric acid or a peptic ulcer breaks a blood vessel
- **Perforation**—when a peptic ulcer forms a hole in the duodenal wall
- **Obstruction**—when a peptic ulcer blocks the path of food trying to leave the stomach

How Is Zollinger-Ellison Syndrome Diagnosed?

A healthcare provider diagnoses ZES based on the following:

- Medical history
- Physical exam
- Signs and symptoms
- Blood tests
- Upper gastrointestinal (GI) endoscopy
- Imaging tests to look for gastrinomas
- Measurement of stomach acid

Medical History

Taking a medical and family history is one of the first things a healthcare provider may do to help diagnose ZES. The healthcare provider may ask about family cases of MEN1 in particular.

Physical Exam

A physical exam may help diagnose ZES. During a physical exam, a healthcare provider usually:

- Examines a person's body

- Uses a stethoscope to listen to bodily sounds

- Taps on specific areas of the person's body

Signs and Symptoms

A healthcare provider may suspect ZES if:

- Diarrhea accompanies peptic ulcer symptoms or if peptic ulcer treatment fails.

- A person has peptic ulcers without the use of nonsteroidal anti-inflammatory drugs (NSAIDs) such as aspirin and ibuprofen or a bacterial *helicobacter pylori* (*H. Pylori*) infection. NSAID use and *H. Pylori* infection may cause peptic ulcers.

- A person has severe ulcers that bleed or cause holes in the duodenum or stomach.

- A healthcare provider diagnoses a person or the person's family member with MEN1 or a person has symptoms of MEN1.

Blood Tests

The healthcare provider may use blood tests to check for an elevated gastrin level. A technician or nurse draws a blood sample during an office visit or at a commercial facility and sends the sample to a lab for analysis. A healthcare provider will ask the person to fast for several hours prior to the test and may ask the person to stop acid-reducing medications for a period of time before the test. A gastrin level that is 10 times higher than normal suggests ZES

A healthcare provider may also check for an elevated gastrin level after an infusion of secretin. Secretin is a hormone that causes gastrinomas to release more gastrin. A technician or nurse places an intravenous (IV) needle in a vein in the arm to give an infusion of secretin. A healthcare provider may suspect ZES if blood drawn after the infusion shows an elevated gastrin level.

Upper Gastrointestinal Endoscopy

The healthcare provider uses an upper GI endoscopy to check the esophagus, stomach, and duodenum for ulcers and esophagitis—a general term used to describe irritation and swelling of the esophagus. This procedure involves using an endoscope—a small, flexible tube with a light—to see the upper GI tract, which includes the esophagus, stomach, and duodenum. A gastroenterologist—a doctor who specializes in digestive diseases—performs the test at a hospital or an outpatient center. The gastroenterologist carefully feeds the endoscope down the esophagus and into the stomach and duodenum. A small camera mounted on the endoscope transmits a video image to a monitor, allowing close examination of the intestinal lining. A person may receive a liquid anesthetic that is gargled or sprayed on the back of the throat. A technician or nurse inserts an IV needle in a vein in the arm if anesthesia is given.

Imaging Tests

To help find gastrinomas, a healthcare provider may order one or more of the following imaging tests:

- **Computerized tomography (CT) scan.** A CT scan is an x-ray that produces pictures of the body. A CT scan may include the injection of a special dye, called "contrast medium." CT scans use a combination of x-rays and computer technology to create images. CT scans require the person to lie on a table that slides into a tunnel-shaped device where an x-ray technician takes x-rays. A computer puts the different views together to create a model of the pancreas, stomach, and duodenum. The x-ray technician performs the procedure in an outpatient center or a hospital, and a radiologist—a doctor who specializes in medical imaging—interprets the images. The person does not need anesthesia. CT scans can show tumors and ulcers.

- **Magnetic resonance imaging (MRI).** MRI is a test that takes pictures of the body's internal organs and soft tissues without using x-rays. A specially trained technician performs the procedure in an outpatient center or a hospital, and a radiologist interprets the images. The person does not need anesthesia, though people with a fear of confined spaces may receive light sedation, taken by mouth. An MRI may include the injection of contrast medium. With most MRI machines, the person will lie on a table that slides into a tunnel-shaped device that may be open ended or closed at one end. Some machines allow the person to lie in a more open space. During an MRI, the person, although usually awake, remains perfectly still while the technician takes the images, which usually takes only a few minutes. The technician will take a sequence of images from different angles to create a detailed picture of the upper GI tract. During sequencing, the person will hear loud mechanical knocking and humming noises.

- **Endoscopic ultrasound.** This procedure involves using a special endoscope called an "endo echoscope" to perform ultrasound of the pancreas. The endo echoscope has a built-in miniature ultrasound probe that bounces safe, painless sound waves off organs to create an image of their structure. A gastroenterologist performs the procedure in an outpatient center or a hospital, and a radiologist interprets the images. The gastroenterologist carefully feeds the endo echoscope down the esophagus, through the stomach and duodenum, until it is near the pancreas. A person may receive a liquid anesthetic that is gargled or sprayed on the back of the throat. A sedative helps the person stay relaxed and comfortable. The images can show gastrinomas in the pancreas.

- **Angiogram.** An angiogram is a special kind of x-ray in which an interventional radiologist—a specially trained radiologist—threads a thin, flexible tube called a "catheter" through the large arteries, often from the groin, to the artery of interest. The radiologist injects contrast medium through the catheter so the images show up more clearly on the x-ray. The interventional radiologist performs the procedure and interprets the images in a hospital or an outpatient center. A person does not need anesthesia, though a light sedative may help reduce a person's anxiety during the procedure. This test can show gastrinomas in the pancreas.

- **Somatostatin receptor scintigraphy.** An x-ray technician performs this test, also called "OctreoScan," at a hospital or an outpatient center, and a radiologist interprets the images. A person does not need anesthesia. A radioactive compound called a "radiotracer," when injected into the bloodstream, selectively labels tumor cells. The labeled cells light up when scanned with a device called a "gamma camera." The test can show gastrinomas in the duodenum, pancreas, and other parts of the body.

Small gastrinomas may be hard to see; therefore, healthcare providers may order several types of imaging tests to find gastrinomas.

Stomach-Acid Measurement

Using a sample of stomach juices for analysis, a healthcare provider may measure the amount of stomach acid a person produces. During the exam, a healthcare provider puts in a nasogastric tube—a tiny tube inserted through the nose and throat that reaches into the stomach. A person may receive a liquid anesthetic that is gargled or sprayed on the back of the throat. Once the tube is placed, a healthcare provider takes samples of the stomach acid. High acid levels in the stomach indicate ZES.

How Is Zollinger-Ellison Syndrome Treated?

A healthcare provider treats ZES with medications to reduce gastric acid secretion and with surgery to remove gastrinomas. A healthcare provider sometimes uses chemotherapy—medications to shrink tumors—when tumors are too widespread to remove with surgery.

Medications

A class of medications called "proton pump inhibitors" (PPIs) includes:

- Esomeprazole (Nexium®)
- Lansoprazole (Prevacid®)
- Pantoprazole (Protonix®)
- Omeprazole (Prilosec® or Zegerid®)
- Dexlansoprazole (Dexilant®)

Proton pump inhibitors stop the mechanism that pumps acid into the stomach, helping to relieve peptic ulcer pain and promote healing. A healthcare provider may prescribe people who have ZES higher-than-normal doses of PPIs to control the acid production. Studies show that PPIs may increase the risk of hip, wrist, and spine fractures when a person takes them long-term or in high doses, so it is important for people to discuss risks versus benefits with their healthcare provider.

Surgery

Surgical removal of gastrinomas is the only cure for ZES. Some gastrinomas spread to other parts of the body, especially the liver and bones. Finding and removing all gastrinomas before they spread is often challenging because many of the tumors are small.

Chemotherapy

Healthcare providers sometimes use chemotherapy drugs to treat gastrinomas that cannot be surgically removed, including:

- Streptozotocin (Zanosar®)

- 5-fluorouracil (Adrucil®)

- Doxorubicin (Doxil®)

Part Six

Disorders of
the Ovaries and Testes

Chapter 42

Hypogonadism

Hypogonadism is a condition in which the sex glands either under-perform or, in some cases, are absent altogether. In women, this means the ovaries produce little or no estrogen, a hormone that, among other functions, is responsible for sexual development, helps regulate the menstrual cycle, assists in the maintenance of uterine function during pregnancy, plays a role in blood clotting and brain function, helps build healthy bones, and affects mood. Hypogonadism may result in infertility and an increased risk of osteoporosis, as well other effects on overall health and quality of life (QOL).

Causes of Hypogonadism

There are two types of hypogonadism, primary and secondary. Primary hypogonadism, which under normal circumstances occurs naturally as a result of menopause, may be caused by a chromosomal disorder, such as Turner syndrome, in which the X chromosome is partially or completely missing, by surgical removal of the ovaries, or by autoimmune disorders. The causes of secondary hypogonadism include problems with the hypothalamus or pituitary gland, infection, head injury, inflammatory diseases, rapid weight loss, or drug use.

"Hypogonadism," © 2017 Omnigraphics. Reviewed September 2019.

Symptoms of Hypogonadism

The signs and symptoms of hypogonadism may include:

- Lack of development secondary sex characteristics during puberty
- Lack of (or reduced) menstruation
- Absent or decreased libido
- Reduction in vaginal lubrication
- Reduced fertility
- Hot flashes
- Loss of body hair
- Changes in energy and mood
- Sleep disturbance
- Loss of bone mass
- Frequent urination or urinary tract infections
- Inability or reduced ability to smell

Diagnosis of Hypogonadism

Diagnosing hypogonadism begins with a physical exam in which the doctor will ask about family history and the extent of symptoms, examine the genitalia, assess the development of secondary sex characteristics, and evaluate overall health. Depending on the results of the examination, tests may include:

- Measurement of estrogen levels
- Follicle-stimulating hormone (FSH) and luteinizing hormone (LH) tests to evaluate pituitary function
- Tests for anemia and iron deficiency
- Evaluation of levels of prolactin (a hormone that, among a wide range of other functions, promotes milk production)
- Thyroid tests
- Genetic tests
- Ultrasound of the ovaries
- Magnetic resonance imaging (MRI) of the head to examine the pituitary gland

Treatment of Hypogonadism

The treatment of hypogonadism depends on its cause. For example, if the problem were a tumor in the pituitary gland, surgical removal might be recommended. However, in most cases it is a chronic condition that requires lifelong management. The most common treatment involves hormone-replacement therapy to restore development and function. Estrogen and progesterone (a hormone that plays a role in maintaining pregnancy) may be administered via injection, pills, a topical gel, or slow-release skin patches.

Possible Complications of Hypogonadism

If untreated, the risks and complications of hypogonadism can include:

- Delayed puberty

- Infertility

- Sexual dysfunction

- Weakness

- Osteoporosis

- Heart disease

In addition, hormone replacement therapy, although the most effective means of treating hypogonadism, does carry some risks. These may include blood clots, stroke, heart disease, breast and endometrial cancer, and gallbladder disease.

References

1. "Hypogonadism in Females," The Woman's Clinic, n.d.

2. "Hypogonadotropic Hypogonadism," Women Health & Lifestyle, n.d.

3. Martel, Janelle. "Hypogonadism," Healthline.com, November 19, 2015.

4. Vogiatzi, Maria G., MD. "Hypogonadism," Medscape.com, October 14, 2016.

5. Wisse, Brent, MD. "Hypogonadism," MedlinePlus, National Institutes of Health (NIH), October 25, 2014.

Chapter 43

Gynecomastia

What Is Gynecomastia?

Gynecomastia is the enlargement of male breast tissue, most often due to an imbalance of the hormones estrogen and testosterone. The condition can affect one or both breasts and can make the breast tender. It is usually not permanent or dangerous; however, affected males can experience a considerable amount of social embarrassment and psychological distress.

Pseudogynecomastia (false gynecomastia) can sometimes be confused with gynecomastia; but, the former is caused by an excessive amount of fat tissue on the chest, while the latter is an above-average growth of the breast tissue itself.

Prevalence of Gynecomastia

Gynecomastia can occur at any stage of a man's life, depending on the degree of hormonal change. Newborn babies often have this condition for a short time immediately after birth when the mother's estrogen remains in their bloodstreams. In infants, it usually disappears within the first year of life. Teenage boys may experience gynecomastia during puberty starting from as early as the age of 10, with aggressive growth between the ages of 13 and 14, and slowly regressing in the later teen years.

"Gynecomastia," © 2018 Omnigraphics. Reviewed September 2019.

Statistically, only about 4 percent of males between the ages of 10 and 19 are found to have gynecomastia. The condition is most prevalent among older adults between the ages of 50 and 80. 1 in every 4 men in this age group is affected, and in these cases, there may be other medical problems associated with the condition.

Causes and Risk Factors of Gynecomastia

The exact cause of gynecomastia is unclear; however, in most cases, it is thought to be the result of an imbalance between estrogen and testosterone. These hormones are responsible for the development and control of sex characteristics in both males and females. In general, testosterone helps create typically male characteristics, such as facial hair, muscle mass, body hair, and a deep voice. Estrogen aids in the development of what are commonly regarded as feminine characteristics, including breast development. Since men have both hormones in their systems, if an imbalance favors estrogen, gynecomastia can result.

Some other causes and risk factors of gynecomastia include:

- Medication, such as antibiotics, anti-anxiety drugs, anabolic steroids, heart medications, anti-androgens, tricyclic antidepressants, gastric motility medications, and ulcer medications

- Cancer and acquired immunodeficiency syndrome (AIDS) treatments

- The use of substances, such as alcohol, heroin, methadone, marijuana, and amphetamines

- A variety of physical conditions, including hypogonadism, tumors, kidney failure, liver failure, cirrhosis, malnutrition, and starvation

- The use of tea tree oil or lavender oil, herbal products that contain natural estrogen

- Obesity or the lack of a proper diet and nutrition

Diagnosis of Gynecomastia

To begin evaluating a patient for gynecomastia, a healthcare provider will ask for a medical history, including such information as the symptoms being experienced, how long they have persisted, if tenderness is present around the breast area, type of medication being taken, general health condition, drug history, and family health history. The healthcare provider will then perform a careful examination of the breast tissue, genitals, and abdomen.

Tests a doctor may order to help confirm a diagnosis of gynecomastia include:

- Computerized tomography (CT) scans

- Blood tests

- Mammograms

- Magnetic resonance imaging (MRI) scans

- Tissue biopsies

- Testicular ultrasounds

Treatment of Gynecomastia

In young patients, treatment is often not necessary, since in such cases, gynecomastia usually resolves on its own. For older individuals, a number of treatment methods can be recommended by healthcare providers. For example, medications may be prescribed to help restore hormone balance. Certain medications, such as tamoxifen, aromatase inhibitors (Arimidex), and raloxifene (Evista)—while not specifically approved for the treatment of gynecomastia—may help in some cases. If any health condition is causing the gynecomastia, it will need to be addressed through specific treatment. If gynecomastia has been resulted from the use of certain drugs, doctors may prescribe a different medication that may help improve the condition.

In rare cases, surgery may be an option if medication and other treatment prove to be ineffective. Surgical options include liposuction, a procedure that removes the breast fat but not the breast gland tissue, and mastectomy, a procedure that removes the breast gland tissue.

In order to make good decisions and ensure the best possible outcome, before beginning any treatment, the patient should ask the following questions of the healthcare provider:

- Is the breast enlargement likely to resolve on its own?

- What types of treatments are available?

- How long will treatment last?

- Are there any health conditions that are triggering the gynecomastia?

- Should I avoid any particular substance or medication to improve the condition?

- Should I be tested for breast cancer?

- If my breasts are hurting, what can I do to stop the pain?

Treatment options also include getting psychological counseling, as well as help and support from family. The condition can cause stress and embarrassment; therefore, counseling, group therapy, and help explaining the condition to family and friends can have a major impact on the recovery process.

References

1. Booth, Stephanie. "Enlarged Breasts in Men: Causes and Treatments," WebMD, December 13, 2015.

2. "Enlarged Breasts in Men (Gynecomastia)," Mayo Clinic, August 29, 2017.

3. "Gynecomastia," Cleveland Clinic, n.d.

4. "Gynecomastia," Familydoctor.org, March 2014.

5. Lemaine, Valerie, M.D., Cenk Cayci, M.D., Patricia S. Simmons, M.D., and Paul Petty, M.D. "Gynecomastia in Adolescent Males," U.S. National Library of Medicine (NLM), February 27, 2013.

Chapter 44

Menstrual Problems

Chapter Contents

Section 44.1

Premenstrual Syndrome

This section includes text excerpted from "Premenstrual Syndrome
(PMS)," Office on Women's Health (OWH), U.S. Department of
Health and Human Services (HHS), March 16, 2018.

What Is Premenstrual Syndrome?

Premenstrual syndrome (PMS) is a combination of physical and
emotional symptoms that many women get after ovulation and before
the start of their menstrual period. Researchers think that PMS happens in the days after ovulation because estrogen and progesterone levels begin falling dramatically if you are not pregnant. PMS symptoms
go away within a few days after a woman's period starts as hormone
levels begin rising again.

Some women get their periods without any signs of PMS or only
very mild symptoms. For others, PMS symptoms may be so severe
that it makes it hard to do everyday activities such as going to work or
school. Severe PMS symptoms may be a sign of premenstrual dysphoric
disorder (PMDD). PMS goes away when you no longer get a period,
such as after menopause. After pregnancy, PMS might come back, but
you might have different PMS symptoms.

Who Gets Premenstrual Syndrome

As many as three in four women say they get PMS symptoms at
some point in their lifetime. For most women PMS symptoms are mild.

Less than five percent of women of childbearing age get a more
severe form of PMS, called "PMDD."

Premenstrual syndrome may happen more often in women who:

• Have high levels of stress

• Have a family history of depression

• Have a personal history of either postpartum depression or
depression

Does Premenstrual Syndrome Change with Age?

Yes. PMS symptoms may get worse as you reach your late 30s or
40s and approach menopause and are in the transition to menopause,
called "perimenopause."

This is especially true for women whose moods are sensitive to changing hormone levels during the menstrual cycle. In the years leading up to menopause, your hormone levels also go up and down in an unpredictable way as your body slowly transitions to menopause. You may get the same mood changes, or they may get worse.

Premenstrual syndrome stops after menopause when you no longer get a period.

What Are the Symptoms of Premenstrual Syndrome?

Premenstrual syndrome symptoms are different for every woman. You may get physical symptoms, such as bloating or gassiness, or emotional symptoms, such as sadness, or both. Your symptoms may also change throughout your life.

Physical symptoms of PMS can include:

- Swollen or tender breasts
- Constipation or diarrhea
- Bloating or a gassy feeling
- Cramping
- Headache or backache
- Clumsiness
- Lower tolerance for noise or light

Emotional or mental symptoms of PMS include:

- Irritability or hostile behavior
- Feeling tired
- Sleep problems (sleeping too much or too little)
- Appetite changes or food cravings
- Trouble with concentration or memory
- Tension or anxiety
- Depression, feelings of sadness, or crying spells
- Mood swings
- Less interest in sex

Talk to your doctor or nurse if your symptoms bother you or affect your daily life.

What Causes Premenstrual Syndrome

Researchers do not know exactly what causes PMS. Changes in hormone levels during the menstrual cycle may play a role. These changing hormone levels may affect some women more than others.

How Is Premenstrual Syndrome Diagnosed?

There is no single test for PMS. Your doctor will talk with you about your symptoms, including when they happen and how much they affect your life.

You probably have PMS if you have symptoms that:

- Happen in the five days before your period for at least three menstrual cycles in a row

- End within four days after your period starts

- Keep you from enjoying or doing some of your normal activities

Keep track of which PMS symptoms you have and how severe they are for a few months. Write down your symptoms each day on a calendar or with an app on your phone. Take this information with you when you see your doctor.

How Does Premenstrual Syndrome Affect Other Health Problems?

About half of women who need relief from PMS also have another health problem, which may get worse in the time before their menstrual period. These health problems share many symptoms with PMS and include:

- **Depression and anxiety disorders.** These are the most common conditions that overlap with PMS. Depression and anxiety symptoms are similar to PMS and may get worse before or during your period.

- **Myalgic encephalomyelitis (ME)/chronic fatigue syndrome (CFS).** Some women report that their symptoms often get worse right before their period. Research shows that women with ME/CFS may also be more likely to have heavy menstrual bleeding and early or premature menopause.

- **Irritable bowel syndrome (IBS).** IBS causes cramping, bloating, and gas. Your IBS symptoms may get worse right before your period.

- **Bladder pain syndrome.** Women with bladder pain syndrome are more likely to have painful cramps during PMS.

Premenstrual syndrome symptoms may also worsen some health problems, such as asthma, allergies, and migraines.

What You Can Do at Home to Relieve Premenstrual Syndrome Symptoms

These tips will help you be healthier in general, and may relieve some of your PMS symptoms.

- **Get regular aerobic physical activity throughout the month.** Exercise can help with symptoms such as depression, difficulty concentrating, and fatigue.

- **Choose healthy foods most of the time.** Avoiding foods and drinks with caffeine, salt, and sugar in the two weeks before your period may lessen many PMS symptoms.

- **Get enough sleep.** Try to get about eight hours of sleep each night. Lack of sleep is linked to depression and anxiety and can make PMS symptoms such as moodiness worse.

- **Find healthy ways to cope with stress.** Talk to your friends or write in a journal. Some women also find yoga, massage, or meditation helpful.

- **Do not smoke.** In one large study, women who smoked reported more PMS symptoms and worse PMS symptoms than women who did not smoke.

Over-the-counter (OTC) and prescription medicines can help treat some PMS symptoms. OTC pain relievers you can buy in most stores may help lessen physical symptoms, such as cramps, headaches, backaches, and breast tenderness. These include:

- Ibuprofen

- Naproxen

- Aspirin

Some women find that taking an OTC pain reliever right before their period starts to lessen the amount of pain and bleeding they have during their period.

Prescription medicines may help if OTC pain medicines do not work:

- **Hormonal birth control** may help with the physical symptoms of PMS, but it may make other symptoms worse. You may need to try several different types of birth control before you find one that helps your symptoms.

- **Antidepressants** can help relieve emotional symptoms of PMS for some women when other medicines do not help. Selective serotonin reuptake inhibitors, or SSRIs, are the most common type of antidepressant used to treat PMS.

- **Diuretics** ("water pills") may reduce symptoms of bloating and breast tenderness.

- **Antianxiety medicine** may help reduce feelings of anxiousness.

All medicines have risks. Talk to your doctor or nurse about the benefits and risks.

Intake of Vitamins or Minerals to Treat Premenstrual Syndrome Symptoms

Studies show that certain vitamins and minerals may help relieve some PMS symptoms. The U.S. Food and Drug Administration (FDA) does not regulate vitamins or minerals and herbal supplements in the same way they regulate medicines. Talk to your doctor before taking any supplement.

Studies have found benefits for:

- **Calcium.** Studies show that calcium can help reduce some PMS symptoms, such as fatigue, cravings, and depression. Calcium is found in foods such as milk, cheese, and yogurt. Some foods, such as orange juice, cereal, and bread, have calcium added (fortified). You can also take a calcium supplement.

- **Vitamin B$_6$.** Vitamin B$_6$ may help with PMS symptoms, including moodiness, irritability, forgetfulness, bloating, and anxiety. Vitamin B$_6$ can be found in foods such as fish, poultry, potatoes, fruit (except for citrus fruits), and fortified cereals. You can also take it as a dietary supplement.

Studies have found mixed results for:

- **Magnesium.** Magnesium may help relieve some PMS symptoms, including migraines. If you get menstrual migraines, talk to your doctor about whether you need more magnesium. Magnesium is found in green, leafy vegetables such as spinach, as well as in nuts, whole grains, and fortified cereals. You can also take a supplement.

- **Polyunsaturated fatty acids (omega-3 and omega-6).** Studies show that taking a supplement with 1 to 2 grams of polyunsaturated fatty acids may help reduce cramps and other PMS symptoms. Good sources of polyunsaturated fatty acids include flaxseed, nuts, fish, and green leafy vegetables.

Some women report relief from their PMS symptoms with yoga or meditation. Others say herbal supplements help relieve symptoms. Talk with your doctor or nurse before taking any of these supplements. They may interact with other medicines you take, making your other medicine not work or cause dangerous side effects. The FDA does not regulate herbal supplements at the same level that it regulates medicines.

Some research studies show relief from PMS symptoms with these herbal supplements, but other studies do not. Many herbal supplements should not be used with other medicines. Some herbal supplements women use to ease PMS symptoms include:

- **Black cohosh.** The underground stems and roots of black cohosh are used fresh or dried to make tea, capsules, pills, or liquid extracts. Black cohosh is most often used to help treat menopausal symptoms, and some women use it to help relieve PMS symptoms.

- **Chasteberry.** Dried ripe chasteberry is used to prepare liquid extracts or pills that some women take to relieve PMS symptoms. Women taking hormonal birth control or hormone therapy for menopausal symptoms should not take chasteberry.

- **Evening primrose oil.** The oil is taken from the plant's seeds and put into capsules. Some women report that the pill helps relieve PMS symptoms, but the research results are mixed.

Researchers continue to search for new ways to treat PMS.

Section 44.2

Premenstrual Dysphoric Disorder

This section includes text excerpted from "Premenstrual
Dysphoric Disorder (PMDD)," Office on Women's Health (OWH),
U.S. Department of Health and Human Services (HHS), March 16, 2018.

Premenstrual dysphoric disorder (PMDD) is a health problem that
is similar to premenstrual syndrome (PMS) but is more serious. PMDD
causes severe irritability, depression, or anxiety in a week or two before
your period starts. Symptoms usually go away two to three days after
your period starts. You may need medicine or other treatment to help
with your symptoms.

What Is Premenstrual Dysphoric Disorder?

Premenstrual dysphoric disorder is a condition similar to PMS that
also happens in a week or two before your period starts as hormone
levels begin to fall after ovulation. PMDD causes more severe symptoms than PMS, including severe depression, irritability, and tension.

Who Gets Premenstrual Dysphoric Disorder

Premenstrual dysphoric disorder affects up to five percent of women
of childbearing age. Many women with PMDD may also have anxiety
or depression.

What Are the Symptoms of Premenstrual Dysphoric Disorder?

Symptoms of PMDD include:

- Lasting irritability or anger that may affect other people
- Feelings of sadness or despair, or even thoughts of suicide
- Feelings of tension or anxiety
- Panic attacks
- Mood swings or crying often
- Lack of interest in daily activities and relationships
- Trouble thinking or focusing

- Tiredness or low energy

- Food cravings or binge eating

- Trouble sleeping

- Feeling out of control

- Physical symptoms, such as cramps, bloating, breast tenderness, headaches, and joint or muscle pain

What Causes Premenstrual Dysphoric Disorder

Researchers do not know for sure what causes PMDD or PMS. Hormonal changes throughout the menstrual cycle may play a role. A brain chemical called "serotonin" may also play a role in PMDD. Serotonin levels change throughout the menstrual cycle. Some women may be more sensitive to these changes.

How Is Premenstrual Dysphoric Disorder Diagnosed?

Your doctor will talk to you about your health history and do a physical examination. You will need to keep a calendar or diary of your symptoms to help your doctor diagnose PMDD. You must have five or more PMDD symptoms, including one mood-related symptoms, to be diagnosed with PMDD.

What Are the Treatment Options for Premenstrual Dysphoric Disorder?

Selective serotonin reuptake inhibitors (SSRIs). SSRIs are a type of antidepressants that can change serotonin levels in the brain. The U.S. Food and Drug Administration (FDA) approved three SSRIs to treat PMDD:

- Sertraline

- Fluoxetine

- Paroxetine Hydrochloride (HCI)

Birth control pills. The FDA has approved a birth control pill containing drospirenone and ethinyl estradiol, to treat PMDD.

Over-the-counter (OTC) pain relievers may help relieve physical symptoms, such as cramps, joint pain, headaches, backaches, and breast tenderness. These include:

- Ibuprofen

- Naproxen

- Aspirin

Stress management, such as relaxation techniques and spending time on activities you enjoy can be helpful.

Making healthy changes, such as eating a healthy combination of foods across the food groups, cutting back on salty and sugary foods, and getting more physical activity, may also help relieve some PMDD symptoms.

But PMDD can be serious enough that some women should go to a doctor or nurse to discuss treatment options. And, if you are thinking of hurting yourself or others, call 911 right away.

Section 44.3

Menstrual Irregularities

This section includes text excerpted from "What Are Menstrual Irregularities?" *Eunice Kennedy Shriver* National Institute of Child Health and Human Development (NICHD), January 31, 2017.

What Are Menstrual Irregularities?

For most women, a normal menstrual cycle ranges from 21 to 35 days. However, 14 to 25 percent of women have irregular menstrual cycles, meaning the cycles are shorter or longer than normal; they are heavier or lighter than normal; or are experienced with other problems, such as abdominal cramps. Irregular cycles can be ovulatory, meaning that ovulation occurs, or anovulatory, meaning ovulation does not occur.

The most common menstrual irregularities include:

- **Amenorrhea** or **absent menstrual periods.** When a woman does not get her period by age 16, or when she stops getting her period for at least 3 months and is not pregnant.

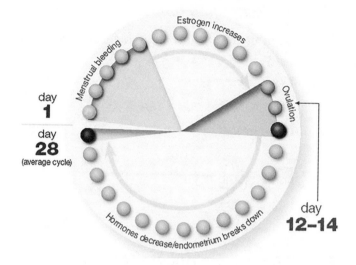

Figure 44.1. *The Menstrual Cycle* (Source: "About Menstruation," *Eunice Kennedy Shriver* National Institute of Child Health and Human Development (NICHD).)

- **Oligomenorrhea or infrequent menstrual periods.** Periods that occur more than 35 days apart.

- **Menorrhagia or heavy menstrual periods.** Also called "excessive bleeding." Although anovulatory bleeding and menorrhagia are sometimes grouped together, they do not have the same cause and require different diagnostic testing.

- **Prolonged menstrual bleeding.** Bleeding that exceeds eight days in duration on a regular basis.

- **Dysmenorrhea.** Painful periods that may include severe menstrual cramps.

    Additional menstrual irregularities include:

- **Polymenorrhea.** Frequent menstrual periods occurring less than 21 days apart.

- **Irregular menstrual periods** with a cycle-to-cycle variation of more than 20 days.

- **Shortened menstrual bleeding** of less than 2 days in duration.

- **Intermenstrual bleeding.** Episodes of bleeding that occur between periods, also known as "spotting."

What Are the Symptoms of Menstruation?

The primary sign of menstruation is bleeding from the vagina. Additional symptoms include:

- Abdominal or pelvic cramping
- Lower back pain
- Bloating and sore breasts
- Food cravings
- Mood swings and irritability
- Headache
- Fatigue

How Many Women Are Affected by Menstrual Irregularities?

Menstrual irregularities occur in an estimated 14 to 25 percent of women of childbearing age.

Estimates of the number of women with menstrual irregularities may differ by the cause or nature of the irregularity. For example, if a woman experiences severe cramps, she might be included in the tally of women with endometriosis rather than in the tally of women with menstrual irregularities.

What Causes Menstrual Irregularities

Menstrual irregularities can have a variety of causes, including pregnancy, hormonal imbalances, infections, diseases, trauma, and certain medications.

Causes of Irregular Periods

- Perimenopause (generally in the late 40s and early 50s)
- Primary ovarian insufficiency (POI)
- Eating disorders (anorexia nervosa or bulimia)
- Excessive exercise
- Thyroid dysfunction (too much or too little thyroid hormone)
- Elevated levels of the hormone prolactin, which is made by the pituitary gland to help the body produce milk

- Uncontrolled diabetes
- Cushing syndrome (elevated levels of the hormone cortisol, used in the body's response to stress)
- Late-onset congenital adrenal hyperplasia (problem with the adrenal gland)
- Hormonal birth control (birth control pills, injections, or implants)
- Hormone-containing intrauterine devices (IUDs)
- Scarring within the uterine cavity (Asherman syndrome)
- Medications, such as those to treat epilepsy or mental-health problems

Causes of Heavy or Prolonged Menstrual Bleeding

- Adolescence (during which cycles may not be associated with ovulation)
- Polycystic ovary syndrome (PCOS) (bleeding irregular but heavy)
- Uterine fibroids (benign growths of uterine muscle)
- Endometrial polyps (benign overgrowth of the lining of the uterus)
- Adenomyosis (the presence of uterine lining in the wall of the uterus)
- Nonhormonal IUDs
- Bleeding disorders, such as leukemia, platelet disorders, clotting factor deficiencies, or (less common) von Willebrand disease
- Pregnancy complications (miscarriage)

Causes of Dysmenorrhea

- Endometriosis (uterine lining grows outside the uterus)
- Uterine abnormalities (fibroids or adenomyosis)
- Intrauterine devices (IUDs)
- Pelvic scarring due to sexually transmitted infections (STIs), such as chlamydia or gonorrhea
- Heavy menstrual flow

How Do Healthcare Providers Diagnose Menstrual Irregularities?

A healthcare provider diagnoses menstrual irregularities using a combination of the following:

- Medical history

- Physical examination

- Blood tests

- Ultrasound examination

- Endometrial biopsy—a small sample of the uterus's endometrial lining is taken to be examined under a microscope

- Hysteroscopy—a diagnostic scope that allows a healthcare provider to examine the inside of the uterus, typically done as an outpatient procedure

- Saline infusion sonohysterography—ultrasound imaging of the uterine cavity while it is filled with sterile saline solution

- Transvaginal ultrasonography—ultrasound imaging of the pelvic organs, including the ovaries and uterus, using an ultrasound transducer that is inserted into the vagina

What Are the Common Treatments for Menstrual Irregularities?

Treatments for menstrual irregularities often vary based on the type of irregularity and certain lifestyle factors, such as whether a woman is planning to get pregnant.

Treatment for menstrual irregularities that are due to anovulatory bleeding (absent periods, infrequent periods, and irregular periods) include:

- Oral contraceptives

- Cyclic progestin

Treatments for an underlying disorder that is causing the menstrual problem, such as counseling and nutritional therapy for an eating disorder

Treatment for menstrual irregularities that are due to ovulatory bleeding (heavy or prolonged menstrual bleeding) include:

- Insertion of a hormone-releasing intrauterine device
- Use of various medications (such as those containing progestin or tranexamic acid) or nonsteroidal anti-inflammatory medications (NSAIDs)

If the cause is structural or if medical management is ineffective, then the following may be considered:

- Surgical removal of polyps or uterine fibroids
- Uterine artery embolization, a procedure to block blood flow to the uterus
- Endometrial ablation, a procedure to cauterize (remove or close off by burning) blood vessels in the endometrial lining of the uterus
- Hysterectomy

Treatment for dysmenorrhea (painful periods) include:

- Applying a heating pad to the abdomen
- Taking NSAIDs
- Taking contraceptives, including injectable hormone therapy or birth control pills, using varied or less common treatment regimens

Chapter 45

Polycystic Ovarian Syndrome

Polycystic ovary syndrome (PCOS) is a health problem that affects 1 in 10 women of childbearing age. Women with PCOS have a hormonal imbalance and metabolism problems that may affect their overall health and appearance. PCOS is also a common and treatable cause of infertility.

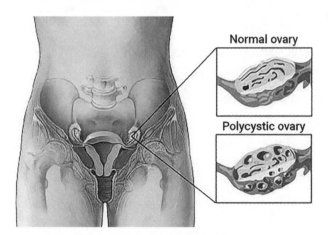

Figure 45.1. *Normal Ovary and Polycystic Ovary*

This chapter includes text excerpted from "Polycystic Ovary Syndrome," Office on Women's Health (OWH), U.S. Department of Health and Human Services (HHS), April 1, 2019.

What Is Polycystic Ovary Syndrome?

Polycystic ovary syndrome, also known as "polycystic ovarian syndrome," is a common health problem caused by an imbalance of reproductive hormones. The hormonal imbalance creates problems in the ovaries. The ovaries make the egg that is released each month as part of a healthy menstrual cycle. With PCOS, the egg may not develop as it should or it may not be released during ovulation as it should be.

Polycystic ovary syndrome can cause missed or irregular menstrual periods. Irregular periods can lead to:

• Infertility (inability to get pregnant). In fact, PCOS is one of the most common causes of infertility in women.

• Development of cysts (small fluid-filled sacs) in the ovaries

Who Gets Polycystic Ovary Syndrome

Between 5 and 10 percent of women between 15 and 44, or during the years you can have children, have PCOS. Most women find out they have PCOS in their twenties and thirties, when they have problems getting pregnant and see their doctor. But, PCOS can happen at any age after puberty.

Women of all races and ethnicities are at risk of PCOS. Your risk of PCOS may be higher if you have obesity or if you have a mother, sister, or aunt with PCOS.

What Are the Symptoms of Polycystic Ovary Syndrome?

Some of the symptoms of PCOS include:

• **Irregular menstrual cycle.** Women with PCOS may miss periods or have fewer periods (fewer than eight in a year). Or, their periods may come every 21 days or more often. Some women with PCOS stop having menstrual periods.

• **Too much hair** on the face, chin, or parts of the body where men usually have hair. This is called "hirsutism." Hirsutism affects up to 70 percent of women with PCOS.

• **Acne** on the face, chest, and upper back

• **Thinning hair** or hair loss on the scalp; male-pattern baldness

• **Weight gain** or difficulty losing weight

- **Darkening of skin,** particularly along neck creases, in the groin, and underneath breasts

- **Skin tags,** which are small excess flaps of skin in the armpits or neck area

What Causes of Polycystic Ovary Syndrome

The exact cause of PCOS is not known. Most experts think that several factors, including genetics, play a role:

- **High levels of androgens.** Androgens are sometimes called "male hormones," although all women make small amounts of androgens. Androgens control the development of male traits, such as male-pattern baldness. Women with PCOS have more androgens than normal. Higher than normal androgen levels in women can prevent the ovaries from releasing an egg (ovulation) during each menstrual cycle, and can cause extra hair growth and acne, two signs of PCOS.

- **High levels of insulin.** Insulin is a hormone that controls how the food you eat is changed into energy. Insulin resistance is when the body's cells do not respond normally to insulin. As a result, your insulin blood levels become higher than normal. Many women with PCOS have insulin resistance, especially those who have overweight or obesity, have unhealthy eating habits, do not get enough physical activity, and have a family history of diabetes (usually type 2 diabetes). Over time, insulin resistance can lead to type 2 diabetes.

Can You Still Get Pregnant If You Have Polycystic Ovary Syndrome?

Yes. Having PCOS does not mean you cannot get pregnant. PCOS is one of the most common, but treatable, causes of infertility in women. In women with PCOS, the hormonal imbalance interferes with the growth and release of eggs from the ovaries (ovulation). If you do not ovulate, you cannot get pregnant.

Your doctor can talk with you about ways to help you ovulate and to raise your chance of getting pregnant. You can also use ovulation calculator to see which days in your menstrual cycle you are most likely to be fertile.

Will Your Polycystic Ovary Syndrome Symptoms Go Away at Menopause?

Yes and no. PCOS affects many systems in the body. Many women with PCOS find that their menstrual cycles become more regular as they get closer to menopause. However, their PCOS hormonal imbalance does not change with age, so they may continue to have symptoms of PCOS.

Also, the risks of PCOS-related health problems, such as diabetes, stroke, and heart attack, increase with age. These risks may be higher in women with PCOS than those without.

How Is Polycystic Ovary Syndrome Diagnosed?

There is no single test to diagnose PCOS. To help diagnose PCOS and rule out other causes of your symptoms, your doctor may talk to you about your medical history and do a physical exam and different tests:

- **Physical exam.** Your doctor will measure your blood pressure, body mass index (BMI), and waist size. They will also look at your skin for extra hair on your face, chest or back, acne, or skin discoloration. Your doctor may look for any hair loss or signs of other health conditions (such as an enlarged thyroid gland).

- **Pelvic exam.** Your doctor may do a pelvic exam for signs of extra male hormones (for example, an enlarged clitoris) and check to see if your ovaries are enlarged or swollen.

- **Pelvic ultrasound (sonogram).** This test uses sound waves to examine your ovaries for cysts and check the endometrium (lining of the uterus or womb).

- **Blood tests.** Blood tests check your androgen hormone levels, sometimes called "male hormones." Your doctor will also check for other hormones related to other common health problems that can be mistaken for PCOS, such as thyroid disease. Your doctor may also test your cholesterol levels and test you for diabetes.

Once other conditions are ruled out, you may be diagnosed with PCOS if you have at least two of the following symptoms:

- Irregular periods, including periods that come too often, not often enough, or not at all

- Signs that you have high levels of androgens:
  - Extra hair growth on your face, chin, and body (hirsutism)
  - Acne
  - Thinning of scalp hair
- Higher than normal blood levels of androgens
- Multiple cysts on one or both ovaries

How Is Polycystic Ovary Syndrome Treated?

There is no cure for PCOS, but you can manage the symptoms of PCOS. You and your doctor will work on a treatment plan based on your symptoms, your plans for having children, and your risk of long-term health problems, such as diabetes and heart disease. Many women will need a combination of treatments, including:

- Steps you can take at home to help relieve your symptoms
- Medicines

What You Can Do to Improve Your Polycystic Ovary Syndrome Symptoms

You can take steps at home to help your PCOS symptoms, including:

- **Losing weight.** Healthy eating habits and regular physical activity can help relieve PCOS-related symptoms. Losing weight may help to lower your blood glucose levels, improve the way your body uses insulin, and help your hormones reach normal levels. Even a 10 percent loss in body weight (for example, a 150-pound woman losing 15 pounds) can help make your menstrual cycle more regular and improve your chances of getting pregnant.

- **Removing hair.** You can try facial hair removal creams, laser hair removal, or electrolysis to remove excess hair. You can find hair-removal creams and products at drugstores. Procedures, such as laser hair removal or electrolysis must be done by a doctor and may not be covered by health insurance.

- **Slowing hair growth.** A prescription skin treatment (eflornithine HCl cream) can help slow down the growth rate of new hair in unwanted places.

What Types of Medicines Treat Polycystic Ovary Syndrome?

The types of medicines that treat PCOS and its symptoms include:

- **Hormonal birth control, including the pill, patch, shot, vaginal ring, and hormone intrauterine device (IUD).** For women who do not want to get pregnant, hormonal birth control can:

  - Make your menstrual cycle more regular

  - Lower your risk of endometrial cancer

  - Help improve acne and reduce extra hair on the face and body (Ask your doctor about birth control with both estrogen and progesterone.)

- **Antiandrogen medicines.** These medicines block the effect of androgens and can help reduce scalp hair loss, facial and body hair growth, and acne. They are not approved by the U.S. Food and Drug Administration (FDA) to treat PCOS symptoms. These medicines can also cause problems during pregnancy.

- **Metformin.** Metformin is often used to treat type 2 diabetes and may help some women with PCOS symptoms. It is not approved by the FDA to treat PCOS symptoms. Metformin improves insulin's ability to lower your blood sugar and can lower both insulin and androgen levels. After a few months of use, metformin may help restart ovulation, but it usually has little effect on acne and extra hair on the face or body. Research shows that metformin may have other positive effects, including lowering body mass and improving cholesterol levels.

What Are the Treatment Options for Polycystic Ovary Syndrome If You Want to Get Pregnant?

You have several options to help your chances of getting pregnant if you have PCOS:

- **Losing weight.** If you have overweight or obesity, losing weight through healthy eating and regular physical activity can help make your menstrual cycle more regular and improve your fertility.

- **Medicine.** After ruling out other causes of infertility in you and your partner, your doctor might prescribe a medicine to help you ovulate, such as clomiphene (Clomid).

- **In vitro fertilization (IVF).** IVF may be an option if medicine does not work. In IVF, your egg is fertilized with your partner's sperm in a laboratory and then placed in your uterus to implant and develop. Compared to medicine alone, IVF has higher pregnancy rates and better control over your risk of having twins and triplets (by allowing your doctor to transfer a single fertilized egg into your uterus).

- **Surgery.** Surgery is also an option, usually only if the other options do not work. The outer shell (called the "cortex") of ovaries is thickened in women with PCOS and thought to play a role in preventing spontaneous ovulation. Ovarian drilling is a surgery in which the doctor makes a few holes in the surface of your ovary using lasers or a fine needle heated with electricity. Surgery usually restores ovulation, but only for 6 to 8 months.

How Does Polycystic Ovary Syndrome Affect Pregnancy?

PCOS can cause problems during pregnancy for you and for your baby. Women with PCOS have higher rates of:

- Miscarriage
- Gestational diabetes
- Preeclampsia
- Cesarean section (C-section)

Your baby also has a higher risk of being heavy (macrosomia) and of spending more time in a neonatal intensive care unit (NICU).

How You Can Prevent Problems from Polycystic Ovary Syndrome during Pregnancy?

You can lower your risk of problems during pregnancy by:

- **Reaching a healthy weight before you get pregnant.**

- **Reaching healthy blood sugar levels before you get pregnant.** You can do this through a combination of healthy eating habits, regular physical activity, weight loss, and medicines such as metformin.

- **Taking folic acid.** Talk to your doctor about how much folic acid you need.

Is Polycystic Ovary Syndrome Linked to Other Health Problems?

Yes, studies have found links between PCOS and other health problems, including:

- **Diabetes.** More than half of women with PCOS will have diabetes or prediabetes (glucose intolerance) before the age of 40.

- **High blood pressure.** Women with PCOS are at greater risk of having high blood pressure compared with women of the same age without PCOS. High blood pressure is a leading cause of heart disease and stroke.

- **Unhealthy cholesterol.** Women with PCOS often have higher levels of LDL (bad) cholesterol and low levels of HDL (good) cholesterol. High cholesterol raises your risk of heart disease and stroke.

- **Sleep apnea.** This is when momentary and repeated stops in breathing interrupt sleep. Many women with PCOS have overweight or obesity, which can cause sleep apnea. Sleep apnea raises your risk of heart disease and diabetes.

- **Depression and anxiety.** Depression and anxiety are common among women with PCOS.

- **Endometrial cancer.** Problems with ovulation, obesity, insulin resistance, and diabetes (all common in women with PCOS) increase the risk of developing cancer of the endometrium (lining of the uterus or womb).

Researchers do not know if PCOS causes some of these problems, if these problems cause PCOS, or if there are other conditions that cause PCOS and other health problems.

Chapter 46

Primary Ovarian Insufficiency

What Is Primary Ovarian Insufficiency?

Healthcare providers use the term "primary ovarian insufficiency" (POI) when a woman's ovaries stop working normally before she is 40 years of age.

Many women naturally experience reduced fertility when they are around 40-years-old. This age may mark the start of irregular menstrual periods that signal the onset of menopause. For women with POI, irregular periods and reduced fertility occur before the age of 40, sometimes as early as the teenage years.

In the past, POI used to be called "premature menopause" or "premature ovarian failure," but those terms do not accurately describe what happens in a woman with POI. A woman who has gone through menopause will never have another normal period and cannot get pregnant. A woman with POI may still have periods, even though they might not come regularly, and she may still get pregnant.

This chapter contains text excerpted from "Primary Ovarian Insufficiency (POI): Condition Information," *Eunice Kennedy Shriver* National Institute of Child Health and Human Development (NICHD), December 1, 2016. Reviewed September 2019.

Who Is at Risk for Primary Ovarian Insufficiency?

Several factors can affect a woman's risk for POI:

- **Family history.** Women who have a mother or sister with POI are more likely to have the disorder. About 10 to 20 percent of women with POI have a family history of the condition.

- **Genes.** Some changes to genes and genetic conditions put women at higher risk for POI. Research suggests that these disorders and conditions cause as much as 28 percent of POI cases. For example:

  - Women who carry a variation of the gene for fragile X syndrome are at higher risk for fragile X-associated POI (FXPOI). Fragile X syndrome is the most common inherited form of intellectual and developmental disability, but women with FXPOI do not have fragile X syndrome itself. Instead, they have a change or mutation in the same gene that causes Fragile X syndrome, and this change is linked to FXPOI.

  - Most women who have Turner syndrome develop POI. Turner syndrome is a condition in which a girl or woman is partially or completely missing an X chromosome. Most women are XX, meaning they have two X chromosomes. Women with Turner syndrome are X_0, meaning one of the X chromosomes is missing.

- **Other factors.** Autoimmune diseases, viral infections, chemotherapy, and other treatments also may put a woman at higher risk of POI.

What Are the Symptoms of Primary Ovarian Insufficiency?

The first sign of POI is usually menstrual irregularities or missed periods, which is sometimes called "amenorrhea."

In addition, some women with POI have symptoms similar to those experienced by women who are going through natural menopause, including:

- Hot flashes

- Night sweats

- Irritability

- Poor concentration

- Decreased sex drive

- Pain during sex

- Vaginal dryness

For many women with POI, trouble getting pregnant or infertility is the first symptom they experience and is what leads them to visit their healthcare provider. This is sometimes called "occult" (hidden) or "early POI."

What Causes Primary Ovarian Insufficiency

In most cases, the exact cause of POI is unknown. Research shows that POI is related to problems with the follicles—the small sacs in the ovaries in which eggs grow and mature.

Follicles start out as microscopic seeds called "primordial follicles." These seeds are not yet follicles, but they can grow into them. Normally, a woman is born with approximately 2 million primordial follicles, typically enough to last until she goes through natural menopause, usually around age 50.

For a woman with POI, there are problems with the follicles:

- **Follicle depletion.** A woman with follicle depletion runs out of working follicles earlier than normal or expected. In the case of POI, the woman runs out of working follicles before natural menopause occurs around age 50. As of now, there is no safe way for scientists to make primordial follicles.

- **Follicle dysfunction.** A woman with follicle dysfunction has follicles remaining in her ovaries, but the follicles are not working properly. Scientists do not have a safe and effective way to make follicles start working normally again.

Although the exact cause is unknown in a majority of cases, some causes of follicle depletion and dysfunction have been identified:

- **Genetic and chromosomal disorders.** Disorders such as fragile X syndrome and Turner syndrome can cause follicle depletion.

- **Low number of follicles.** Some women are born with fewer primordial follicles, so they have a smaller pool of follicles to use throughout their lives. Even though only one mature follicle releases an egg each month, less mature follicles usually develop along with that mature follicle and egg. Scientists do not understand exactly why this happens, but these "supporting" follicles seem to help the mature follicle function normally. If these extra follicles are missing, the main follicle will not mature and release an egg properly.

- **Autoimmune diseases.** Typically, the body's immune cells protect the body from invading bacteria and viruses. However, in autoimmune diseases, immune cells turn on healthy tissue. In the case of POI, the immune system may damage developing follicles in the ovaries. It could also damage the glands that make the hormones needed for the ovaries and follicles to work properly. Several studies suggest that about one-fifth of women with POI have an autoimmune disease.

  - **Thyroiditis** is an autoimmune disorder most commonly associated with the POI. It is an inflammation of the thyroid gland, which makes hormones that control metabolism, or the pace of body processes.

  - **Addison disease** is also associated with POI. Addison disease affects the adrenal glands, which produce hormones that help the body respond to physical stress, such as illness and injury; the hormones also affect ovary function. A small percentage of women with POI have Addison disease.

- **Chemotherapy or radiation therapy.** These strong treatments for cancer may damage the genetic material in cells, including follicle cells.

- **Metabolic disorders.** These disorders affect the body's ability to create, store, and use the energy it needs. For example, galactosemia affects how your body processes galactose, a type of sugar. A majority of women with galactosemia also have POI.

- **Toxins.** Cigarette smoke, chemicals, and pesticides can speed up follicle depletion. In addition, viruses have been shown to affect follicle function.

How Do Healthcare Providers Diagnose Primary Ovarian Insufficiency?

The key signs of POI are:

- Missed or irregular periods for four months, typically after having had regular periods for a while

- High levels of follicle-stimulating hormone (FSH)

- Low levels of estrogen

If a woman is younger than age 40 and begins having irregular periods or stops having periods for 4 months or longer, her healthcare provider may take these steps to diagnose the problem:

- **Do a pregnancy test.** This test will rule out an unexpected pregnancy as the reason for missed periods.

- **Do a physical exam.** During the physical exam, the healthcare provider looks for signs of other disorders. In some cases, the presence of these other disorders will rule out POI. Or, if the other disorders are associated with POI, such as Addison disease, a healthcare provider will know that POI may be present.

- **Collect blood.** The healthcare provider will collect your blood and send it to a lab, where a technician will run several tests, including:

  - **Follicle-stimulating hormone test.** FSH signals the ovaries to make estrogen, sometimes called the "female hormone" because women need high levels of it for fertility and overall health. If the ovaries are not working properly, as is the case in POI, the level of FSH in the blood increases. The healthcare provider may do two FSH tests, at least a month apart. If the FSH level in both tests is as high as it is in women who have gone through menopause, then POI is likely.

  - **Luteinizing hormone test.** LH signals a mature follicle to release an egg. Women with POI have high LH levels, more evidence that the follicles are not functioning normally.

  - **Estrogen test.** In women with POI, estrogen levels are usually low, because the ovaries are not functioning properly in their role as estrogen producers.

  - **Karyotype test.** This test looks at all 46 of your chromosomes to check for abnormalities. The karyotype test could reveal genetic changes in the structure of chromosomes that might be associated with POI and other health problems.

- **Do a pelvic ultrasound.** In this test, the healthcare provider uses a sound wave (sonogram) machine to create and view pictures of the inside of a woman's pelvic area. A sonogram can show whether or not the ovaries are enlarged or have multiple follicles.

The healthcare provider will also ask questions about a woman's medical history. She or he may ask about:

- A blood relative with POI or its symptoms

- A blood relative with fragile X syndrome or an unidentified intellectual or developmental disability

- Ovarian surgery

- Radiation or chemotherapy treatment

- Pelvic inflammatory disease (PID) or other sexually transmitted infections (STIs)

- An endocrine disorder, such as diabetes

If they do not do tests to rule out POI, some healthcare providers might assume missed periods are related to stress. However, this approach is problematic because it will lead to a delay in diagnosis; further evaluation is needed.

What Disorders or Conditions Associated with Primary Ovarian Insufficiency?

Because POI results in lower levels of certain hormones, women with POI are at greater risk for a number of health conditions, including:

- **Osteoporosis.** The hormone estrogen helps keep bones strong. Without enough estrogen, women with POI often develop osteoporosis. Osteoporosis is a bone disease that causes weak, brittle bones that are more likely to break and fracture.

- **Low thyroid function.** This problem is also called "hypothyroidism." The thyroid is a gland that makes hormones that control your body's metabolism and energy level. Low levels of the hormones made by the thyroid can affect your metabolism and can cause very low energy and mental sluggishness. Cold feet and constipation are also features of low thyroid function. Some women with POI also have low thyroid function.

- **Anxiety and depression.** Hormonal changes caused by POI can contribute to anxiety or lead to depression. Women diagnosed with POI can be shy, anxious in social settings, and may have low self-esteem more often than women without POI. It is possible that depression may contribute to POI.

- **Cardiovascular disease (CVD).** Lower levels of estrogen, as seen in POI, can affect the muscles lining the arteries and can increase the buildup of cholesterol in the arteries. Both factors increase the risk of atherosclerosis—or hardening of the arteries—which can slow or block the flow of blood to the heart. Women with POI have higher rates of illness and death from heart disease than do women without POI.

- **Dry eye syndrome and ocular surface disease.** Some women with POI have one of these conditions, which cause discomfort and may lead to blurred vision. If not treated, these conditions can cause permanent eye damage.

Addison disease is also associated with the POI. Addison disease is a life-threatening condition that affects the adrenal glands, which produce hormones that help the body respond to physical stress, such as illness and injury. These hormones also affect ovary function. A small percentage of women with POI have Addison disease.

What Are the Treatments for Primary Ovarian Insufficiency?

There is no proven treatment to restore normal function to a woman's ovaries. But, there are treatments for some of the symptoms of POI, as well as treatments and behaviors to reduce health risks and conditions associated with the POI.

It is also important to note that between 5 and 10 percent of women with POI get pregnant without medical intervention after they are diagnosed with POI. Some research suggests that these women go into what is known as "spontaneous remission" of POI, meaning that the ovaries begin to function normally on their own. When the ovaries are working properly, fertility is restored and the women can get pregnant

Hormone Replacement Therapy

Hormone replacement therapy (HRT) is the most common treatment for women with POI. It gives the body estrogen and other hormones that the ovaries are not making. HRT improves sexual health and decreases the risks for cardiovascular disease (CVD) (including heart attacks, stroke, and high blood pressure) and osteoporosis.

If a woman with POI begins HRT, she is expected to start having regular periods again. In addition, HRT is expected to reduce other symptoms, such as hot flashes and night sweats, and help maintain bone health. HRT will not prevent pregnancy, and evidence suggests it might improve pregnancy rates for women with POI by lowering high levels of luteinizing hormone—which stimulates ovulation—to normal in some women.

Hormone replacement therapy is usually a combination of an estrogen and a progestin. A progestin is a form of progesterone. Sometimes, the combination might also include testosterone, although this approach is controversial. HRT comes in several forms: pills, creams, gels, patches that stick onto the skin, an intrauterine device, or a vaginal ring. Estradiol is the natural form of human estrogen. The optimal method of providing estradiol to women with POI is by a skin patch or vaginal ring. These methods are linked with a lower risk of potentially fatal blood clots developing. Most women require a dose of 100 micrograms of estradiol per day. It is important to take a progestin along with estradiol to balance out the effect of estrogen on the lining of the womb. Women who do not take a progestin along with estradiol are at increased risk of developing endometrial cancer. The progestin with the best evidence available to support use in women with POI is 10 mg of medroxyprogesterone acetate by mouth per day for the first 12 calendar days of each month.

A healthcare provider may suggest that a woman with POI take HRT until she is about 50 years old, the age at which menopause usually begins.

After that time, she should talk with her healthcare provider about stopping the treatment because of risks associated with using this type of therapy in the years after the normal age of menopause.

Is it Safe for Women with Primary Ovarian Insufficiency to Take Hormone Replacement Therapy?

In general, HRT treatment for women with POI is safe and is associated with only minimal side effects. Women with POI take HRT to replace hormones their bodies would normally be making if they did not have POI.

The HRT taken by women with POI is different from the hormone therapies taken by women who are going through or have gone through natural menopause, which are often called "menopausal" or "post-menopausal hormone therapy" (PMHT).

A large, long-term study—called the "Women's Health Initiative"—examined the effects of a specific type of PMHT, taken for more than 5 years, by women ages 50 to 79 who had already gone through menopause. This study showed that PMHT was associated with an increased risk of stroke, blood clots, heart disease, heart attacks, and breast cancer in these women.

These results do not apply to young women with POI who take HRT. The type and amount of HRT prescribed to women with POI is different from the PMHT taken by older women.

A woman should talk to her healthcare provider if she has questions about HRT as a treatment for POI. Also, she should tell her healthcare provider about any side effects she experiences while taking HRT. There are many different types of HRT. Women should work with their healthcare providers to find out the best type of treatment.

Calcium and Vitamin D Supplements

Because women with POI are at higher risk for osteoporosis, they should get at least 1,200 to 1,500 mg of elemental calcium and 1000 international units (IU) of vitamin D, which helps the body absorb calcium, every day. These nutrients are important for bone health. A healthcare provider may do a bone mineral density test to check for bone loss.

Regular Physical Activity and Healthy Body Weight

Weight-bearing physical activity, such as walking, jogging, and stair climbing, helps build bone strength and prevents osteoporosis. Maintaining a healthy body weight and getting regular physical activity are also important for reducing the risk of heart disease. These factors can affect cholesterol levels, which in turn can change the risk for heart disease.

Treatments for Associated Conditions

Primary ovarian insufficiency is associated with other health conditions, including (but not limited to) Addison disease, fragile X permutation, thyroid dysfunction, depression, anxiety, and certain other genetic, metabolic, and autoimmune disorders.

Women who have POI, as well as one of these associated conditions, will require additional treatment for the associated condition. In some cases, treatment involves medication or hormone therapy. Other types of treatments might also be needed.

Emotional Support

For many women who experience infertility, including those with POI, feelings of loss are common. In one study, almost 9 out of 10 women reported feeling moderate to severe emotional distress when they learned of their POI diagnosis. Several organizations offer help finding these types of professionals.

Primary Ovarian Insufficiency in Teens

Receiving a diagnosis of POI can be emotionally difficult for teenagers and their parents. A teen may have a similar emotional experience as an adult who receives the diagnosis, but there are many aspects of the experience that are unique to being a teenager. It is important for parents, the teenager, and healthcare providers to work closely together to ensure that the teenager gets the right treatment and maintains her emotional and physical health in the long term. There are resources to provide advice and support for parents, teenagers, and healthcare providers.

Chapter 47

Precocious Puberty and Delayed Puberty

What Is Puberty?

Puberty is the body's natural process of sexual maturation. Puberty trigger lies in a small part of the brain called the "hypothalamus," a gland that secretes a gonadotropin-releasing hormone (GnRH). GnRH stimulates the pituitary gland, a pea-sized organ connected to the bottom of the hypothalamus, to emit two hormones: luteinizing hormone (LH) and follicle-stimulating hormone (FSH). These two hormones signal the female and male sex organs (ovaries and testes, respectively) to begin releasing the appropriate sex hormones, including estrogens and testosterone, which launch the other signs of puberty in the body.

What Are the Symptoms of Puberty?
In Girls

The signs of puberty include:

- Growth of pubic and other body hair

- Growth spurt

This chapter includes text excerpted from "Puberty and Precocious Puberty: Condition Information," *Eunice Kennedy Shriver* National Institute of Child Health and Human Development (NICHD), December 1, 2016. Reviewed September 2019.

- Breast development

- Onset of menstruation (after puberty is well advanced)

- Acne

In Boys

The signs of puberty include:

- Growth of pubic hair, other body hair, and facial hair

- Enlargement of testicles and penis

- Muscle growth

- Growth spurt

- Acne

- Deepening of the voice

How Do Healthcare Providers Diagnose Puberty?

To identify whether a child is entering puberty, a pediatrician (a physician specializing in the treatment of children) will carefully examine the following:

- In girls, the growth of pubic hair and breasts

- In boys, the increase in size of the testicles and penis and the growth of pubic hair

The pediatrician will compare what she or he finds against the Tanner scale, a five-point scale that gauges the extent of puberty development in children.

What Is Precocious Puberty?

In the majority of cases of precocious puberty, no underlying cause can be identified. When a cause cannot be identified, the condition is called "idiopathic precocious puberty."

Sometimes the cause is an abnormality involving the brain. In other children, the signs of puberty occur because of a problem such as a tumor or genetic abnormality in the ovaries, testes, or adrenal glands, causing overproduction of sex hormones.

How Many Children Are at Risk of Precocious Puberty?

Precocious puberty is rare, meaning it affects about 1 percent or less of the United States population. Girls are more affected than boys. One study suggests that African American girls have some early breast development or some early pubic hair more often than white girls or Hispanic girls. There is a greater chance of being affected by precocious puberty if a child is:

- Female

- African American

- Obese

Types of Precocious Puberty

Precocious puberty can be divided into two categories, depending on where in the body the abnormality occurs—central precocious puberty and peripheral precocious puberty.

Central Precocious Puberty

This type of early puberty, also known as "gonadotropin-dependent precocious puberty," occurs when the abnormality is located in the brain. The brain signals the pituitary gland to begin puberty at an early age. Central precocious puberty is the most common form of precocious puberty and affects many more girls than boys.

The causes of central precocious puberty include:

- Brain tumors

- Prior radiation to the brain

- Prior infection of the brain

- Other brain abnormalities

Peripheral Precocious Puberty

This form of early puberty is also called "gonadotropin-independent precocious puberty." In peripheral precocious puberty, the abnormality is not in the brain but in the testicles, ovaries, or adrenal glands, causing overproduction of sex hormones, such as testosterone and estrogens.

411

Peripheral precocious puberty may be caused by:

- Tumors of the ovary, testis, or adrenal gland

- In boys, tumors that secrete a hormone called "hCG," or "human chorionic gonadotropin"

- Certain rare genetic syndromes, such as McCune-Albright syndrome or familial male precocious puberty

- Severe hypothyroidism, in which the thyroid gland secretes abnormally low levels of hormones

- Disorders of the adrenal gland, such as congenital adrenal hyperplasia

- Exposure of the child to medicines or creams that contain estrogens or androgens

Diagnosis of Precocious Puberty

After giving a child a complete physical examination and analyzing his or her medical history, a healthcare provider may perform tests to diagnose precocious puberty, including:

- A **blood test** to check the level of hormones, such as the gonadotropins (LH and FSH), estradiol, testosterone, dehydroepiandrosterone sulfate (DHEAS), and thyroid hormones

- A **gonadotropin-releasing hormone agonist (GnRHa) stimulation test** can tell whether a child's precocious puberty is gonadotropin-dependent or gonadotropin-independent

- Measuring **blood 17-hydroxyprogesterone** to test for congenital adrenal hyperplasia

- A **"bone age" x-ray** to determine if bones are growing at a normal rate

The healthcare provider may also use imaging techniques to rule out a tumor or other organ abnormality as a cause. These imaging methods may include:

- **Ultrasound (sonography) to examine the gonads.** An ultrasound painlessly creates an image on a computer screen of blood vessels and tissues, allowing a healthcare provider to monitor organs and blood flow in real time.

- A **magnetic resonance imaging (MRI) scan** of the brain and pituitary gland using an instrument that produces detailed images of organs and bodily structures.

Treatment of Precocious Puberty

There are a number of reasons to treat precocious puberty.

Treatment for precocious puberty can help stop puberty until the child is closer to the normal time for sexual development. One reason to consider treating precocious puberty is that rapid growth and bone maturation, caused by precocious puberty, can prevent a child from reaching his or her full height potential. Children grow rapidly in height during puberty and reach their final adult height after puberty. Children who go through puberty too early may not reach their full adult height potential because their growth stops too soon.

Another reason to consider treating precocious puberty is that a young child may not be psychologically ready for the physical and hormonal changes that occur in puberty.

However, not all children with precocious puberty require treatment, particularly if the onset of puberty is only slightly early. The goal of treatment is to prevent the production of sex hormones to prevent the early halt of growth, short stature in adulthood, emotional effects, social problems, and problems with libido (especially in boys).

If precocious puberty is caused by a specific medical problem, treating the underlying problem can often stop the progression of precocious puberty. In addition, precocious puberty can often be stopped by medical treatment to block the hormones that cause puberty. For example, medications called "GnRHa" are used to treat central precocious puberty. These medications, some of which are injected, suppress production of LH and FSH.

What Is Delayed Puberty?

Many children with delayed puberty will eventually go through an otherwise normal puberty, just at a late age. Sometimes, this delay occurs because the child is just maturing more slowly than average, a condition called "constitutional delay of puberty." This condition often runs in families.

Puberty can be delayed in children who have not gotten proper nutrition due to long-term illnesses. Also, some young girls who undergo intense physical training for a sport, such as running or gymnastics, start puberty later than normal.

In other cases, the delay in puberty is not just due to slow maturation but occurs because the child has a long-term medical condition known as "hypogonadism," in which the sex glands (the testes in men and the ovaries in women) produce few or no hormones.

In primary hypogonadism, the problem lies in the ovaries or testes, which fail to make sex hormones normally. Some causes include:

- Genetic disorders, especially Turner syndrome (in women) and Klinefelter syndrome (in men)

- Certain autoimmune disorders

- Developmental disorders

- Radiation or chemotherapy

- Infection

- Surgery

Treatment of Delayed Puberty

With delayed puberty or hypogonadism, treatment varies with the origin of the problem but may involve:

- In males, testosterone injections, skin patches, or gel

- In females, estrogen and/or progesterone given as pills or skin patches

Part Seven

Other Disorders of Endocrine and Metabolic Functioning

Chapter 48

Inborn Errors of Metabolism

Chapter Contents

Section 48.1

Understanding Inborn Errors of Metabolism

This section includes text excerpted from "About Inborn Errors of Metabolism," National Human Genome Research Institute (NHGRI), February 23, 2013. Reviewed September 2019.

Metabolism is a sequence of chemical reactions that take place in cells in the body. These reactions are responsible for the breakdown of nutrients and the generation of energy in our bodies. Inborn errors of metabolism (IEM) are a group of disorders that causes a block in a metabolic pathway leading to clinically significant consequences.

What Are the Different Forms of Inborn Errors of Metabolism?

The different IEM are usually named for the enzyme that is not working properly. For example, if the enzyme carbamoyl phosphate synthetase 1 (CPS1) is not working, the IEM is called "CPS1 deficiency."

Table 48.1. Categories of Inborn Errors of Metabolism

Inborn Errors of Metabolism	Examples
Urea cycle disorders	Ornithine transcarbamylase deficiency, citrullinemia, argininosuccinic aciduria, argininemia
Organic acidemias	Propionic acidemia, methylmalonic aciduria, isovaleric acidemia, glutaric acidemia, maple syrup urine disease
Fatty acid oxidation defects	Medium-chain acyl-CoA dehydrogenase deficiency, carnitine palmitoyltransferase 1 deficiency, long chain hydroxyacyl-CoA dehydrogenase deficiency
Amino acidopathies	Tyrosinemia, phenylketonuria, homocystinuria
Carbohydrate disorders	Galactosemia, fructosemia
Mitochondrial disorders	MELAS, MERFF, pyruvate dehydrogenase deficiency

What Causes the Inborn Errors of Metabolism

The IEM are caused by mutations (or alterations) in the genes that tell our cells how to make the enzymes and cofactors for metabolism.

A mutation causes a gene to not function at all or not to function as well as it should. Most often these altered genes are inherited from parents, but they may also occur spontaneously.

How Are the Different Forms of Inborn Errors of Metabolism Inherited?

Humans have two copies of most genes, with one copy inherited from our mother and one copy inherited from our father. This is not the case for the genes that are on our sex chromosomes (the "X" and "Y" chromosomes). These are different in men and women: men have only one X chromosome, and, therefore, only one copy of the genes on that chromosome, while women have two X chromosomes and, therefore, have two copies of the genes on that chromosome. A father passes on his X chromosome to all of his daughters and his Y chromosome on to all of his sons. A mother passes on an X chromosome to each child.

What Is the Chance of Having Inborn Errors of Metabolism If Someone Else in the Family Has It?

The chance that someone else in the family has the same IEM as their relative depends on the inheritance pattern of the IEM, whether the at-risk family member is male or female, and the rest of the family history (how many relatives have been diagnosed with the disorder already and whether genetic testing has been performed in other relatives). In some cases, the age of the at-risk family member and whether or not they have shown any signs or symptoms of the disorder is helpful in estimating the chances that they also have the disorder.

Talk to your metabolic specialist and/or genetic counselor to determine those relatives who may be at risk for having an IEM and for coordination of genetic testing, when appropriate.

What Are the Symptoms of Inborn Errors of Metabolism and How Are They Diagnosed?

In general, the earlier someone develops symptoms of an IEM, the more severe their disorder. The severity of symptoms is generally based on:

- The position of the defective enzyme within the metabolic pathway

- Whether or not there is any functional enzyme or cofactor being produced

However, other environmental and genetic factors may play a role in determining the severity of symptoms for a given patient.

Inborn errors of metabolism are multisystemic diseases and thus patients may present with a variety of symptoms, many of which depend on the specific metabolic pathways involved. Some findings in patients with IEM may include elevated acid levels in the blood, low blood sugar, high blood ammonia, abnormal liver function tests, and blood cell abnormalities. Certain patients may also have neurologic abnormalities, such as seizures and developmental delays. Growth may also be affected.

How Are Inborn Errors of Metabolism Treated?

Treatment of IEM is tailored to the specific disorder once a diagnosis is made. In general, the goals of treatment are to minimize or eliminate the buildup of toxic metabolites that result from the block in metabolism while maintaining growth and development. This may be accomplished by special modified diets, supplements and medications.

A doctor who specializes in metabolic disorders should see IEM patients on a regular basis. Severely affected patients will likely be seen on a more frequent basis than mild or moderately affected patients.

Section 48.2

Galactosemia

This section includes text excerpted from "Galactosemia," Genetic and Rare Diseases Information Center (GARD), National Center for Advancing Translational Sciences (NCATS), October 11, 2018.

What Is Galactosemia?

Galactosemia, which means "galactose in the blood," refers to a group of inherited disorders that impair the body's ability to process and produce energy from a sugar called "galactose." When people with galactosemia injest foods or liquids containing galactose, undigested sugars build up in the blood. Galactose is present in many foods, including all dairy products (milk and anything made from milk), many baby formulas, and some fruits and vegetables. The impaired ability to process galactose can be due to the deficiency of any of 3 enzymes, caused by mutations in different genes. There are three main types of galactosemia which are distinguished based on their genetic causes, signs and symptoms, and severity:

- **Classic galactosemia (type 1)**—the most common and severe type, caused by mutations in the *GALT* gene, and characterized by a complete deficiency of an enzyme called "galactose-1-phosphate uridyl transferase" (GALT). Early signs and symptoms include liver dysfunction, susceptibility to infections, failure to thrive, and cataracts. These can usually be prevented or improved by early diagnosis and treatment, but other progressive or long-term problems are common despite treatment. These include intellectual deficits, movement disorders, and premature ovarian failure (in females).

- **Galactokinase deficiency (type 2)**—caused by mutations in the *GALK1* gene and characterized by a deficiency of the enzyme galactokinase 1. This type typically causes only the development of cataracts, which may be prevented or resolved with treatment. Rarely, this type causes pseudotumor cerebri (a condition which mimics the symptoms of a large brain tumor when no brain tumor is present).

- **Galactose epimerase deficiency (type 3)**—caused by mutations in the *GALE* gene and characterized by a deficiency of the enzyme UDP-galactose-4-epimerase. Symptoms and severity of this type depend on whether the deficiency is confined to certain types of blood cells or is present in all tissues. Some people with this type have no signs or symptoms, while others have symptoms similar to those with classic galactosemia. Like in classic galactosemia, many symptoms can be prevented or improved with treatment.

There is also a "variant" of classic galactosemia called "Duarte variant galactosemia," in which a person has mutations in the *GALT* gene but has only partial deficiency of the enzyme. Infants with this form may have jaundice, which resolves when switched to a low-galactose formula. Some studies have found that people with this form are at increased risk for mild neurodevelopmental problems, but other studies have found there is no increased risk. The risk may depend on the extent of the deficiency.

Inheritance of all types of galactosemia is autosomal recessive. The diagnosis may be suspected based on symptoms or results of newborn screening tests, and can be confirmed by measuring enzyme activity and genetic testing. Depending on the type of galactosemia, treatment may involve removing galactose from the diet (as soon as the disorder is suspected), calcium supplementation, and individualized care for any additional symptoms. The long-term outlook for people with galactosemia varies depending on the type, symptoms present, and commitment to the diet.

Symptoms of Galactosemia

For most diseases, symptoms will vary from person to person. People with the same disease may not have all the symptoms listed.

Diagnosis of Galactosemia

Making a diagnosis for a genetic or rare disease can often be challenging. Healthcare professionals typically look at a person's medical history, symptoms, physical exam, and laboratory test results in order to make a diagnosis. The following resources provide information relating to diagnosis and testing for this condition. If you have questions about getting a diagnosis, you should contact a healthcare professional.

Testing Resources

- The Genetic Testing Registry (GTR) provides information about the genetic tests for this condition. The intended audience for the GTR is healthcare providers and researchers. Patients and consumers with specific questions about a genetic test should contact a healthcare provider or a genetics professional.

Newborn Screening

- The Newborn Screening Coding and Terminology Guide has information on the standard codes used for newborn screening tests. Using these standards helps compare data across different laboratories.

Section 48.3

Maple Syrup Urine Disease

This section includes text excerpted from "Maple Syrup Urine Disease," U.S. Social Security Administration (SSA), March 28, 2018.

What Is Maple Syrup Urine Disease?

Maple syrup urine disease (MSUD) is an inherited metabolic disorder in which the body is unable to process certain protein building blocks (amino acids) properly. Because these amino acids are not metabolized, they, along with their various byproducts, abnormally accumulate in the cells and fluids of the body. The condition gets its name from the distinctive sweet odor of the affected infant's earwax, sweat and urine. Mutations in the branched-chain keto acid dehydrogenase E1, alpha polypeptide (BCKDHA), branched-chain keto acid dehydrogenase E1, beta polypeptide (BCKDHB), dihydrolipoamide branched chain transacylase E2 (DBT), and *dihydrolipoamide dehydrogenase (DLD)* genes cause MSUD. Because of an enzyme defect, individuals with this condition cannot break down the branched chained amino acids (BCAA) leucine, isoleucine, and valine. This leads to a build-up of these chemicals in the blood. There are four common forms:

- Classic MSUD that occurs in infants, usually in the first two weeks of life

- Intermediate MSUD

- Intermittent MSUD

- Thiamine-responsive MSUD

In the classic form, the disorder presents after the infant has had milk containing protein. This causes an increase in the offending amino acids which become toxic to the brain. Early signs and symptoms are poor feeding, vomiting, lethargy, hypo or hypertonia, dystonia, seizures and encephalopathy which can lead to early death or permanent neurologic damage. Later in infancy or childhood, developmental delays are noted. In the intermittent form, MSUD can damage the brain during times of physical stress (such as infection, fever, or not eating for a long time) which leads to metabolic decompensation.

Diagnosis of Maple Syrup Urine Disease

Diagnostic testing for MSUD includes blood and urine amino acid tests that measure the levels of leucine, isoleucine, alloisoleucine, and valine. If MSUD is found, there will be signs of ketosis and excess acid (acidosis). These are measured in the usual newborn screening test.

Onset and Progression

If the disease is not treated, MSUD can lead to seizures, coma, and death at any age. In the intermittent type, symptoms become apparent later in infancy or childhood and are typically milder. Long-term sequelae may include developmental delays, learning problems, seizures, and motor difficulties. Even with dietary treatment, stressful situations and illnesses can still cause high levels of certain amino acids. Death may occur during these episodes.

Treatment of Maple Syrup Urine Disease

If the disease is not treated, MSUD can lead to seizures, coma, and death at any age. In the intermittent type, symptoms become apparent later in infancy or childhood and are typically milder. Long-term sequelae may include developmental delays, learning problems, seizures, and motor difficulties. Even with dietary treatment, stressful situations and illnesses can still cause high levels of certain amino acids. Death may occur during these episodes.

Section 48.4

Phenylketonuria

This section includes text excerpted from "Phenylketonuria (PKU): Condition Information," *Eunice Kennedy Shriver* National Institute of Child Health and Human Development (NICHD), December 1, 2016. Reviewed September 2019.

What Is Phenylketonuria?

Phenylketonuria, often called "PKU," is an inherited disorder that can cause intellectual and developmental disabilities (IDDs) if not treated. In PKU, the body cannot process a portion of a protein called "phenylalanine," which is in all foods containing protein. If the phenylalanine level gets too high, the brain can become damaged.

All children born in the U.S. hospitals are tested routinely for PKU soon after birth, making it easier to diagnose and treat affected children early.

Children and adults who are treated early and consistently develop normally.

Depending on the level of phenylalanine and tolerance for phenylalanine in the diet, PKU is classified into two different types: classic, which is the severe form, and moderate. Therefore, each patient needs an individualized treatment plan. Some people may benefit from a medication called "sapropterin dihydrochloride" (brand name Kuvan®) that treats the disorder.

Who Is at Risk for Phenylketonuria?

Some genetic disorders, including PKU, develop more often among people whose ancestors come from a particular region. People originally from the same region frequently share versions of their genes that have been passed down from common ancestors. These can include genes with mutations or changes that can cause PKU.

In the United States, PKU is most common in people of European or Native American ancestry. It is much less common among people of African, Hispanic, or Asian ancestry.

What Are Common Symptoms of Phenylketonuria?

Children with untreated PKU appear normal at birth. But, by age three to six months, they begin to lose interest in their surroundings.

By age one year, children are developmentally delayed and their skin has less pigmentation than someone without the condition. If people with PKU do not restrict the phenylalanine in their diet, they develop severe intellectual and developmental disabilities.

Other symptoms include:

- Behavioral or social problems

- Seizures, shaking, or jerking movements in the arms and legs

- Stunted or slow growth

- Skin rashes, such as eczema

- Small head size, called "microcephaly"

- A musty odor in urine, breath, or skin that is a result of the extra phenylalanine in the body

- Fair skin and blue eyes, due to the body's failure to transform phenylalanine into melanin, the pigment responsible for a person's coloring

What Causes Phenylketonuria

Phenylketonuria is caused by mutations in the gene that helps make an enzyme called "phenylalanine hydroxylase," or "PAH." This enzyme is needed to convert the amino acid phenylalanine into other substances the body needs. When this gene, known as the *"PAH* gene," is defective, the body cannot break down phenylalanine.

Amino acids help build protein, but phenylalanine can cause harm when it builds up in a person's body. In particular, nerve cells in the brain are sensitive to phenylalanine.

Many different PAH mutations result in problems with breaking down phenylalanine. Some mutations cause PKU, others cause non-phenylketonuria hyperphenylalaninemia and others are silent mutations that do not have an effect.

Is Phenylketonuria Inherited?

Phenylketonuria is inherited from a person's parents. The disorder is passed down in a recessive pattern, which means that for a child to develop PKU, both parents have to contribute a mutated version of the *PAH* gene. If both parents have PKU, their child will have PKU as well.

Sometimes, a parent does not have PKU but is a carrier, which means the parent carries a mutated *PAH* gene. If only one parent carries the mutated gene, the child will not develop PKU.

Even if both parents carry the mutated *PAH* gene, their child still may not develop PKU. This is because a child's parents each carry two versions of the *PAH* gene, only one of which they will pass on during conception.

If both of a child's parents are carriers, there is a 25 percent chance that each parent will pass on the normal *PAH* gene. In this case, the child will not have the disorder. Conversely, there is also a 25 percent chance that the carrier parents will both pass along the mutated gene, causing the child to have PKU. However, there is a 50 percent chance that a child will inherit one normal gene from one parent and one abnormal gene from the other, making the child a carrier.

What Are Common Treatments for Phenylketonuria?

There is no cure for PKU, but treatment can prevent intellectual disabilities and other health problems. A person with PKU should receive treatment at a medical center that specializes in the disorder.

The Phenylketonuria Diet

People with PKU need to follow a diet that limits foods with phenylalanine. The diet should be followed carefully and be started as soon after birth as possible. In the past, experts believed that it was safe for people to stop following the diet as they got older. However, they recommend that people with PKU stay on the diet throughout their lives for better physical and mental health.

It is especially important for a pregnant woman with PKU to strictly follow the low-phenylalanine diet throughout her pregnancy to ensure the healthy development of her infant.

People with PKU need to avoid various high-protein foods, including:

- Milk and cheese

- Eggs

- Nuts

- Soybeans

- Beans

- Chicken, beef, or pork

- Fish

- Peas

- Beer

People with PKU also need to avoid the sweetener aspartame, which is in some foods, drinks, medications, and vitamins. Aspartame releases phenylalanine when it is digested, so it raises the level of phenylalanine in a person's blood.

Often, people with PKU also have to limit their intake of lower-protein foods, such as certain fruits and vegetables. However, a PKU diet can include low-protein noodles and other special products.

The amount of phenylalanine that is safe to consume differs for each person. Therefore, a person with PKU needs to work with a healthcare professional to develop an individualized diet. The goal is to eat only the amount of phenylalanine necessary for healthy growth and body processes but not any extra. Frequent blood tests and doctor visits are necessary to help determine how well the diet is working. Some relaxation of the diet may be possible as a child gets older, but the recommendation is lifelong adherence to the diet. Following the diet is especially important during pregnancy.

However, the PKU diet can be very challenging. Getting support from friends and family or a support group can help. Sticking with the diet ensures better functioning and improved overall health.

A Phenylketonuria Formula

People who follow the PKU diet will not get enough essential nutrients from food. Therefore, they must drink a special formula.

A newborn who is diagnosed with PKU should receive special infant formula. The formula may be mixed with a small amount of breast milk or regular infant formula to make sure the child gets enough phenylalanine for normal development but not enough to cause harm.

Older children and adults receive a different formula to meet their nutritional needs. This formula should be consumed every day throughout a person's life.

In addition to the formula, healthcare professionals may recommend other supplements. For example, fish oil may be recommended to help with fine motor coordination and other aspects of development.

Medication for Phenylketonuria

The U.S. Food and Drug Administration (FDA) has approved the drug sapropterin dihydrochloride (Kuvan®) for the treatment of PKU. Kuvan® is a form of BH4, which is a substance in the body that helps break down phenylalanine. However, having too little BH4 is only one reason a person may not break down phenylalanine. Therefore, Kuvan® only helps some people reduce the phenylalanine in their blood. Even if the medication helps, it will not decrease the phenylalanine to the desired amount and must be used together with the PKU diet.

When the FDA approved Kuvan®, the agency suggested that research on the medication continue to determine its long-term safety and effectiveness.

Other Treatments for Phenylketonuria

Other treatments include large neutral amino acid supplementation, which may help prevent phenylalanine from entering the brain, and enzyme replacement therapy, which uses a substance similar to the enzyme that usually breaks down phenylalanine. Researchers are also investigating the possibility of using gene therapy, which involves injecting new genes to break down phenylalanine. That would result in the breakdown of phenylalanine and decreased blood phenylalanine levels.

If Phenylketonuria Is Not Treated, What Problems Occur?

Children and adults who do not receive treatment for PKU may develop a variety of symptoms.

- **Children with PKU** who are not treated may develop symptoms including behavioral problems, seizures, and severe intellectual and developmental disabilities.

- **Adults with PKU** who do not follow a special diet may develop unstable moods and take longer to process information. Adults with high phenylalanine levels who go back on a PKU diet may be able to improve their mental functioning and slow down any damage to their central nervous systems.

- **Pregnant women with PKU** who do not strictly follow a low-phenylalanine diet may give birth to a child with serious problems, including intellectual and developmental disabilities, a head that is too small (microcephaly), heart defects, and low birth weight.

Section 48.5

Urea Cycle Disorders

This section includes text excerpted from "Urea Cycle Disorders," Genetic and Rare Diseases Information Center (GARD), National Center for Advancing Translational Sciences (NCATS), September 10, 2013. Reviewed September 2019.

What Is Urea Cycle Disorder?

A urea cycle disorder is a genetic disorder that results in a deficiency of one of the six enzymes in the urea cycle. These enzymes are responsible for removing ammonia from the bloodstream. The urea cycle involves a series of biochemical steps in which nitrogen, a waste product of protein metabolism, is changed to a compound called "urea" and removed from the blood. Normally, the urea is removed from the body through the urine.

In urea cycle disorders, nitrogen builds up in the blood in the form of ammonia, a highly toxic substance, resulting in hyperammonemia (elevated blood ammonia). Ammonia then reaches the brain through the blood, where it can cause irreversible brain damage, coma and/or death. The onset and severity of urea cycle disorders is highly variable. The severity correlates with the amount of urea cycle enzyme function.

Treatment of Urea Cycle Disorders

The medications listed have been approved by the U.S. Food and Drug Administration (FDA) as orphan products for treatment of this condition:

- **Benzoate and phenylacetate (Brand name: Ammonul®)**—
  Manufactured by Ucyclyd Pharma, Inc.

  FDA-approved indication: Adjunctive therapy in the treatment of acute hyperammonemia and associated encephalopathy in patients with deficiencies in enzymes of the urea cycle.

- **Sodium phenylbutyrate (Brand name: Buphenyl®)**—
  Manufactured by Ucyclyd Pharma, Inc.

  FDA-approved indication: Adjunctive therapy in the chronic management of patients with urea cycle disorders involving deficiencies of carbamyl phosphate synthetase, ornithine transcarbamylase, or argininosuccinic acid synthetase.

- **Glycerol phenylbutyrate (Brand name: Ravicti®)** —
  Manufactured by Horizon Pharma, Inc.

  FDA-approved indication: Use as a nitrogen-binding adjunctive therapy for chronic management of adult and pediatric patients at least two months of age with urea cycle disorders (UCDs) that cannot be managed by dietary protein restriction and/or amino acid supplementation alone. RAVICTI must be used with dietary protein restriction and, in some cases, dietary supplements (e.g., essential amino acids, arginine, citrulline, protein-free calorie supplements).

- **Benzoate and phenylacetate (Brand name: Ucephan®)** —
  Manufactured by Immunex Immunex

  FDA-approved indication: For adjunctive therapy in the prevention and treatment of hyperammonemia in patients with urea cycle enzymopathy due to carbamoyl phosphate synthetase, ornithine, transcarbamylase, or argininosuccinate synthetase deficiency.

Living with Urea Cycle Disorders

Living with a genetic or rare disease can impact the daily lives of patients and families.

Chapter 49

Glycogen-Storage Diseases

Chapter Contents

Section 49.1

GSD Type 0 (GSD 0)

This section includes text excerpted from "Glycogen Storage Disease Type 0," Genetics Home Reference (GHR), National Institutes of Health (NIH), January 2014. Reviewed September 2019.

What Is GSD Type 0?

Glycogen storage disease type 0 (GSD 0) is a condition caused by the body's inability to form a complex sugar called "glycogen," which is a major source of stored energy in the body. GSD 0 has two types: in muscle GSD 0, glycogen formation in the muscles is impaired, and in liver GSD 0, glycogen formation in the liver is impaired.

The signs and symptoms of muscle GSD 0 typically begin in early childhood. Affected individuals often experience muscle pain and weakness or episodes of fainting (syncope) following moderate physical activity, such as walking upstairs. The loss of consciousness that occurs with fainting typically lasts up to several hours. Some individuals with muscle GSD 0 have a disruption of the heart's normal rhythm (arrhythmia) known as "long QT syndrome." In all affected individuals, muscle GSD 0 impairs the heart's ability to effectively pump blood and increases the risk of cardiac arrest and sudden death, particularly after physical activity. Sudden death from cardiac arrest can occur in childhood or adolescence in people with muscle GSD 0.

Individuals with liver GSD 0 usually show signs and symptoms of the disorder in infancy. People with this disorder develop low blood sugar (hypoglycemia) after going long periods of time without food (fasting). Signs of hypoglycemia become apparent when affected infants begin sleeping through the night and stop late-night feedings; these infants exhibit extreme tiredness (lethargy), pale skin (pallor), and nausea. During episodes of fasting, ketone levels in the blood may increase (ketosis). Ketones are molecules produced during the breakdown of fats, which occurs when stored sugars (such as glycogen) are unavailable. These short-term signs and symptoms of liver GSD 0 often improve when food is eaten and sugar levels in the body return to normal. The features of liver GSD 0 vary; they can be mild and go unnoticed for years, or they can include developmental delay and growth failure.

There are other names too for glycogen-storage diseases which include:

- Glycogen synthase deficiency

- Glycogen synthetase deficiency

- GSD 0

- GSD type 0

- Hypoglycemia with deficiency of glycogen synthetase

Frequency of Glycogen Storage Disease Type 0

The prevalence of GSD 0 is unknown; fewer than 10 people with the muscle type and fewer than 30 people with the liver type have been described in the scientific literature. Because some people with muscle GSD 0 die from sudden cardiac arrest early in life before a diagnosis is made and many with liver GSD 0 have mild signs and symptoms, it is thought that GSD 0 may be underdiagnosed.

Causes of Glycogen Storage Disease Type 0

Mutations in the *GYS1* gene cause muscle GSD 0, and mutations in the *GYS2* gene cause liver GSD 0. These genes provide instructions for making different versions of an enzyme called "glycogen synthase." Both versions of glycogen synthase have the same function, to form glycogen molecules by linking together molecules of the simple sugar glucose, although they perform this function in different regions of the body.

The *GYS1* gene provides instructions for making muscle glycogen synthase; this form of the enzyme is produced in most cells, but it is especially abundant in heart (cardiac) muscle and the muscles used for movement (skeletal muscles). During cardiac muscle contractions or rapid or sustained movement of skeletal muscle, glycogen stored in muscle cells is broken down to supply the cells with energy.

The *GYS2* gene provides instructions for making liver glycogen synthase, which is produced solely in liver cells. Glycogen that is stored in the liver can be broken down rapidly when glucose is needed to maintain normal blood sugar levels between meals.

Mutations in the *GYS1* or *GYS2* gene lead to a lack of functional glycogen synthase, which prevents the production of glycogen from glucose. Mutations that cause GSD 0 result in a complete absence of glycogen in either liver or muscle cells. As a result, these cells do not have glycogen as a source of stored energy to draw upon following physical activity or fasting. This shortage of glycogen leads to the signs and symptoms of GSD 0.

Section 49.2

von Gierke Disease (GSD1)

This section includes text excerpted from "Glycogen Storage Disease
Type 1A," Genetic and Rare Diseases Information Center (GARD),
National Center for Advancing Translational Sciences (NCATS),
December 19, 2010. Reviewed September 2019.

What Is Glycogen Storage Disease Type 1A?

Glycogen storage disease type 1 (GSD1) is an inherited disorder
caused by the buildup of a complex sugar called "glycogen" in the body's
cells. The accumulation of glycogen in certain organs and tissues, especially the liver, kidneys, and small intestines, impairs their ability to
function normally. Researchers have described two types of glycogen
storage disease type 1, which differ in their signs and symptoms and
genetic cause. These types are known as "glycogen storage disease
type IA" and "glycogen storage disease type IB."

Glycogen storage disease type 1A is characterized by growth retardation leading to short stature and accumulation of glycogen and fat
in the liver and kidneys. Although some newborns present with severe
hypoglycemia, it is more common for infants to present at age three to
four months with hepatomegaly, lactic acidosis, hyperuricemia, hyperlipidemia, and/or hypoglycemic seizures. Untreated children typically
have doll-like faces with fat cheeks and relatively thin extremities.
Xanthoma and diarrhea may be present. Impaired platelet function
can lead to a bleeding tendency, making epistaxis a frequent problem. Glycogen storage disease type 1A is caused by the deficiency of
glucose-6-phosphatase (G6Pase) catalytic activity which results from
mutations in the *G6PC* gene. This condition is inherited in an autosomal recessive pattern.

Section 49.3

Pompe Disease (GSD 2)

This section includes text excerpted from "Pompe Disease," Genetics
Home Reference (GHR), National Institutes of Health (NIH),
February 2016. Reviewed September 2019.

What Is Pompe Disease?

Pompe disease is an inherited disorder caused by the buildup of a
complex sugar called "glycogen" in the body's cells. The accumulation
of glycogen in certain organs and tissues, especially muscles, impairs
their ability to function normally.

There are other names for Pompe disease, which include:

- Acid maltase deficiency

- Acid maltase deficiency disease

- Alpha-1,4-glucosidase deficiency

- AMD

- Deficiency of alpha-glucosidase

- GAA deficiency

- Glycogen storage disease type II

- Glycogenosis type II

- GSD II

- GSD2

Types of Pompe Disease

Researchers have described three types of Pompe disease, which
differ in severity and the age at which they appear. These types are
known as "classic infantile-onset," "nonclassic infantile-onset," and
"late-onset."

The classic form of infantile-onset Pompe disease begins within
a few months of birth. Infants with this disorder typically experience muscle weakness (myopathy), poor muscle tone (hypotonia), an
enlarged liver (hepatomegaly), and heart defects. Affected infants may
also fail to gain weight and grow at the expected rate (failure to thrive)

and have breathing problems. If untreated, this form of Pompe disease leads to death from heart failure in the first year of life.

The nonclassic form of infantile-onset Pompe disease usually appears by age one. It is characterized by delayed motor skills (such as rolling over and sitting) and progressive muscle weakness. The heart may be abnormally large (cardiomegaly), but affected individuals usually do not experience heart failure. The muscle weakness in this disorder leads to serious breathing problems, and most children with nonclassic infantile-onset Pompe disease live only into early childhood.

The late-onset type of Pompe disease may not become apparent until later in childhood, adolescence, or adulthood. Late-onset Pompe disease is usually milder than the infantile-onset forms of this disorder and is less likely to involve the heart. Most individuals with late-onset Pompe disease experience progressive muscle weakness, especially in the legs and the trunk, including the muscles that control breathing. As the disorder progresses, breathing problems can lead to respiratory failure.

Frequency of Pompe Disease

Pompe disease affects about 1 in 40,000 people in the United States. The incidence of this disorder varies among different ethnic groups.

Causes of Pompe Disease

Mutations in the *GAA* gene cause Pompe disease. The *GAA* gene provides instructions for producing an enzyme called "acid alpha-glucosidase" (also known as "acid maltase"). This enzyme is active in lysosomes, which are structures that serve as recycling centers within cells. The enzyme normally breaks down glycogen into a simpler sugar called "glucose," which is the main energy source for most cells.

Mutations in the *GAA* gene prevent acid alpha-glucosidase from breaking down glycogen effectively, which allows this sugar to build up to toxic levels in lysosomes. This buildup damages organs and tissues throughout the body, particularly the muscles, leading to the progressive signs and symptoms of Pompe disease.

Inheritance Pattern of Pompe Disease

This condition is inherited in an autosomal recessive pattern, which means both copies of the gene in each cell have mutations. The parents of an individual with an autosomal recessive condition each carry one copy of the mutated gene, but they typically do not show signs and symptoms of the condition.

Section 49.4

Forbes Disease (GSD 3)

This section includes text excerpted from "Glycogen Storage Disease Type 3," Genetic and Rare Diseases Information Center (GARD), National Center for Advancing Translational Sciences (NCATS), February 13, 2012. Reviewed September 2019.

What Is Forbes Disease?

Glycogen storage disease type 3 (GSDIII) is an inherited disorder caused by the buildup of glycogen in the body's cells. This buildup impairs the function of certain organs and tissues, especially the liver and muscles. Symptoms typically begin in infancy and may include hypoglycemia, hyperlipidemia (excess of fats in the blood), and elevated blood levels of liver enzymes; later symptoms may include hepatomegaly, chronic liver disease (cirrhosis), and liver failure later in life. Some individuals have short stature and noncancerous (benign) tumors called "adenomas" in the liver. GSDIII is caused by mutations in the *AGL* gene and is inherited in an autosomal recessive manner. Treatment typically includes a high-protein diet with cornstarch supplementation to maintain a normal level of glucose in the blood. GSDIII is divided into types IIIa, IIIb, IIIc, and IIId; types IIIa and IIIc mainly affects the liver and muscles, and GSD types IIIb and IIId typically affect only the liver.

There are other names for Forbes disease, which include:

- Cori disease

- Limit dextrinosis

- Amylo-1,6-glucosidase deficiency

- Glycogen debrancher deficiency

439

Symptoms of Forbes Disease

In infancy, individuals with GSDIII may have low blood sugar (hypoglycemia), increased amounts of fats in the blood (hyperlipidemia), and elevated levels of liver enzymes in the blood. Hypoglycemia may cause occasional seizures in some individuals. As they age, children usually develop an enlarged liver (hepatomegaly), which can cause the abdomen to protrude. Liver size may return to normal during adolescence, but some affected individuals develop chronic liver disease and subsequent liver failure years later. Individuals often have delayed growth due to their liver problems, which can lead to short stature. They may also have difficulty fighting infections, and may experience unusually frequent nosebleeds. A small percentage of individuals develop benign (noncancerous) tumors in the liver called "adenomas."

Glycogen storage disease types IIIa and IIIc typically affect both the liver and muscles, while types IIIb and IIId typically affect only the liver. Individuals with type IIIa may develop myopathy in both the heart and skeletal muscles later in life. The first signs and symptoms of this are typically poor muscle tone (hypotonia) and mild myopathy in early childhood. The myopathy may become severe by early to mid-adulthood.

Causes of Forbes Disease

Glycogen storage disease type 3 is caused by changes (mutations) in the *AGL* gene. This gene provides instructions for making the glycogen debranching enzyme, which is involved in the breakdown of glycogen—an important source of stored energy in the body. Most mutations in the *AGL* gene lead to production of a nonworking form of the glycogen debranching enzyme; these mutations are usually responsible for causing GSD types IIIa and IIIb. The mutations in the *AGL* gene that cause types IIIc and IIId presumably lead to the production of glycogen debranching enzyme with reduced function. All *AGL* mutations, however, lead to the increased buildup of abnormal, partially broken down glycogen within cells. This buildup damages tissues and organs in the body, thereby causing the signs and symptoms of GSDIII.

Inheritance of Forbes Disease

Glycogen storage disease type 3 is inherited in an autosomal recessive manner. This means that mutations in both copies of the disease-causing gene (usually 1 inherited from each parent) are necessary to cause the condition. Individuals with 1 abnormal copy of the gene are referred to as carriers; carriers are unaffected and typically do not show any signs or symptoms of the condition. When 2 carriers for an autosomal recessive condition have children together, each child has a 25 percent (1 in 4) risk to have the condition, a 50 percent (1 in 2) risk to be a carrier like each of her/his parents, and a 25 percent chance to not be a carrier and not have the condition.

Diagnosis of Forbes Disease

Glycogen storage disease type 3 should be suspected when three main features are present: hepatomegaly (enlarged liver), ketotic hypoglycemia (low blood sugar accompanied by ketosis), and elevated serum concentration of transaminases (a type of enzyme) and CK. Debranching enzyme activity (which is deficient in individuals with the condition) can be measured in a liver biopsy, but this is now not typically necessary for diagnosis. Genetic testing of the *AGL* gene, the only gene known to be associated with GSDIII, confirms the diagnosis.

Treatment of Forbes Disease

There is no cure for GSDIII as of now. In some cases, diet therapy is helpful. Strict adherence to a dietary regimen may reduce liver size, prevent hypoglycemia (low blood sugar), help to reduce symptoms, and allow for growth and development. Management typically includes a high-protein diet with cornstarch supplementation to maintain a normal level of glucose in the blood. In infancy, feeding every three to four hours is typically recommended. Toward the end of the first year of life, cornstarch is usually tolerated and can be used to avoid hypoglycemia. A high-protein diet prevents breakdown of muscle protein in times of glucose need and preserves skeletal and cardiac muscles. Skeletal and cardiac myopathies may be improved with high-protein diet and avoiding excessive carbohydrate intake. Liver transplantation may be indicated for patients with hepatic cancers.

Individuals seeking personal treatment advice should speak with their healthcare provider.

Section 49.5

Andersen Disease (GSD 4)

This section includes text excerpted from "Glycogen Storage Disease Type 4," Genetic and Rare Diseases Information Center (GARD), National Center for Advancing Translational Sciences (NCATS), December 23, 2012. Reviewed September 2019.

What Is Andersen Disease?

Glycogen storage disease type 4 (GSD 4) is part of a group of disorders which lead to abnormal accumulation of glycogen (a storage form of glucose) in various parts of the body. Symptoms of GSD 4 usually begin in infancy and typically include failure to thrive; enlarged liver and spleen (hepatosplenomegaly); and in many cases, progressive liver cirrhosis and liver failure. In rare cases individuals may have a form with nonprogressive liver disease, or a severe neuromuscular form. GSD 4 is caused by mutations in the *GBE1* gene and is inherited in an autosomal recessive manner. Treatment typically focuses on the specific symptoms that are present in each individual.

Symptoms of Andersen Disease

The signs and symptoms of GSD 4 can vary greatly between affected individuals, and several forms of GSD 4 have been described. Most affected individuals have a "classic" form characterized by progressive cirrhosis of the liver, eventually leading to liver failure. In these individuals, signs and symptoms typically begin in infancy and include failure to grow and gain weight appropriately (failure to thrive); enlargement of the liver and spleen (hepatosplenomegaly); abnormal fluid build-up in the abdomen (ascites); and enlargement of veins in the wall of the esophagus (esophageal varices) which may rupture and cause coughing up of blood. Progressive liver disease in affected children can lead to the need for a liver transplant or life-threatening complications by approximately five years of age. There have been some reports of affected individuals having nonprogressive liver disease; very mildly affected individuals may not show signs and symptoms of the disease.

There have also been reports of neuromuscular forms of GSD 4, most of which become apparent in late childhood. These may be characterized by skeletal muscle or heart muscle disease (myopathy or cardiomyopathy) caused by the accumulation of glycogen in the muscle tissue. Signs and symptoms in these cases may include muscle weakness or fatigue, exercise intolerance, and muscle wasting (atrophy). Complications with these forms may include heart failure.

A more severe neuromuscular form that is apparent at birth has also been reported; this form may be characterized by generalized edema (swelling caused by fluid); decreased muscle tone (hypotonia); muscle weakness and wasting; joints having fixed positions (contractures); and neurologic involvement, which can cause life-threatening complications early in life.

Causes of Andersen Disease

Glycogen storage disease type 4 is caused by mutations in the *GBE1* gene. The *GBE1* gene normally provides instructions for making the glycogen branching enzyme. This enzyme is necessary for making glycogen, a major source of stored energy in the body. Glycogen is formed by assembling many molecules of glucose. The glycogen branching enzyme is involved in the formation of "branches" of glucose chains, which help to make glycogen more compact for storage and allows it to break down more easily when it is needed for energy. The *GBE1* gene mutations that cause GSD 4 lead to a decrease in the amount or functionality of the glycogen branching enzyme. Glycogen is then not formed properly, and substances called "polyglucosan" bodies build up in cells throughout the body, causing the signs and symptoms of the condition.

Inheritance of Andersen Disease

Glycogen storage disease type 4 is inherited in an autosomal recessive manner. This means that an individual must have two abnormal copies of the *GBE1* gene to be affected (1 abnormal copy inherited from each parent). Individuals with one abnormal copy of the *GBE1* gene, such as the parents of an affected individual, are referred to as carriers. Carriers typically do not have signs or symptoms of an autosomal recessive condition. When two carriers of an autosomal recessive condition are having children, each of their children has a 25 percent (1 in 4) risk to be affected, a 50 percent (1 in 2) risk to be a carrier like each parent, and a 25 percent chance to not be a carrier and not be affected.

Diagnosis of Andersen Disease

Making a diagnosis for a genetic or rare disease can often be challenging. Healthcare professionals typically look at a person's medical history, symptoms, physical exam, and laboratory test results in order to make a diagnosis. If you have questions about getting a diagnosis, you should contact a healthcare professional.

Treatment of Andersen Disease

Management of GDS 4 typically focuses on the signs and symptoms that are present in each individual. Studies have shown that in some cases, strict dietary therapy can help to maintain normal levels of glucose in the blood, reduce liver size, reduce symptoms, and allow for improved growth and development. Growing evidence indicates that a high-protein diet may improve muscle function in individuals with weakness or exercise intolerance and slow disease progression. Supportive care is typically needed for complications, such as liver failure, heart failure, and neurologic dysfunction. Liver transplantation may be necessary for individuals with progressive liver disease. Individuals with cardiomyopathy may require the use of certain medications.

Chapter 50

Inherited Metabolic Storage Disorders

Chapter Contents

Section 50.1

Lipid Storage Diseases

This section includes text excerpted from "Lipid Storage
Diseases Fact Sheet," National Institute of Neurological
Disorders and Stroke (NINDS), August 13, 2019.

What Are Lipid Storage Diseases?

Lipid storage diseases, or the lipidoses, are a group of inherited
metabolic disorders in which harmful amounts of fatty materials (lipids) accumulate in various cells and tissues in the body. People with
these disorders either do not produce enough of one of the enzymes
needed to break down (metabolize) lipids or they produce enzymes
that do not work properly. Over time, this excessive storage of fats
can cause permanent cellular and tissue damage, particularly in the
brain, peripheral nervous system (the nerves from the spinal cord to
the rest of the body), liver, spleen, and bone marrow.

What Are Lipids?

Lipids are fat-like substances that are important parts of the membranes found within and between cells and in the myelin sheath that
coats and protects the nerves. Lipids include oils, fatty acids, waxes,
steroids (such as cholesterol and estrogen), and other related compounds.

These fatty materials are stored naturally in the body's cells, organs,
and tissues. Tiny bodies within cells called "lysosomes" regularly convert or metabolize, the lipids and proteins into smaller components to
provide energy for the body. Disorders in which intracellular material
that cannot be metabolized is stored in the lysosomes are called "lysosomal storage diseases." In addition to lipid storage diseases, other
lysosomal storage diseases include the mucolipidoses, in which excessive amounts of lipids with attached sugar molecules are stored in the
cells and tissues, and the mucopolysaccharidoses, in which excessive
amounts of large, complicated sugar molecules are stored.

How Are Lipid Storage Diseases Inherited?

Lipid storage diseases are inherited from one or both parents who
carry a defective gene that regulates a particular lipid-metabolizing
enzyme in a class of the body's cells. They can be inherited in two
ways:

- **Autosomal recessive inheritance** occurs when both parents carry and pass on a copy of the faulty gene, but neither parent is affected by the disorder. Each child born to these parents has a 25 percent chance of inheriting both copies of the defective gene, a 50 percent chance of being a carrier like the parents, and a 25 percent chance of not inheriting either copy of the defective gene. Children of either gender can be affected by an autosomal recessive pattern of inheritance.

- **X-linked (or sex-linked) recessive inheritance** occurs when the mother carries the affected gene on the X chromosome. The X and Y chromosomes are involved in gender determination. Females have two X chromosomes and males have one X chromosome and one Y chromosome. Sons of female carriers have a 50 percent chance of inheriting and being affected with the disorder, as the sons receive one X chromosome from the mother and a Y chromosome from the father. Daughters have a 50 percent chance of inheriting the affected X chromosome from the mother and are carriers or mildly affected. Affected men do not pass the disorder to their sons but their daughters will be carriers for the disorder.

What Are the Types of Lipid Storage Disease?

The types of lipid storage diseases include:

- Gaucher disease
- Niemann-Pick disease
- Fabry disease
- Farber disease
- Gangliosidoses
- Krabbe disease
- Metachromatic leukodystrophy
- Wolman disease

How Are Lipid Storage Diseases Diagnosed?

In some states, some of these disorders (most notably and contro-versially Krabbe disease) are screened for at birth.

In older children, diagnosis is made through clinical examination, enzyme assays (laboratory tests that measure enzyme activity), genetic testing, biopsy, and molecular analysis of cells or tissues. In some forms of the disorder, urine analysis can identify the presence of stored material. In others, the abnormality in enzyme activity can be detected in white blood cells without a tissue biopsy. Some tests can also determine if a person carries the defective gene that can be passed on to her or his children. This process is known as "genotyping."

Biopsy for lipid storage disease involves removing a small sample of the liver or other tissue and studying it under a microscope. In this procedure, a physician will administer a local anesthetic and then remove a small piece of tissue either surgically or by needle biopsy (a small piece of tissue is removed by inserting a thin, hollow needle through the skin).

Genetic testing can help individuals who have a family history of lipid storage disease determine if they are carrying a mutated gene that causes the disorder. Other genetic tests can determine if a fetus has the disorder or is a carrier of the defective gene. Prenatal testing is usually done by chorionic villus sampling (CVS), in which a very small sample of the placenta is removed and tested during early pregnancy. The sample, which contains the same deoxyribonucleic acid (DNA) as the fetus, is removed by a catheter inserted through the cervix or by a fine needle inserted through the abdomen. Results are usually available within two to four weeks.

How Are Lipid Storage Diseases Treated?

There is no specific treatment available for most of the lipid storage disorders but highly effective enzyme replacement therapy is available for type 1 and type 3 Gaucher disease. Enzyme replacement therapy is also available for Fabry disease, although it is not as effective as for Gaucher disease. However, antiplatelet medications can help prevent strokes and medications that lower blood pressure can slow the decline of kidney function in people with Fabry disease. The U.S. Food and Drug Administration (FDA) has approved the drug migalastat (Galafold) as an oral medication for adults with Fabry disease who have a certain genetic mutation. Eliglustat tartrate, an oral drug approved for Gaucher treatment, works by administering small molecules that reduce the action of the enzyme that catalyzes glucose to ceramide. Medications such as gabapentin and carbamazepine may be prescribed to help treat pain (including bone pain). Restricting one's diet does not prevent lipid build-up in cells and tissues.

Section 50.2

Gaucher Disease

This section includes text excerpted from "Gaucher Disease
Information Page," National Institute of Neurological
Disorders and Stroke (NINDS), March 27, 2019.

What Is Gaucher Disease?

Gaucher disease is one of the inherited metabolic disorders
known as lipid storage diseases. Lipids are fatty materials that
include oils, fatty acids, waxes, and steroids (such as cholesterol
and estrogen). People with Gaucher disease either do not produce
enough of the enzyme glucocerebrosidase needed to break down
lipids or have enzymes that do not work properly. Fatty materials
can accumulate in the brain and other organs. General symptoms
may begin in early life or adulthood and include skeletal disorders
and bone lesions that may cause pain and fractures, enlarged
spleen and liver, liver malfunction, anemia, and yellow spots in
the eyes.

There are three common clinical subtypes of Gaucher disease:

- **Type 1** (or nonneuropathic) typically does not affect the brain.
  Symptoms may begin early in life or in adulthood. People in
  this group usually bruise easily due to low blood platelets
  and experience fatigue due to anemia They also may have an
  enlarged liver and spleen. Many individuals with a mild form of
  the disorder may not show any symptoms.

- **Type 2 Gaucher disease** (acute infantile neuropathic Gaucher
  disease) symptoms usually begin by three months of age and
  includes extensive brain damage, seizures, spasticity, poor
  ability to suck and swallow, and enlarged liver and spleen.
  Affected children usually die before two years of age.

- **Type 3** (or chronic neuropathic Gaucher disease) includes
  signs of brain involvement, seizures, skeletal irregularities,
  eye movement disorders, cognitive deficit, poor coordination,
  enlarged liver and spleen, respiratory problems, and blood
  disorders.

Treatment of Gaucher Disease

Treatment can prevent or lessen some symptoms of the disease.

Enzyme replacement therapy is available for most people with types 1 and 3 Gaucher disease. Given intravenously every two weeks, this therapy decreases liver and spleen size, reduces skeletal abnormalities, and reverses other symptoms of the disorder. The U.S. Food and Drug Administration (FDA) has approved eliglustat tartrate for Gaucher treatment, which works by administering small molecules that reduce the action of the enzyme that catalyzes glucose to ceramide.

Surgery to remove the whole or part of the spleen may be required on rare occasions, and blood transfusions may benefit some anemic individuals. Other individuals may require joint replacement surgery to improve mobility and quality of life (QOL).

There is no effective treatment for severe brain damage that may occur in persons with types 2 and 3 Gaucher disease.

Prognosis of Gaucher Disease

Enzyme replacement therapy is very beneficial for type 1 and most type 3 individuals with this condition. Successful bone marrow transplantation can reverse the nonneurological effects of the disease, but the procedure carries a high risk and is rarely performed in individuals with Gaucher disease. People with Gaucher disease type 1 are at increased risk for Parkinson disease and Lewy Body Dementia. Gaucher disease type 2 is usually fatal by age two. People with Gaucher type 3 may have a shortened life expectancy.

Section 50.3

Hurler Syndrome

This section includes text excerpted from "Hurler Syndrome," Genetic
and Rare Diseases Information Center (GARD), National Center
for Advancing Translational Sciences (NCATS), March 17, 2014.
Reviewed September 2019.

What Is Hurler Syndrome?

Hurler syndrome is the most severe form of mucopolysaccharidosis type
1, a rare lysosomal storage disease, characterized by skeletal abnormalities, cognitive impairment, heart disease, respiratory problems, enlarged
liver and spleen, characteristic facies and reduced life expectancy.

Epidemiology of Hurler Syndrome

The prevalence of the Hurler subtype of Mucopolysaccharidosis
type 1 (MPS1) is estimated at 1/200,000 in Europe.

Clinical Description of Hurler Syndrome

Patients present within the first year of life with musculoskel-
etal alterations including short stature, dysostosis multiplex,
thoracic-lumbar kyphosis, progressive coarsening of the facial features
(including large head with bulging frontal bones, depressed nasal
bridge with broad nasal tip and anteverted nostrils, full cheeks and
enlarged lips), cardiomyopathy and valvular abnormalities, neurosen-
sorial hearing loss, enlarged tonsils and adenoids, and nasal secretion.

Developmental delay is usually observed between 12 and 24 months
of life and is primarily in the realm of speech with progressive cognitive
and sensorial deterioration.

Hydrocephaly can occur after the age of two. Diffuse corneal compromise leading to corneal opacity becomes detectable from three years
of age onwards. Other manifestations include organomegaly, hernias,
and hirsutism.

Etiology of Hurler Syndrome

Hurler syndrome is caused by mutations in the *IDUA* gene leading
to a complete deficiency in the alpha-L-iduronidase enzyme and lysosomal accumulation of dermatan sulfate and heparan sulfate.

Diagnostic Methods of Hurler Syndrome

Early diagnosis is difficult as the first clinical manifestations are not specific. Diagnosis is based on detection of increased urinary excretion of heparan and dermatan sulfate and confirmed by demonstration of an enzymatic deficiency in leukocytes or fibroblasts. Genetic testing is available.

Differential Diagnosis of Hurler Syndrome

Differential diagnoses include the milder form of mucopolysaccharidosis type 1, the Hurler-Scheie syndrome, although this form is associated with only slight cognitive impairment. Differential diagnoses also include mucopolysaccharidosis type 6 and type 2 and mucolipidosis type 2.

Antenatal Diagnosis of Hurler Syndrome

Antenatal diagnosis is possible by measurement of enzymatic activity in cultivated chorionic villus or amniocytes and by genetic testing if the disease-causing mutation is known.

Genetic Counseling of Hurler Syndrome

Transmission is autosomal recessive. Genetic counseling and testing should be offered to couples with a positive family history.

Management and Treatment of Hurler Syndrome

Management is multidisciplinary. Hematopoietic stem cell transplantation (HSCT) is the treatment of choice for patients with Hurler syndrome under 2.5 years of age (and in selected patients over this age limit) as it can prolong survival, preserve neurocognition, and ameliorate some somatic features. HSCT should be performed early in the disease course before developmental deterioration begins. Enzyme replacement therapy (ERT) with laronidase is recommended for all Hurler patients and is a lifelong therapy that alleviates nonneurological symptoms. The early use of ERT has been shown to delay or even prevent the development of some of the clinical features of this condition. Additional management of Hurler syndrome is largely supportive, and includes surgical interventions (e.g., adenotonsillectomy, hernia repair, ventriculoperitoneal shunt, cardiac valve replacement, carpal tunnel release, spinal decompression); physical, occupational, and speech therapies; respiratory support (e.g., continuous positive pressure ventilation with oxygen supplementation); hearing aids; and medications for pain and gastrointestinal disturbances.

Prognosis of Hurler Syndrome

Patients often succumb to the condition in the first decade from respiratory and cardiac complications but ERT and HSCT can improve life expectancy. The timing of diagnosis, and therefore, of treatment initiation, is an important factor for the success of both HSCT and laronidase.

Section 50.4

Krabbe Disease

This section includes text excerpted from "Krabbe Disease Information Page," National Institute of Neurological Disorders and Stroke (NINDS), March 27, 2019.

What Is Krabbe Disease?

Globoid-cell leukodystrophy, more popularly known with the name, "Krabbe disease," is a rare, inherited metabolic disorder in which harmful amounts of lipids (fatty materials such as oils and waxes) build up in various cells and tissues in the body and destroy brain cells. Krabbe disease, also called "globoid cell leukodystrophy," is characterized by globoid cells (cells that have more than one nucleus) that break down the nerve's protective myelin coating. Krabbe disease is caused by a deficiency of galactocerebrosidase, an essential enzyme for myelin metabolism. The disease most often affects infants, with onset before age six months, but can occur in adolescence or adulthood.

Symptoms of Krabbe disease include:

- Severe deterioration of mental and motor skills

- Muscle weakness

- Hypertonia (inability of a muscle to stretch)

- Myoclonic seizures (sudden, shock-like contractions of the limbs)

- Spasticity (involuntary and awkward movement)

- Unexplained fever

- Blindness

- Difficulty with swallowing

- Deafness

Treatment of Krabbe Disease

No specific treatment for Krabbe disease has been developed. Generally, treatment for the disorder is symptomatic and supportive. Medicines may be prescribed to help treat pain, and physical therapy may help maintain or increase muscle tone and circulation. Results of a very small clinical trial of children with infantile Krabbe disease found that children who received umbilical cord blood stem cells from unrelated donors prior to symptom onset developed with little neurological impairment. Bone marrow transplantation may help some people.

Prognosis of Krabbe Disease

Krabbe disease in infants is generally fatal before age two. Individuals with a later onset form of the disease generally have a milder course of the disease and live significantly longer.

Section 50.5

Metachromatic Leukodystrophy

This section includes text excerpted from "Metachromatic Leukodystrophy Information Page," National Institute of Neurological Disorders and Stroke (NINDS), March 27, 2019.

What Is Metachromatic Leukodystrophy?

Metachromatic leukodystrophy (MLD) is one of a group of genetic disorders characterized by the toxic buildup of lipids (fatty materials such as oils and waxes) and other storage materials in cells in the white matter of the central nervous system and peripheral nerves. The buildup of storage materials impairs the growth or development of the myelin sheath, the fatty covering that acts as an insulator around nerve fibers. (Myelin, which lends its color to the white matter of the brain, is a complex substance made up of a mixture of fats and proteins. MLD is one of several lipid storage diseases, which result in the harmful buildup of lipids in brain cells and other cells and tissues in the body. People with lipid storage diseases either do not produce enough of one of the enzymes needed to break down (metabolize) lipids or they produce enzymes that do not work properly. MLD, which affects males and females, is caused by a deficiency of the enzyme arylsulfatase A.

Metachromatic leukodystrophy has three characteristic forms:

- **Late infantile MLD** typically begins between 12 and 20-months following birth. Infants appear normal at first but develop difficulty walking after the first year of life and eventually lose the ability to walk. Other symptoms include muscle wasting and weakness, developmental delays, progressive loss of vision leading to blindness, impaired swallowing, and dementia before age 2. Most children with this form of MLD die by age 5.

- **Juvenile form of MLD** (which begins between 3 to 10 years of age) includes impaired school performance, mental deterioration, an inability to control movements, seizures, and dementia. Symptoms continue to get worse, and death eventually occurs 10 to 20 years following disease onset.

- **Adult MLD** commonly begins after age 16, with symptoms that include psychiatric disturbances, seizures, tremors, impaired concentration, depression, and dementia. Death generally occurs within 6 to 14 years after the onset of symptoms.

Treatment of Metachromatic Leukodystrophy

There is no cure for MLD. Bone marrow transplantation may delay the progression of the disease in some infantile-onset cases. Other treatment is symptomatic and supportive. Considerable progress has been made with regard to gene therapy in an animal model of MLD and in clinical trials.

Prognosis of Metachromatic Leukodystrophy

The prognosis for MLD is poor. Most children within the infantile form die by age 5. Symptoms of the juvenile form progress with death occurring 10 to 20 years following onset. Those persons affected by the adult form typically die within 6 to 14 years following the onset of symptoms.

Section 50.6

Cerebral X-Linked Adrenoleukodystrophy

This section includes text excerpted from "Adrenoleukodystrophy Information Page," National Institute of Neurological Disorders and Stroke (NINDS), March 27, 2019.

What Is Cerebral X-Linked Adrenoleukodystrophy?

X-linked adrenoleukodystrophy (ALD) is one of a group of genetic disorders called the "leukodystrophies" that cause damage to the myelin sheath, an insulating membrane that surrounds nerve cells in the brain. Women have two X chromosomes and are the carriers of the disease, but since men only have one X chromosome and lack the protective effect of the extra X chromosome, they are more severely affected. People with X-ALD accumulate high levels of saturated, very-long-chain fatty acids (VLCFA) in the brain and adrenal cortex. The loss of myelin and the progressive dysfunction of the adrenal gland are the primary characteristics of X-ALD.

While nearly all patients with X-ALD suffer from adrenal insufficiency, also known as "Addison disease," the neurological symptoms can begin either in childhood or in adulthood. The childhood cerebral form is the most severe, with onset between ages 4 and 10.

The most common symptoms are usually behavioral changes such as abnormal withdrawal or aggression, poor memory, and poor school performance. Other symptoms include visual loss, learning disabilities, seizures, poorly articulated speech, difficulty swallowing, deafness, disturbances of gait and coordination, fatigue, intermittent vomiting, increased skin pigmentation, and progressive dementia. The milder adult-onset form is also known as "adrenomyeloneuropathy" (AMN), which typically begins between ages 21 and 35. Symptoms may include progressive stiffness, weakness or paralysis of the lower limbs, and ataxia. Although adult-onset ALD progresses more slowly than the classic childhood form, it can also result in deterioration of brain function.

Almost half the women who are carriers of X-ALS will develop a milder form of AMN; such carriers almost never develop symptoms that are seen in boys the X-ALD. X-ALD should not be confused with neonatal adrenoleukodystrophy, which is a disease of newborns and young infants and belongs to the group of peroxisomal biogenesis disorders.

Treatment of Cerebral X-Linked Adrenoleukodystrophy

The adrenal function must be tested periodically in all patients with ALD. Treatment with adrenal hormones can be lifesaving. Symptomatic and supportive treatments for ALD include physical therapy, psychological support, and special education. Evidence suggests that a mixture of oleic acid and erucic acid, known as "Lorenzo's Oil," administered to boys with X-ALD prior to symptom onset can prevent or delay the appearance of the childhood cerebral form It is not known whether Lorenzo's Oil will have any beneficial effects in AMN. Furthermore, Lorenzo's Oil has no beneficial effect on symptomatic boys with X-ALD. Bone marrow transplantations can provide long-term benefits to boys who have early evidence of the childhood cerebral form of X-ALD, but the procedure carries the risk of mortality and morbidity and is not recommended for those whose symptoms are already severe or who have the adult-onset or neonatal forms.

Prognosis of Cerebral X-Linked Adrenoleukodystrophy

The prognosis for patients with childhood cerebral X-ALD is generally poor due to progressive neurological deterioration unless bone marrow transplantation is performed early. Death usually occurs within 1 to 10 years after the onset of symptoms. Adult-onset AMN will progress over decades.

Chapter 51

McCune-Albright Syndrome

What Is McCune-Albright Syndrome?

McCune-Albright syndrome (MAS) is a disorder that affects the skin, skeleton, and certain endocrine organs (hormone-producing tissues). Cafe-au-lait spots of the skin are common and are usually the first apparent sign of MAS. The main skeletal feature is fibrous dysplasia, which ranges in severity and can cause various complications. Early skeletal symptoms may include limping, pain, or fracture. Endocrinous features may include precocious puberty especially in girls (resulting of estrogen excess from ovarian cysts), excess growth hormone; thyroid lesions with possible hyperthyroidism; renal phosphate wasting, and, rarely, Cushing syndrome caused by an excess of the hormone cortisol produced by the adrenal glands, which are small glands located on top of each kidney.

McCune-Albright syndrome is not inherited. MAS is caused by a somatic mutation in a gene called "*GNAS*," which is acquired after an egg is fertilized and only affects some of the body's cells and tissues.

This chapter contains text excerpted from the following sources: Text beginning with the heading "What Is McCune-Albright Syndrome?" is excerpted from "McCune-Albright Syndrome," Genetic and Rare Diseases Information Center (GARD), National Center for Advancing Translational Sciences (NCATS), March 22, 2018; Text under the heading "Treatments of McCune-Albright Syndrome" is excerpted from "What Are the Treatments for McCune-Albright Syndrome (MAS)?" *Eunice Kennedy Shriver* National Institute of Child Health and Human Development (NICHD), December 1, 2016. Reviewed September 2019.

Management depends on the symptoms in each person and may include optimizing function related to fractures and deformities; medications; and surgery.

Symptoms of McCune-Albright Syndrome

Signs and symptoms of MAS relate to the skeleton (bones), the endocrine organs (hormone-producing tissues), and the skin. Symptoms can range from mild to severe.

Skeletal symptoms may include:

- **Fibrous dysplasia**—Normal bone is replaced by softer, fibrous tissue. This may lead to limping, pain, fractures, progressive scoliosis, uneven growth, facial deformity, and loss of mobility.

Endocrine symptoms may include:

- **Early puberty** (also called "precocious puberty")—Girls with MAS can have menstrual bleeding by age two (as early as 4 to 6 months in some), many years before breast enlargement and pubic hair growth begin. Early-onset menstruation is thought to be due to excess estrogen that may be produced by ovarian cysts. Precocious puberty in boys with MAS occurs less frequently and later in life when compared to girls, and presents with penile growth and testes enlargement.

- **Thyroid disease**—The thyroid gland may become enlarged (called a "goiter") or develop masses called "nodules." About half of people with MAS have hyperthyroidism.

- **Increased production of growth hormone**—The pituitary gland may produce too much growth hormone. This can result in acromegaly.

- **Cushing syndrome**—Rarely, people with MAS produce too much cortisol in the adrenal glands. This can cause weight gain in the face and upper body, slowed growth, fragile skin, fatigue, and other health problems.

- **Testicular abnormalities in males**—Testicular abnormalities are seen in the majority of males with MAS (~85%), and typically manifest as abnormally large testes (macroorchidism).

- **Phosphate wasting**—Increased production of the hormone FGF23 can result in renal tubulopathy, impairing the kidneys' ability to function properly.

Skin symptoms may include:

- **Cafe-au-lait spots**—People with MAS usually have light brown patches of skin. These spots often appear on one side of the body and may be present from birth.

Less common features of MAS may include hepatitis; gastroesophageal reflux or gastrointestinal polyps; pancreatic complications such as pancreatitis; intramuscular myxomas (benign tumors); and cancers. Cancers that have been associated with MAS include bone, thyroid, testicular, and breast. Precocious puberty and growth hormone excess may contribute to an increased risk of cancer.

Causes of McCune-Albright Syndrome

McCune-Albright syndrome is caused by somatic mutations in the *GNAS* gene. This gene provides instructions for making part of a protein that influences many cell functions by regulating hormone activity. *GNAS* mutations that cause MAS result in a protein that causes the enzyme adenylate cyclase to always be "on." This leads to overproduction of several hormones, resulting in the signs and symptoms of MAS.

Precocious puberty in MAS is gonadotropin-independent. This means that it is not caused by early release of gonadotropins (luteinizing hormone and follicle-stimulating hormone), but, instead, the cause is the early secretion of high levels of sex hormones (male androgens and female estrogens). Precocious puberty caused by this condition is much more common in girls than in boys, resulting from an excess of estrogen produced by cysts in the ovaries.

Other endocrine problems that may also occur in people with MAS are hyperthyroidism, acromegaly, and Cushing syndrome. The hyperthyroidism in the MAS is caused by an enlarged thyroid gland (goiter) or by thyroid masses called "nodules." Acromegaly results from an excess of growth hormone produced by the pituitary gland (a structure at the base of the brain that makes several hormones). Cushing syndrome results from an excess of the hormone cortisol produced by the adrenal glands.

Inheritance of McCune-Albright Syndrome

McCune-Albright syndrome is not inherited. It is caused by a random, somatic mutation in the *GNAS* gene. Mutations that cause MAS occur very early in development, after an egg is fertilized (conception).

These mutations are not present in the egg or sperm of the parents of affected children. Because these mutations are acquired after conception, some of the body's cells have a normal *GNAS* gene, while other cells have the mutated gene. This phenomenon is called "mosaicism."

Diagnosis of McCune-Albright Syndrome

The diagnosis of MAS can be made in people who have two or more of the following typical clinical features of MAS:

- Café-au-lait skin spots with characteristic features (jagged, irregular borders; distribution respecting the midline of the body; and following the developmental lines of Blaschko)

- Polyostotic fibrous dysplasia (involving more than one bone) or *GNAS* mutation-proven monostotic fibrous dysplasia (involving a single bone)

- Any of the following endocrine abnormalities (each with specific characteristics):

  - Gonadotropin-independent precocious puberty

  - Testicular lesions

  - Thyroid lesions

  - Growth hormone excess

  - Phosphate wasting

  - Neonatal hypercortisolism (Cushing syndrome)

McCune-Albright syndrome may be suspected at birth based upon identifying the characteristic cafe-au-lait spots. However, in many cases, it may not be suspected until late infancy or childhood when precocious puberty develops or when bone deformities become obvious.

In cases when only one bone has fibrous dysplasia and there are not other symptoms, genetic testing is needed to establish the diagnosis.

Treatments of McCune-Albright Syndrome

Treatment for MAS depends on the extent and the severity of a person's symptoms. For example, healthcare providers may recommend medication for endocrine problems, or surgery for bone issues.

- **Medications,** including agents that block the production of certain hormones, may help address several conditions associated with MAS, including:

  - Cushing syndrome

  - Hyperthyroidism

  - Growth hormone excess

  - Low blood phosphates

  - Precocious puberty

  - Bone pain

- **Surgery** may help address:

  - Bone deformities or uneven growth

  - Cushing syndrome, by removing adrenal glands

  - Hyperthyroidism, by removing the thyroid gland

  - Hearing and vision problems, such as by relieving pinched nerves

Healthcare providers may also recommend bisphosphonates, or drugs that help prevent bone loss. More research is needed to determine the role of these medications in MAS; at present, they are often recommended to treat pain from the PFD caused by MAS. In addition, strengthening exercises may help build muscle around bones affected by PFD, which can reduce the risk of bone fractures.

Chapter 52

Metabolic Diseases of the Muscle

What Are Metabolic Diseases of the Muscle?

"Metabolism" is a term used to describe the system by which the body breaks down food into sugars and acids, which it uses for energy. A metabolic disorder takes place when abnormal chemical reactions interrupt this process causing an individual to have too much or too little of certain substances needed for optimal health. When such disorders affect muscles they can be called "metabolic myopathy" (from the Greek myo—"muscle" and pathos—"suffering"), or simply metabolic muscle diseases.

This group of rare disorders is caused by genetic defects that are usually the result of enzyme defects in the body that make it difficult for the muscles to maintain adequate levels of adenosine triphosphate (ATP) a molecule that stores the energy we need to do work. Some of the metabolic muscle diseases that begin in infancy can be very serious, or even fatal, while those that affect older children or adults are often (although not always) less severe, tend to progress more slowly, and are generally more treatable, sometimes through adjustments in lifestyle, physical activity, or diet.

"Metabolic Diseases of the Muscle," © 2017 Omnigraphics. Reviewed September 2019.

Types of Metabolic Muscle Diseases

Metabolic muscle diseases are a very large and diverse group of conditions. And although some of these disorders do not fit neatly into categories, the majority of them are often organized into three major types:

- **Glycogen metabolic disorders.** The body needs glucose (sugar) to generate energy, and most glucose is stored in the liver and muscles as a substance called "glycogen." When the body is unable to convert sufficient amounts of this material into a usable form of energy, glycogen metabolic disorders are the result. There are numerous glycogen metabolic disorders, some of which include McArdle disease, Pompe disease, and Tarui disease.

- **Lipid metabolic diseases.** Lipids are water-insoluble fatty molecules that, among other biological functions, are responsible for storing energy. When abnormalities occur in the enzymes that break down lipids, the result can be a buildup of fatty acids, which can cause muscle weakness and pain. Some lipid metabolic disorders include carnitine palmitoyltransferase II deficiency (CPT II), very long-chain acyl-CoA dehydrogenase deficiency (VLCAD), and trifunctional protein deficiency (TFP).

- **Mitochondrial myopathies.** Mitochondria are rod-shaped organelles (specialized cell structures) that convert nutrients into ATP and produce energy. Because they are found in all cells, problems with mitochondria, generally caused by genetic mutations, may result in disorders in many systems, including the muscles. Mitochondrial myopathies include myoclonus epilepsy with ragged-red fibers (MERFF), mitochondrial DNA depletion syndrome (MDS), and progressive external ophthalmoplegia (PEO).

Symptoms of Metabolic Diseases of the Muscle

Since the group of metabolic muscle diseases is so large and varied, symptoms may be specific to the particular disorder. But, in general, they can be broken down into two groups.

Dynamic, or **activity-related symptoms**, such as:

- Pain after exercise
- Cramps

- Myoglobinuria (myoglobin in the urine, usually from muscle deterioration)
- Weakness after exercise or in response to cold

Static, or **fixed symptoms**, which include:

- Progressive muscle weakness
- Swollen and tender muscles
- Systemic involvement, such as with disorders of the endocrine system or the brain
- General malaise

Diagnosis of Metabolic Diseases of the Muscle

Because metabolic muscle diseases are both rare and diverse, diagnosing them can be a challenge, especially since many symptoms are common to all three major types. In general, doctors use biopsies and various blood tests to narrow down a diagnosis. And as with most medical conditions, the process begins with a thorough patient history and physical examination, then proceeds to various diagnostic tests.

Blood tests, such as:

- Complete blood count (CBC)
- Serum electrolytes
- Glucose levels
- Ammonia levels
- Liver transaminases (an enzyme whose level may indicate muscle damage)
- Creatinine and blood urea nitrogen levels
- Creatine kinase (an enzyme found in the muscles and brain)
- Thyroid function test

Other diagnostic tests, including:

- Urinalysis
- Forearm ischemic lactate test (which measures lactate and ammonia levels after forearm exercise)
- Electromyography (in which needle electrodes measure electrical currents in a muscle as it contracts)

- Muscle biopsy (the removal of a small piece of muscle tissue for analysis)

- Electrocardiogram, or EKG (a test of heart function)

- DNA analysis (used especially in tests for mitochondrial myopathies)

- Magnetic resonance imaging, or MRI (generally used to test for complications)

Treatments of Metabolic Diseases of the Muscle

Not surprisingly, treatments for metabolic muscle diseases vary widely depending upon the disorder's type and underlying cause. Common treatments include medication, physical therapy, braces and other devices, lifestyle changes, and diet restrictions. More specific treatments are recommended based on the classification of disease.

Glycogen Metabolic Muscular Disorders

- Patients are often advised to engage in regular aerobic exercise while avoiding isometric, or muscle-straining, activities. Studies show that those who follow such an exercise routine have a much better long-term outcome and quality of life, so physical therapy is frequently recommended.

- Maintaining blood glucose levels during the daytime has been shown to help alleviate exercise intolerance. This can be accomplished through diet or by consuming the equivalent of 40 grams of sugar about 30 to 40 minutes before exercise.

- Depending on the specific type of disorder, a high-protein diet may prove beneficial, as will eating several small meals throughout the day, rather fewer large meals.

- Certain medications, such as statins, should be avoided. Typically prescribed to reduce blood pressure, statins are a class of drug that have muscle aches as a known side effect. There is also evidence that patients with an underlying metabolic muscular disorder have a predisposition to even more serious statin myopathy.

- Some glycogen disorders result in a build-up of high levels of uric acid in the body, resulting in muscle and joint pain, as with gout. To counter this, a doctor may prescribe corticosteroids or other medications. In addition, patients are also often advised to increase their water intake, modify their diet, and take citric acid or other supplements.

- In some cases, doctors advise that young children with glycogen metabolic muscular disorders be given a mixture of uncooked cornstarch and water or soy milk.

Lipid Metabolic Muscular Disorders

- Treatment often involves avoiding prolonged strenuous activity, since this can trigger muscle aches or weakness, cramps, and the breakdown of muscle fibers. Exposure to extremes of heat and cold should also be avoided.

- Meals should be eaten frequently to prevent hypoglycemia, or low blood sugar, which can cause headache, nausea, anxiety, impaired judgment, and possibly coma, as well as metabolic crisis, a serious condition that results from the build-up of toxic substances in the blood.

- Doctors often recommend a low-fat, high-carbohydrate diet, which provides the body with sugars that can be readily converted to energy. Long-chain fatty acids should be replaced with medium-chain fatty acids (the so-called "good fat"), which provide a number of health benefits, including lower cholesterol, easier digestion, and improved cardiac health.

- Supplementing the diet with medium-chain triglyceride oil (MCT oil) may be prescribed for some patients. This product, generally made from coconut and palm kernel oils, can help make up for certain deficiencies and provide extra energy.

- L-carnitine supplements may help some individuals with lipid metabolic disorders. These are intended to boost a natural substance responsible for creating energy and helping the body eliminate waste. Riboflavin (vitamin B_2) and coenzyme (a natural antioxidant) supplements are sometimes prescribed, as well.

- Other treatments for some serious cases of certain disorders may include enzyme-replacement therapy, bone-marrow transplant, or LDL apheresis, a procedure in which blood is regularly cleaned of cholesterol by circulating it through a machine.

Mitochondrial Metabolic Muscular Disorders

- Some of the dietary and lifestyle changes recommended for other types of metabolic muscle diseases may also apply to certain mitochondrial disorders, including high-protein food. regular aerobic exercise, and avoiding activities that strain muscles.

- Since these disorders are associated with muscle weakness and problems with balance and coordination, a regimen of physical therapy can help improve muscle tone and range of motion, relieve pain, and help with balance issues.

- As with other types of muscular diseases, supplements are often recommended. These can include coenzyme Q-10, L-carnitine, B-vitamins, and riboflavin, as well as antioxidants to help to reduce free radical accumulation, which in some patients may improve energy and function.

- Other supplements have also been used with some success, including Pyruvate, which helps break down fats, and N-acetylcysteine, which affects glucose levels and works as an antioxidant.

- Since this group of disorders is made up of inherited conditions and genetic mutations, a number of treatments based on gene-therapy are undergoing experimentation. Future therapies could include substituting faulty genetic material with healthy replacements.

References

1. Katirji, Bashar, MD, FACP. "Metabolic Myopathies," Medscape.com, December 10, 2014.

2. Kimpton, Kimberly, PT. "Metabolic Myopathies," The Rheumatologist, December 1, 2007.

3. "Metabolic Diseases of Muscle," Muscular Dystrophy Association (MDA), n.d.

4. "Metabolic Myopathies," Kennedy Krieger Institute, n.d.

5. Wortmann, Robert L., MD. "Metabolic Myopathies," American College of Rheumatology (ACR), August 2013.

Chapter 53

Metabolic Neuropathies

What Are Metabolic Neuropathies?

Metabolic neuropathies are a range of peripheral nerve disorders that have a metabolic origin. "Metabolic" is a term used to describe the process through which the body breaks down food into sugars and acids, which it uses for energy, and "neuropathy" refers to nerve problems.

Some of these conditions are inherited and some are caused by various diseases, but one thing they have in common is nerve damage that results from problems with myelin (the protective coating around nerve fibers) and axons (nerve fibers) as a result of dysfunction of the metabolic pathways within cells.

Causes of Metabolic Neuropathies

There are a very large number of possible origins for metabolic neuropathies but they are generally caused either by the body's inability to use energy (often the result of a nutritional deficiency) or by a buildup of toxins in the body. Some of the most common causes include:

- **Diabetes.** Probably the most common cause of metabolic neuropathy, diabetes refers to a group of disorders characterized by high glucose (blood sugar) levels, either because of inadequate insulin production or the inability to respond to insulin. Glucose

"Metabolic Neuropathies," © 2017 Omnigraphics. Reviewed September 2019.

will be present in large quantities in the blood but they will not reach the cells, and the cells undergo starvation. Some serious long-term complications may include heart disease, kidney failure, stroke, and eye damage.

- **Uremia.** Another common cause of metabolic neuropathy, uremia is a serious condition that results from kidney disease or damage. With this disorder, the kidneys are unable to function normally, causing a buildup of urea and other waste products, which become toxic in high enough concentrations.

- **Hypoglycemia.** Also called "low blood sugar," hypoglycemia is a condition in which the body does not have enough glucose to produce the energy it needs. This can lead to heart palpitations, fatigue, blurred vision, and in extreme cases, seizures and loss of consciousness.

- **Liver disease.** Liver disease can be inherited or may be acquired through such factors as infection, immune system problems, cancer, excessive alcohol or drug use, and exposure to toxins. Untreated, liver disease can progress to liver failure, which could be life-threatening.

- **Polycythemia.** This is a condition in which red-blood-cell count is abnormally high. It can be hereditary or may be caused by long-term cigarette smoking, exposure to carbon monoxide, or hypoxia (oxygen deficiency). It can make the patient susceptible to blood clots, stroke, or heart attack.

- **Chronic obstructive pulmonary disease (COPD).** COPD is a progressive inflammatory lung disorder that makes it hard to breathe. Exposure to cigarette smoke is one of its primary causes, but long-term exposure to other irritants, such as air pollution, dust, or chemical fumes, may also be contributing factors.

There are many other possible causes for metabolic neuropathies, some of which include hypothyroidism, amyloidosis, vitamin deficiency, porphyria, mitochondrial disorders, sepsis, Refsum disease, and Krabbe disease. Note that in many cases no specific cause for the metabolic neuropathy can be found. In these instances, the condition is called "idiopathic," and treatment would focus on relief of symptoms.

Symptoms of Metabolic Neuropathies

The symptoms of metabolic neuropathy, which develop because nerves are damaged and are unable to transmit signals to the brain effectively, can vary considerably depending on the type and location of the affected nerve fibers. Some typical symptoms include:

- Pain, which could arise in any part of the body
- Numbness or a tingling sensation
- Tremors
- Difficult walking
- Loss of balance
- Muscle weakness in any area of the body
- Difficulty using arms or hands
- Cramps
- Tics or twitches

Pain, numbness, or tingling often begin at the ends of the longest nerves in the body, those in the feet and legs, and then progresses upward. At some point, if the condition affects nerves in the autonomous nervous system (which controls unconscious functions such as heartbeat and breathing), symptoms might also include dizziness, difficulty urinating, difficulty swallowing, or constipation.

Diagnosis of Metabolic Neuropathies

Diagnosing metabolic myopathy begins with a discussion, in which the doctor will ask the patient about details of the symptoms and past episodes of similar symptoms. In the physical examination, the doctor will attempt to determine the exact nature, location, and extent of the disorder. Depending on the findings, other diagnostic tests and procedures are likely to be required, including:

- Complete blood count (CBC)
- Blood glucose and glucose tolerance
- Serum protein
- Vitamin B_{12} and vitamin E
- Creatinine level
- Cryoglobulins
- Various antibodies
- Thyroid and liver function

- Ischemic forearm exercise test (measured after forearm exercise)
- Urine tests
- Leukocyte glycogen levels
- Enzyme assays of muscle, platelets, liver, and fibroblasts
- Serum mitochondrial DNA deletion and mutation tests

Treatments of Metabolic Neuropathies

The treatment plan for metabolic neuropathy depends on its underlying cause, but in general the goals include addressing the bothersome and often painful symptoms and attempting to control the originating condition. Treatments may include:

- **Pain management.** Mild pain can be treated with over-the-counter medication, such as nonsteroidal anti-inflammatories. If the pain is more serious, the doctor may prescribe a variety of drugs, including opioids, as necessary. With some patients, topical patches and sprays containing lidocaine or capsaicin might help.

- **Muscle weakness.** Physical therapy is often recommended to help exercise and strengthen muscles. The use of a cane or walker can help some patients who have balance issues, and leg or angle braces may be needed for those experiencing difficulty walking.

- **Nutrition.** Depending on the underlying condition, a nutrition counselor is likely to recommend diet modifications. For example, patients with diabetes will benefit from a low-calorie diet, and those with vitamin deficiencies may be advised to eat certain foods or take supplements.

- **Surgery.** In some cases, surgery may be an option, such as vascular or plastic surgery for patients experiencing foot issues related to diabetes, liver transplants for those with conditions like familial amyloid neuropathy, and kidney transplants to address renal failure.

Treatment for the conditions that cause metabolic neuropathy can vary widely depending on the disorder and may be extremely complicated, especially in the case of systemic diseases. But once the condition is treated, in some cases nerves can regenerate or recover to a large extent and resolve the neuropathy.

References

1. Campellone, Joseph V., MD. "Metabolic Neuropathies," MedlinePlus, National Institutes of Health (NIH), January 5, 2016.

2. Jasmin, Luc, MD, Ph.D., "Metabolic Neuropathies," New York Times Health Guide, February 16, 2012.

3. "Peripheral Neuropathy Fact Sheet," National Institute of Neurological Disorders and Stroke (NINDS), March 9, 2016.

4. Ramachandran, Tarakad S., MBBS, MBA, MPH, FAAN, FACP. "Metabolic Neuropathy," Medscape.com, October 27, 2014.

Chapter 54

Metabolic Syndrome

What Is Metabolic Syndrome?

Metabolic syndrome is the name for a group of risk factors that raises your risk for heart disease and other health problems, such as diabetes and stroke.

The term "metabolic" refers to the biochemical processes involved in the body's normal functioning. Risk factors are traits, conditions, or habits that increase your chance of developing a disease.

Plaque hardens and narrows the arteries, reducing blood flow to your heart muscle. This can lead to chest pain, a heart attack, heart damage, or even death.

Other names of metabolic syndrome include:

- Dysmetabolic syndrome

- Hypertriglyceridemic waist

- Insulin resistance syndrome

- Obesity syndrome

- Syndrome X

This chapter includes text excerpted from "Metabolic Syndrome," National Heart, Lung, and Blood Institute (NHLBI), January 30, 2019.

Causes of Metabolic Syndrome

Metabolic syndrome has several causes that act together. You can control some of the causes, such as overweight and obesity, an inactive lifestyle, and insulin resistance.

You cannot control other factors that may play a role in causing metabolic syndrome, such as growing older. Your risk for metabolic syndrome increases with age.

You also cannot control genetics, which may play a role in causing the condition. For example, genetics can increase your risk for insulin resistance, which can lead to metabolic syndrome.

People who have metabolic syndrome often have two other conditions: excessive blood clotting and constant, low-grade inflammation throughout the body. Researchers do not know whether these conditions cause metabolic syndrome or worsen it.

Risk Factors of Metabolic Syndrome

People at greatest risk for metabolic syndrome have these underlying causes:

- Abdominal obesity (a large waistline)
- An inactive lifestyle
- Insulin resistance

Some people are at risk for metabolic syndrome because they take medicines that cause weight gain or changes in blood pressure, blood cholesterol, and blood sugar levels. These medicines most often are used to treat inflammation, allergies, human immunodeficiency virus (HIV), and depression and other types of mental illness.

Populations Affected

Some racial and ethnic groups in the United States are at higher risk for metabolic syndrome than others. Mexican Americans have the highest rate of metabolic syndrome, followed by whites and blacks.

Other groups at increased risk for metabolic syndrome include:

- People who have a personal history of diabetes
- People who have a sibling or parent who has diabetes
- Women when compared with men
- Women who have a personal history of polycystic ovarian syndrome (a tendency to develop cysts on the ovaries)

Heart Disease Risk

Metabolic syndrome increases your risk for ischemic heart disease. Other risk factors, besides metabolic syndrome, also increase your risk for heart disease. For example, a high LDL "bad cholesterol" level and smoking are major risk factors for heart disease.

Even if you do not have metabolic syndrome, you should find out your short-term risk for heart disease. The National Cholesterol Education Program (NCEP) divides short-term heart disease risk into four categories. Your risk category depends on which risk factors you have and how many you have.

Your risk factors are used to calculate your 10-year risk of developing heart disease. The NCEP has an online calculator that you can use to estimate your 10-year risk of having a heart attack.

- **High risk.** You are in this category if you already have heart disease or diabetes, or if your 10-year risk score is more than 20 percent.

- **Moderately high risk.** You are in this category if you have two or more risk factors and your 10-year risk score is 10 to 20 percent.

- **Moderate risk.** You are in this category if you have two or more risk factors and your 10-year risk score is less than 10 percent.

- **Lower risk.** You are in this category if you have zero or one risk factor.

Even if your 10-year risk score is not high, metabolic syndrome will increase your risk for coronary heart disease over time.

Screening and Prevention of Metabolic Syndrome

The best way to prevent metabolic syndrome is to adopt heart-healthy lifestyle changes. Make sure to schedule routine doctor visits to keep track of your cholesterol, blood pressure, and blood sugar levels. Speak with your doctor about a blood test called a "lipoprotein panel," which shows your levels of total cholesterol, LDL cholesterol, HDL cholesterol, and triglycerides.

Signs, Symptoms, and Complications of Metabolic Syndrome

Metabolic syndrome is a group of risk factors that raises your risk for heart disease and other health problems, such as diabetes and stroke. These risk factors can increase your risk for health problems even if they are only moderately raised (borderline-high risk factors).

Most of the metabolic risk factors have no signs or symptoms, although a large waistline is a visible sign.

Some people may have symptoms of high blood sugar if diabetes—especially type 2 diabetes—is present. Symptoms of high blood sugar often include increased thirst; increased urination, especially at night; fatigue (tiredness); and blurred vision.

High blood pressure usually has no signs or symptoms. However, some people in the early stages of high blood pressure may have dull headaches, dizzy spells, or more nosebleeds than usual.

Diagnosis of Metabolic Syndrome

Your doctor will diagnose metabolic syndrome based on the results of a physical exam and blood tests. You must have at least three of the five metabolic risk factors to be diagnosed with metabolic syndrome.

Metabolic Risk Factors
A Large Waistline

Having a large waistline means that you carry excess weight around your waist (abdominal obesity). This is also called having an "apple-shaped" figure. Your doctor will measure your waist to find out whether you have a large waistline.

A waist measurement of 35 inches or more for women or 40 inches or more for men is a metabolic risk factor. A large waistline means you are at increased risk for heart disease and other health problems.

A High Triglyceride Level

Triglycerides are a type of fat found in the blood. A triglyceride level of 150 mg/dL or higher (or being on medicine to treat high triglycerides) is a metabolic risk factor. (The mg/dL is milligrams per deciliter—the units used to measure triglycerides, cholesterol, and blood sugar.)

A Low High-Density Lipoprotein Cholesterol Level

High-density lipoprotein (HDL) cholesterol sometimes is called "good cholesterol." This is because it helps remove cholesterol from your arteries.

An HDL cholesterol level of less than 50 mg/dL for women and less than 40 mg/dL for men (or being on medicine to treat low HDL cholesterol) is a metabolic risk factor.

High Blood Pressure

A blood pressure of 130/85 mmHg or higher (or being on medicine to treat high blood pressure) is a metabolic risk factor. (mmHg is millimeters of mercury—the units used to measure blood pressure.)

If only one of your two blood pressure numbers is high, you are still at risk for metabolic syndrome.

High Fasting Blood Sugar

A normal fasting blood sugar level is less than 100 mg/dL. A fasting blood sugar level between 100 to 125 mg/dL is considered prediabetes. A fasting blood sugar level of 126 mg/dL or higher is considered diabetes.

A fasting blood sugar level of 100 mg/dL or higher (or being on medicine to treat high blood sugar) is a metabolic risk factor.

About 85 percent of people who have type 2 diabetes—the most common type of diabetes—also have metabolic syndrome. These people have a much higher risk for heart disease than the 15 percent of people who have type 2 diabetes without metabolic syndrome.

Treatment of Metabolic Syndrome

Heart-healthy lifestyle changes are the first line of treatment for metabolic syndrome. If heart-healthy lifestyle changes are not enough, your doctor may prescribe medicines. Medicines are used to treat and control risk factors, such as high blood pressure, high triglycerides, low HDL "good cholesterol," and high blood sugar.

Goals of Treatment

The major goal of treating metabolic syndrome is to reduce the risk of ischemic heart disease. Treatment is directed first at lowering LDL cholesterol and high blood pressure and managing diabetes (if these conditions are present).

The second goal of treatment is to prevent the onset of type 2 diabetes, if it has not already developed. Long-term complications of diabetes often include heart and kidney disease, vision loss, and foot or leg amputation. If diabetes is present, the goal of treatment is to reduce your risk for heart disease by controlling all of your risk factors.

Heart-Healthy Lifestyle Changes

Heart-healthy lifestyle changes include heart-healthy eating, aiming for a healthy weight, managing stress, physical activity, and quitting smoking.

Medicines

Sometimes lifestyle changes are not enough to control your risk factors for metabolic syndrome. For example, you may need statin medications to control or lower your cholesterol. By lowering your blood cholesterol level, you can decrease your chance of having a heart attack or stroke. Doctors usually prescribe statins for people who have:

• Diabetes

• Heart disease or had a prior stroke

• High LDL cholesterol levels

Doctors may discuss beginning statin treatment with those who have an elevated risk for developing heart disease or having a stroke. Your doctor also may prescribe other medications to:

• Decrease your chance of having a heart attack or dying suddenly

• Lower your blood pressure

• Prevent blood clots, which can lead to heart attack or stroke

• Reduce your heart's workload and relieve symptoms of coronary heart disease

Take all medicines regularly, as your doctor prescribes. Do not change the amount of your medicine or skip a dose unless your doctor tells you to. You should still follow a heart-healthy lifestyle, even if you take medicines to treat your risk factors for metabolic syndrome.

Living with Metabolic Syndrome

Metabolic syndrome is a lifelong condition. However, lifestyle changes can help you control your risk factors and reduce your risk for ischemic heart disease and diabetes.

If you already have heart disease or diabetes, lifestyle changes can help you prevent or delay related problems. Examples of these problems include heart attack, stroke, and diabetes-related complications (for example, damage to your eyes, nerves, kidneys, feet, and legs).

Heart-healthy lifestyle changes may include:

- Heart-healthy eating

- Aiming for a healthy weight

- Managing stress

- Physical activity

- Quitting smoking

If lifestyle changes are not enough, your doctor may recommend medicines. Take all of your medicines as prescribed by your doctor. Make realistic short—and long-term goals for yourself when you begin to make healthy lifestyle changes. Work closely with your doctor, and seek regular medical care.

Chapter 55

Multiple Endocrine Neoplasia Type 1

What Is Multiple Endocrine Neoplasia Type 1?

Multiple endocrine neoplasia type 1 (MEN1) is an inherited disorder that causes tumors in the endocrine glands and the duodenum, the first part of the small intestine. MEN1 is sometimes called "multiple endocrine adenomatosis" or "Wermer syndrome," after one of the first doctors to recognize it. MEN1 is rare, occurring in about one in 30,000 people. The disorder affects both sexes equally and shows no geographical, racial, or ethnic preferences.

Endocrine glands release hormones into the bloodstream. Hormones are powerful chemicals that travel through the blood, controlling and instructing the functions of various organs. Normally, the hormones released by endocrine glands are carefully balanced to meet the body's needs.

In people with MEN1, multiple endocrine glands form tumors and become hormonally overactive, often at the same time. The overactive glands may include the parathyroids, pancreas, or pituitary gland. Most people who develop overactivity of only one endocrine gland do not have MEN1.

This chapter includes text excerpted from "Multiple Endocrine Neoplasia Type 1," National Institute of Diabetes and Digestive and Kidney Diseases (NIDDK), April 2012. Reviewed September 2019.

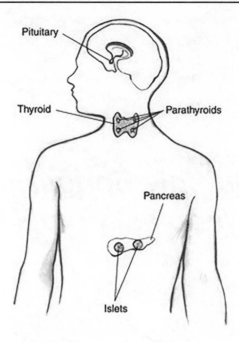

Figure 55.1. *Endocrine Glands*

How Does Multiple Endocrine Neoplasia Type 1 Affect the Endocrine Glands and the Duodenum?
The Parathyroid Glands

The parathyroids are the endocrine glands earliest and most often affected by MEN1. The body normally has four parathyroid glands, which are located close to the thyroid gland in the front of the neck. The parathyroids release into the bloodstream a chemical called "parathyroid hormone" (PTH), which helps maintain a normal supply of calcium in the blood, bones, and urine.

Hyperparathyroidism

In MEN1, all four parathyroid glands tend to be overactive, causing hyperparathyroidism. The parathyroid glands form tumors that release too much PTH, leading to excess calcium in the blood. High blood calcium, known as "hypercalcemia," can exist for many years before it is found by accident or through screening for MEN1. Unrecognized hypercalcemia can cause excess calcium to spill into the urine, leading to kidney stones or kidney damage. Also, the bones may lose calcium and weaken.

Nearly everyone who inherits a susceptibility to MEN1 will develop hyperparathyroidism by age 50, but the disorder can often be detected before age 20. Hyperparathyroidism may cause no problems for many years, or it may cause tiredness, weakness, muscle or bone pain, constipation, indigestion, kidney stones, or thinning of bones.

Doctors must decide whether hyperparathyroidism in MEN1 is severe enough to need treatment, especially in a person who has no symptoms. The usual treatment is an operation to remove most or all of the parathyroid glands. One option is to remove the three largest glands and all but a small part of the fourth. Another is to remove all four glands and at the same time transplant a small part of one gland into the forearm. By maintaining a portion of one gland, the parathyroid transplant continues to release PTH into the bloodstream to do its job.

After parathyroid surgery, regular testing of blood calcium should continue because often the small piece of remaining parathyroid tissue grows larger and causes recurrent hyperparathyroidism. If the remaining piece is in the forearm and additional surgery is needed to remove more parathyroid tissue, the arm operation can be performed under local anesthesia.

Sometimes all four glands are completely removed to prevent recurrence or may be unintentionally removed during parathyroid surgery. People whose parathyroid glands have been completely removed must take daily supplements of calcium and vitamin D or another related treatment to prevent hypocalcemia, or low blood calcium.

The Pancreas and Duodenum

Located behind the stomach, the pancreas has two major roles: to release digestive juices into the intestines and key hormones into the bloodstream. The duodenum is the first part of the small intestine next to the pancreas. The pancreatic hormones are normally produced by small clusters of specialized cells called "pancreatic islets." Some of the major hormones produced by the pancreatic islets are:

- **Insulin**—lowers blood glucose, also called "blood sugar"

- **Glucagon**—raises blood glucose

- **Somatostatin**—inhibits secretion of certain other hormones

- **Vasoactive intestinal peptide (VIP)**—causes intestinal cells to secrete water into the intestine

- **Gastrin**—causes the stomach to produce acid for digestion

Gastrinomas

In MEN1, gastrin may be over secreted by tumors called "gastrinomas" in the pancreas, duodenum, and lymph glands. If exposed to too much gastrin, the stomach releases excess acid, leading to the formation of severe ulcers in the stomach and small intestine. In addition, too much gastrin usually causes serious diarrhea.

People with MEN1 have about a 20 to 60 percent chance of developing gastrinomas. The illness associated with these tumors is called "Zollinger-Ellison syndrome" (ZES). The ulcers caused by untreated gastrinomas are much more dangerous than typical stomach or intestinal ulcers. Left untreated, they can cause rupture of the stomach or intestine and even death.

The gastrinomas associated with MEN1 are not easily cured through tumor surgery because finding the many small gastrinomas in the pancreas, duodenum, and lymph glands is difficult. The mainstay of treatment is powerful medicines called "acid pump inhibitors" that block stomach acid release. Taken by mouth, these medicines have proven effective in controlling the complications of excess gastrin in most cases of ZES.

Rare Pancreatic Complications

Occasionally, a person who has MEN1 develops an islet tumor of the pancreas that secretes high levels of hormones. Insulinomas, for example, produce too much insulin, causing hypoglycemia, or low blood glucose. About 10 percent of adults with MEN1 develop insulinomas. Rare pancreatic tumors may secrete too much glucagon, which can cause diabetes, or too much vasoactive intestinal peptide, also known as "vasoactive intestinal polypeptide" (VIP), which can cause watery diarrhea. Tumors that secrete adrenocorticotropin (ACTH) may also arise in the pancreas. ACTH is normally secreted by the pituitary gland and stimulates the adrenal glands to produce cortisol, a hormone that helps the body respond to stress. Tumors in the pancreas may also infrequently secrete gonadotropin-releasing hormone (GnRH). GnRH is normally secreted by the hypothalamus and stimulates the pituitary gland to release follicle-stimulating hormone (FSH), which regulates fertility in men through sperm production and in women through ovulation. In general, surgery is the mainstay of treatment for these uncommon types of tumors.

The Pituitary Gland

The pituitary gland, a small gland located at the base of the brain, produces many important hormones that regulate basic body functions. The normal major pituitary hormones are:

- **Prolactin**—controls the formation of breast milk and influences fertility and bone strength

- **Growth hormone**—regulates body growth, especially during adolescence

- **Adrenocorticotropic hormone (ACTH)**—stimulates the adrenal glands to produce cortisol

- **Thyrotropin**—stimulates the thyroid gland to produce thyroid hormones, which regulate metabolism

- **Luteinizing hormone**—stimulates the ovaries or testes to produce sex hormones

- **Follicle-stimulating hormone**—regulates fertility

Prolactinomas

The pituitary gland becomes overactive in about one in four people with MEN1. This overactivity can usually be traced to a small tumor in the gland that releases too much prolactin, called a "prolactinoma." High prolactin levels can cause excessive production of breast milk or interfere with fertility in women or with sex drive and fertility in men.

Treatment may not be needed for prolactinomas. If treatment is needed, a medicine known as a "dopamine" agonist can effectively shrink the tumor and lower the production of prolactin. Occasionally, prolactinomas do not respond well to this medication. In such cases, surgery, radiation, or both may be needed.

Rare Pituitary Complications

Rarely, MEN1 creates pituitary tumors that release high amounts of ACTH, which in turn stimulates the adrenal glands to produce excess cortisol. Too much cortisol can lead to muscle weakness, weakened bones and fractures, and thinning skin, among other problems. Pituitary tumors that produce growth hormone cause excessive bone growth or disfigurement. In general, surgery is the mainstay of treatment for these uncommon types of tumors.

Are the Tumors Associated with Multiple Endocrine Neoplasia Type 1 Cancerous?

The tumors associated with MEN1 are usually benign, meaning they are not cancerous. However, they can disrupt normal function by releasing hormones or by crowding nearby tissue. For example, a prolactinoma may become quite large in someone with MEN1. As it grows, the tumor can press against and damage the normal part of the pituitary gland or the nerves for vision. Sometimes impaired vision is the first sign of a pituitary tumor in a person with MEN1.

Another type of benign tumor seen in about one-third of people with MEN1 is a plum-sized, fatty tumor called a "lipoma," which grows under the skin. Lipomas cause no health problems and can be removed by simple cosmetic surgery if desired.

Benign tumors do not spread to or invade other parts of the body. Cancer cells, by contrast, break away from the primary tumor and spread, or metastasize, to other parts of the body through the bloodstream or lymphatic system. The pancreatic islet tumors associated with MEN1 tend to be numerous and small, but most are benign and do not release active hormones into the blood. Over time, gastrinomas may become cancerous but are usually slow-growing.

Eventually, about half of people with MEN1 will develop a cancerous pancreatic or carcinoid tumor. A carcinoid is a slow-growing endocrine tumor inside the chest or stomach of a person with MEN1. Although carcinoids arise from endocrine cells, which are present in many parts of the body, they rarely secrete a hormone in a person with MEN1. Carcinoids of the stomach usually do not require treatment.

Treatment of Pancreatic Endocrine Cancer in Multiple Endocrine Neoplasia Type 1

Because the type of pancreatic endocrine cancer associated with MEN1 can be difficult to recognize, difficult to treat, and slow to progress, doctors have different views about the value of surgery in managing these tumors.

One approach is to "watch and wait," using medical, or nonsurgical, treatments. According to this school of thought, pancreatic surgery has serious complications, so it should not be attempted unless it will cure a tumor or cure a hormone excess state.

Another school advocates early surgery, perhaps when a tumor grows to a certain size, to prevent or treat pancreatic endocrine cancer—even if the tumor does not over secrete a hormone-before the cancer spreads. No clear evidence exists, however, that surgery to prevent pancreatic endocrine cancer from spreading actually leads to longer survival for patients with MEN1.

Doctors agree that excessive release of certain hormones-mainly gastrin-from pancreatic endocrine cancer in MEN1 needs to be treated, and medications are often effective in blocking the effects of these hormones. Some tumors, such as insulinomas, are usually benign and single and are curable by pancreatic surgery. Such surgery needs to be considered carefully in each patient's case.

Is Multiple Endocrine Neoplasia Type 1 the Same in Everyone?

Although MEN1 tends to follow certain patterns, it can affect a person's health in many different ways. Not only do the tumors of MEN1 vary among members of the same family, but some families with MEN1 tend to have a higher rate of prolactin-secreting pituitary tumors and a much lower frequency of gastrin-secreting tumors.

The age at which MEN1 can begin to cause endocrine gland overactivity can differ strikingly from one family member to another. One person may have only mild hyperparathyroidism beginning at age 50, while a relative may develop complications from tumors of the parathyroid, pancreas, and pituitary gland by age 18.

How Is Multiple Endocrine Neoplasia Type 1 Detected?

Multiple endocrine neoplasia type 1 is detected by gene testing or, when gene testing is unavailable or yields a negative result, by laboratory tests that measure hormone levels. Less often, MEN1 is diagnosed based on an individual's medical and family history.

The Genetics of Multiple Endocrine Neoplasia Type 1 and Multiple Endocrine Neoplasia Type 1 Carriers

In a person with MEN1, a mutation, or mistake, exists in the *MEN1* gene in every cell in the person's body. Many different *MEN1* gene mutations have been identified. Each of these mutations can cause the same spectrum of MEN1 tumors. The particular MEN1 mutation in

491

a person's body may be silent, meaning the person has no symptoms, as in a newborn. Or, the MEN1 mutation may be expressed as the MEN1 syndrome. A person with a MEN1 mutation, whether showing symptoms or not, is termed a carrier of the MEN1 mutation or a carrier of the MEN1 syndrome.

Multiple endocrine neoplasia type 1 is an autosomal dominant gene, which means it is inherited by a child from one parent who has the MEN1 mutation.

Gene Testing

Gene testing can identify whether a person is a carrier of the MEN1 mutation. Once identified, carriers undergo approximately yearly testing, a process called "screening," for biochemical indications of a developing tumor. Relatives who are found to lack the known MEN1 mutation in their family can be freed from screening for MEN1. A limited number of laboratories in the United States offer *MEN1* gene testing to locate and identify MEN1 mutations. The gene tests are expensive and can be time-consuming. Once a specific mutation is found in an individual, the gene test for relatives is easier and less expensive.

In 10 to 30 percent of families with MEN1, no mutation is found. However, an undetected MEN1 mutation may still be likely. Sometimes a person with MEN1 knows of no other case of MEN1 among relatives. The most common explanation is that knowledge of the family's health history is incomplete. Less often, the person carries a new *MEN1* gene mutation.

Gene testing may be offered to people who:

- Meet the clinical criteria for MEN1 by having at least two of the following: enlarged parathyroid glands, a pancreatic or duodenal endocrine tumor, or a pituitary tumor

- Do not meet the clinical criteria but are suspected of having MEN1—for example, those who have multiple parathyroid tumors before age 30

- Are first-degree relatives of people with MEN1—children, brothers, or sisters- giving them a 50 percent chance of having inherited the mutation

The Role of Genetic Counseling

Genetic counseling can assist family members in understanding how the test results may affect them individually and as a family.

Genetic counseling may include a review and discussion of the psycho-social benefits and risks of genetic testing. Genetic testing results can affect self-image, self-esteem, and individual and family identity. In genetic counseling, issues related to how and with whom genetic test results will be shared and their possible effect on important matters such as health and life insurance coverage can be addressed. These discussions may occur when a family member is deciding whether to proceed with gene testing and again later when the test results are available. A doctor, nurse, or genetics professional provides the genetic counseling.

Laboratory Tests

Laboratory tests may be performed periodically to screen for MEN1 tumors. Screening can catch tumors in their early stages of development, detect tumors that have come back, and indicate how large they are and where they are located. Catching tumor development early allows doctors to take steps to prevent serious complications from occurring in people with MEN1. Types of tests used for tumor screening can include:

- **Blood tests**—for example, to measure insulin or PTH to detect excess hormone production by a MEN1 tumor

- **Other biochemical tests**—for example, to measure urinary calcium to detect the results of excess hormone production

- **Immunoradiometric assays**, a type of blood test—for example, to measure PTH to detect parathyroid tumors

- **Imaging tests**—for example, ultrasound, computerized tomography (CT), and magnetic resonance imaging (MRI) to allow the doctor to detect tumors that are not secreting hormones. Because imaging tests are more expensive, they are typically done less often than blood tests

The types of tests performed depend on the purpose of the screening. Periodic screening for MEN1 tumors can have two different purposes:

- **To recognize possible carriers of MEN1.** First, screening may be performed to determine if an individual is a carrier of the MEN1 mutation. This screening includes close relatives of a person known to carry MEN1. Although gene testing is one way to identify a carrier of MEN1, sometimes these other methods are used due to a lack of resources, or when the underlying

493

mutation cannot be identified. For this screening purpose, tests are directed at tumors that are most frequent and develop the earliest. Examples of these tests include PTH, calcium, and prolactin tests.

• **To detect early tumors in known carriers of MEN1.** Second, screening may be performed in known carriers of MEN1 to look for any tumor that could develop as a result of the mutation. This periodic testing can recognize a tumor early to optimize its treatment. When an individual is a known carrier of MEN1, more detailed testing is performed to screen for some of the less likely but still harmful tumors.

Laboratory tests for MEN1 tumors can be repeated yearly without waiting for symptoms to appear. This testing can begin at age five. In known carriers, imaging tests may be performed every three years to locate tumors that cannot be found with other laboratory testing.

If an individual's tests are normal, periodic tumor testing should continue indefinitely. However, an unproven carrier with normal tests beyond age 50 is unlikely to have inherited a *MEN1* gene mutation.

Can Multiple Endocrine Neoplasia Type 1 Be Cured?

Multiple endocrine neoplasia type 1 cannot be cured, but regular testing can detect many of the problems caused by MEN1 tumors many years before serious complications develop. Finding these tumors early enables doctors to begin preventive treatment, reducing the chances that MEN1 will cause problems later.

Even after treatment, residual tissue can grow back or different glands may become affected. Periodic and careful monitoring enables doctors to adjust an individual's treatment as needed and to check for any new problems caused by MEN1. Most people with MEN1 have a long and productive life.

Should a Person Who Has Multiple Endocrine Neoplasia Type 1 Avoid Having Children?

A person who has MEN1 or who has a *MEN1* gene mutation may have a hard time deciding whether to have a child. Some facts to consider include the following:

• A man or a woman with MEN1 has a 50 to 50 risk with each pregnancy of having a child with MEN1.

- MEN1 tends to fit a broad pattern within a given family, but the severity of the disorder varies widely from one family member to another. In particular, a parent's experience with MEN1 cannot be used to predict the eventual severity of MEN1 in a child.

- The tumors that result from MEN1 do not usually develop until adulthood. Treatment may require regular monitoring and considerable expense, but the disease usually does not prevent an active, productive adulthood.

- Prolactin-releasing tumors in a man or woman with MEN1 may inhibit fertility and make it difficult to conceive.

- Hyperparathyroidism during pregnancy may raise the risks of complications for mother and child.

- Pregnancy is usually normal for the mother or child who is a carrier of MEN1.

Genetic counselors and other professionals can provide information to help with the decision-making process, but they will not tell individuals or couples what decision to make or how to make it.

Part Eight

Additional Help and Information

Chapter 56

Glossary of Terms Related to Endocrine and Metabolic Disorders

acquired immunodeficiency syndrome (AIDS): A medical condition in which the immune system cannot function properly and protect the body from disease; as a result, the body cannot defend itself against infectious diseases.

acute: A short-term, intense health effect.

adenoma: A noncancerous tumor.

adrenal gland: A small gland that makes steroid hormones, adrenaline, and noradrenaline. These hormones help control heart rate, blood pressure, and other important body functions.

adverse reaction: An untoward (unfavorable) effect caused by a vaccine that is extraneous to (not in keeping with) the vaccine's primary purpose of production of immunity.

amino acid: One of several molecules that join together to form proteins. There are 20 common amino acids found in proteins.

anemia: A condition in which the number of red blood cells is below normal.

This glossary contains terms excerpted from documents produced by several sources deemed reliable.

anesthetic: A drug that causes insensitivity to pain and is used for surgeries and other medical procedures.

antibodies: Special proteins made by the body in response to antigens (foreign substances).

antigen: Foreign substances (e.g., bacteria or viruses) in the body that are capable of causing disease; the presence of antigens in the body triggers an immune response, usually the production of antibodies.

anxiety: Feelings of fear, dread, and uneasiness that may occur as a reaction to stress. A person with anxiety may sweat, feel restless and tense, and have a rapid heart beat.

arthritis: Inflammation of the joints that causes swelling, stiffness, and pain.

asthma: A chronic respiratory disease characterized by constriction of the bronchial tubes to the lungs, which causes sudden and recurring breathing problems, coughing, and chest tightness and wheezing.

benign: Not cancerous. Benign tumors may grow larger but do not spread to other parts of the body.

bladder: The organ in the human body that stores urine. It is found in the lower part of the abdomen.

blood chemistry study: A procedure in which a sample of blood is examined to measure the amounts of certain substances made in the body.

bone marrow: Soft tissue located within bones that produces all blood cells, including the ones that fight infection.

breast cancer: Cancer that forms in tissues of the breast. The most common type of breast cancer is ductal carcinoma, which begins in the lining of the milk ducts (thin tubes that carry milk from the lobules of the breast to the nipple).

calcium: A mineral found in teeth, bones, and other body tissues.

cancer: A term for diseases in which abnormal cells divide without control. Cancer cells can invade nearby tissues and can spread through the bloodstream and lymphatic system to other parts of the body.

cardiovascular: Related to the heart and blood vessels.

caregiver: A caregiver is anyone who helps care for an elderly individual or person with a disability who lives at home. Caregivers usually provide assistance with activities of daily living and other essential activities like shopping, meal preparation, and housework.

cataracts: Clouding of the lens of the eye that reduces the ability to see clearly; can lead to blindness.

catheter: A flexible tube used to deliver fluids into or withdraw fluids from the body.

central nervous system (CNS): The brain and spinal cord.

chemotherapy: Treatment with drugs that kill cancer cells.

chronic pain: Pain that can range from mild to severe, and persists or progresses over a long period of time.

chronological age: The age of a person as measured from her or his birth.

clinical trial: A research study in which one or more human subjects are prospectively assigned to one or more interventions (which may include placebo or other control) to evaluate the effects of those interventions on health-related biomedical or behavioral outcomes.

computed tomography (CT) scan: A series of detailed pictures of areas inside the body taken from different angles; the pictures are created by a computer linked to an x-ray machine.

corticosteroids: A steroid hormone; when given as a medication, it suppresses the body's normal inflammatory reactions to infection. This increases the risk for serious infection.

craniotomy: An operation in which an opening is made in the skull.

de novo: A chromosome abnormality that occurred in the individual and was not inherited from the parents.

dehydration: Inadequate amount of water in the body; can occur from illness or from decreased or lack of fluid intake.

deoxyribonucleic acid (DNA): The double-helix molecule that provides the basis of genetic heredity, about two nanometers in diameter but often several millimeters in length.

depression: A mental condition marked by ongoing feelings of sadness, despair, loss of energy, and difficulty dealing with normal daily life. Other symptoms of depression include feelings of worthlessness

501

and hopelessness, loss of pleasure in activities, changes in eating or sleeping habits, and thoughts of death or suicide.

diabetes: A chronic health condition in which the body is unable to produce insulin and properly break down sugar (glucose) in the blood.

diarrhea: Abnormally watery bowel movements.

diet: What a person eats and drinks. Any type of eating plan.

drug: Any substance, other than food, that is used to prevent, diagnose, treat, or relieve symptoms of a disease or abnormal condition.

enzyme: A protein that speeds up chemical reactions in the body.

fatigue: Extreme tiredness or weariness.

frequency: The number of times an exercise or activity is performed. Frequency is generally expressed in sessions, episodes, or bouts per week.

functioning tumor: A tumor that is found in endocrine tissue and makes hormones.

gland: An organ that makes one or more substances, such as hormones, digestive juices, sweat, tears, saliva, or milk.

glucocorticoid: A compound that belongs to the family of compounds called "corticosteroids" (steroids). Glucocorticoids affect metabolism and have anti-inflammatory and immunosuppressive effects.

glucose: A major source of energy for our bodies and a building block for many carbohydrates. The food digestion process breaks down carbohydrates in foods and drinks into glucose. After digestion, glucose is carried in the blood and goes to body cells where it is used for energy or stored.

heart disease: A number of abnormal conditions affecting the heart and the blood vessels in the heart. The most common type of heart disease is coronary artery disease, which is the gradual buildup of plaques in the coronary arteries, the blood vessels that bring blood to the heart. This disease develops slowly and silently, over decades. It can go virtually unnoticed until it produces a heart attack.

high blood pressure: Your blood pressure rises and falls throughout the day. An optimal blood pressure is less than 120/80 mmHg. When blood pressure stays high—greater than or equal to 140/90 mmHg— you have high blood pressure, also called "hypertension." With high blood pressure, the heart works harder, your arteries take a beating, and your chances of a stroke, heart attack, and kidney problems are greater.

hormone: A chemical made by glands in the body. Hormones circulate in the bloodstream and control the actions of certain cells or organs.

human immunodeficiency virus (HIV): A virus that infects and destroys the body's immune cells and causes a disease called AIDS, or acquired immunodeficiency syndrome.

hydration: The amount of fluid in your body. It is important to replace any fluid your body loses during physical activity.

hypercalcemia: Abnormally high blood calcium.

hyperparathyroidism: A condition in which the parathyroid gland (one of four pea-sized organs found on the thyroid) makes too much parathyroid hormone.

imaging: Tests that produce pictures of areas inside the body.

immune system: A complex system of cellular and molecular components having the primary function of distinguishing self from not self and defense against foreign organisms or substances.

impotence: In medicine, refers to the inability to have an erection of the penis adequate for sexual intercourse.

inherited: Transmitted through genes that have been passed from parents to their offspring (children).

laboratory test: A medical procedure that involves testing a sample of blood, urine, or other substance from the body. Tests can help determine a diagnosis, plan treatment, check to see if treatment is working, or monitor the disease over time.

lymph node: A rounded mass of lymphatic tissue that is surrounded by a capsule of connective tissue. Lymph nodes filter lymph (lymphatic fluid), and they store lymphocytes (white blood cells).

magnetic resonance imaging (MRI): A noninvasive procedure that uses magnetic fields and radio waves to produce three-dimensional computerized images of areas inside the body.

medicare: Federal program that provides hospital and medical expense benefits for people over age 65, or those meeting specific disability standards. Benefits for nursing home and home health services are limited.

medication: A legal drug that is used to prevent, treat, or relieve symptoms of a disease or abnormal condition. Also called "medicine."

menstrual cycle: The monthly cycle of hormonal changes from the beginning of one menstrual period to the beginning of the next one.

metabolic: Relates to metabolism or processes in an organism that make energy.

metastasectomy: Surgery to remove one or more metastases (tumors formed from cells that have spread from the primary tumor).

metastasize: To spread from one part of the body to another. When cancer cells metastasize and form secondary tumors, the cells in the metastatic tumor are like those in the original (primary) tumor.

mosaicism: Abnormal chromosome division resulting in two or more kinds of cells, each containing different numbers of chromosomes.

multiple endocrine neoplasia type 1 syndrome (MEN1 syndrome): A rare, inherited disorder that affects the endocrine glands and can cause tumors in the parathyroid and pituitary glands and the pancreas.

nutrition: The taking in and use of food and other nourishing material by the body. Nutrition is a two-part process. First, food or drink is consumed. Second, the body breaks down the food or drink into nutrients.

obesity: Refers to excess body fat. Because body fat is usually not measured directly, a ratio of body weight to height is often used instead.

ovary: One of a pair of female reproductive glands in which the ova, or eggs, are formed.

pancreas: A glandular organ located in the abdomen. It makes pancreatic juices, which contain enzymes that aid in digestion, and it produces several hormones, including insulin.

parathyroid cancer: A rare cancer that forms in tissues of one or more of the parathyroid glands.

parathyroid gland: One of four pea-sized glands found on the thyroid. The parathyroid hormone produced by these glands increases the calcium level in the blood.

parathyroid hormone (PTH): A substance made by the parathyroid gland that helps the body store and use calcium.

physical activity: Any bodily movement that is produced by the contraction of skeletal muscle and that substantially increases energy expenditure.

pituitary gland: A pea-sized organ in the center of the brain above the back of the nose. It produces hormones that control other glands and many body functions, especially growth.

pituitary tumor: A tumor that forms in the pituitary gland. Most pituitary tumors are benign (not cancer).

prognosis: The likely outcome or course of a disease; the chance of recovery or recurrence.

progression: The process of increasing the intensity, duration, frequency, or amount of activity or exercise as the body adapts to a given activity pattern.

protein: A molecule made up of amino acids. Proteins are needed for the body to function properly. They are the basis of body structures, such as skin and hair, and of other substances such as enzymes, cytokines, and antibodies.

radiation therapy: The use of high-energy radiation from x-rays, gamma rays, neutrons, and other sources to kill cancer cells and shrink tumors.

resection: A procedure that uses surgery to remove tissue or part or all of an organ.

side effect: A problem that occurs when treatment affects healthy tissues or organs. Some common side effects of cancer treatment are fatigue, pain, nausea, vomiting, decreased blood cell counts, hair loss, and mouth sores.

sonogram: A computer picture of areas inside the body created by bouncing high-energy sound waves (ultrasound) off internal tissues or organs.

staging: Performing exams and tests to learn the extent of the cancer within the body, especially whether the disease has spread from the original site to other parts of the body.

steroid: Any of a group of lipids (fats) that have a certain chemical structure. Steroids occur naturally in plants and animals or they may be made in the laboratory.

stroke: Caused by a lack of blood to the brain, resulting in the sudden loss of speech, language, or the ability to move a body part, and, if severe enough, death.

supportive care: Care given to improve the quality of life of patients who have a serious or life-threatening diseases.

thyroid gland: A gland located beneath the voice box (larynx) that produces thyroid hormone. The thyroid helps regulate growth and metabolism.

thyroid hormone: A hormone that affects heart rate, blood pressure, body temperature, and weight.

toxic: Causing temporary or permanent effects detrimental to the functioning of a body organ or group of organs.

tumor debulking: Surgically removing as much of the tumor as possible.

tumor: An abnormal mass of tissue that results when cells divide more than they should or do not die when they should. Tumors may be benign (not cancerous), or malignant (cancerous).

x-ray: A type of high-energy radiation. In low doses, x-rays are used to diagnose diseases by making pictures of the inside of the body.

yoga: An ancient system of practices used to balance the mind and body through exercise, meditation (focusing thoughts), and control of breathing and emotions.

Chapter 57

Additional Resources for Information about Endocrine and Metabolic Disorders

Government Agencies That Provide Information about Endocrine and Metabolic Disorders

Agency for Healthcare Research and Quality (AHRQ)
Office of Communications
5600 Fishers Ln.
Seventh Fl.
Rockville, MD 20857
Phone: 301-427-1104
Website: www.ahrq.gov

Association for Neuro-Metabolic Disorders (ANMD)
5223 Brookfield Ln.
Sylvania, OH 43560-1809
Phone: 419-885-1809
Website: www.healthfinder.gov/
FindServices/Organizations/
Organization.aspx?code=HR2289

Eunice Kennedy Shriver *National Institute of Child Health and Development (NICHD)*
Information Resource Center (IRC)
P.O. Box 3006
Rockville, MD 20847
Toll-Free: 800-370-2943
Toll-Free Fax: 866-760-5947
Website: www.nichd.nih.gov
E-mail: NICHDInformation ResourceCenter@mail.nih.gov

Resources in this chapter were compiled from several sources deemed reliable; all contact information was verified and updated in September 2019.

Genetic and Rare Diseases Information Center (GARD)
P.O. Box 8126
Gaithersburg, MD 20898-8126
Toll-Free: 888-205-2311
Toll-Free TTY: 888-205-3223
Fax: 301-251-4911
Website: www.rarediseases.info.nih.gov

National Cancer Institute (NCI)
9609 Medical Center Dr.
BG 9609, MSC 9760
Bethesda, MD 20892-9760
Toll-Free: 800-4-CANCER
(800-422-6237)
Website: www.cancer.gov
E-mail: NCIinfo@nih.gov

National Heart, Lung, and Blood Institute (NHLBI)
NHLBI Center for Health Information
P.O. Box 30105
Bethesda, MD 20824-0105
Phone: 301-592-8573
Website: www.nhlbi.nih.gov
E-mail: nhlbiinfo@nhlbi.nih.gov

National Human Genome Research Institute (NHGRI)
Communications and Public Liaison Branch (CPLB)
9000 Rockville Pike
31 Center Dr., MSC 2152, Bldg. 31, Rm. 4B09
Bethesda, MD 20892-2152
Phone: 301-402-0911
Fax: 301-402-2218
Website: www.genome.gov

National Institute of Diabetes and Digestive and Kidney Diseases (NIDDK)
Health Information Center
Toll-Free: 800-860-8747
Toll-Free TTY: 866-569-1162
Website: www.niddk.nih.gov
E-mail: healthinfo@niddk.nih.gov

National Institute of Environmental Health Sciences (NIEHS)
P.O. Box 12233, MD K3-16
Research Triangle Park, NC 27709
Phone: 919-541-3345
Fax: 919-541-4395
Website: www.niehs.nih.gov
E-mail: webcenter@niehs.nih.gov

National Institute of Neurological Disorders and Stroke (NINDS)
NIH Neurological Institute
P.O. Box 5801
Bethesda, MD 20824
Toll-Free: 800-352-9424
Website: www.ninds.nih.gov

National Kidney and Urologic Diseases Information Clearinghouse (NKUDIC)
Three Information Way
Bethesda, MD 20892-3580
Toll-Free: 800-891-5390
Phone: 301-654-4415
Website: www.niddk.nih.gov/health-information/communication-programs/information-clearinghouses
E-mail: nkudic@info.niddk.nih.gov

NIH Clinical Center
Office of Communications
10 Center Dr.
Bethesda, MD 20892
Phone: 301-496-2563
Fax: 301-402-9033
Website: www.clinicalcenter.nih.
gov

U.S. National Library of Medicine (NLM)
8600 Rockville Pike
Bethesda, MD 20894
Toll-Free: 888-FIND-NLM
(888-346-3656)
Phone: 301-594-5983
Website: www.nlm.nih.gov

Office on Women's Health (OWH)
U.S. Department of Health and Human Services (HHS)
200 Independence Ave., S.W.
Rm. 712E
Washington, DC 20201
Toll-Free: 800-994-9662
Phone: 202-690-7650
Fax: 202-205-2631
Website: www.womenshealth.
gov

U.S. Social Security Administration (SSA)
Office of Public Inquiries and Communications Support (OPICS)
1100 W. High Rise
6401 Security Blvd.
Baltimore, MD 21235
Toll-Free: 800-772-1213
Toll-Free TTY: 800-325-0778
Website: www.ssa.gov

Private Agencies That Provide Information about Endocrine and Metabolic Disorders

American Academy of Otolaryngology—Head and Neck Surgery (AAO—HNS)
1650 Diagonal Rd.
Alexandria, VA 22314-2857
Phone: 703-836-4444
Website: www.entnet.org
E-mail: memberservices@entnet.
org

American Association of Clinical Endocrinologists (AACE)
245 Riverside Ave.
Ste. 200
Jacksonville, FL 32202
Toll-Free: 800-393-2223
Phone: 904-353-7878
Fax: 240-547-0026
Website: www.aace.com

American Autoimmune-Related Diseases Association, Inc. (AARDA)
22100 Gratiot Ave.
Eastpointe, MI 48021
Toll-Free: 888-852-3456
Phone: 586-776-3900
Fax: 586-776-3903
Website: www.aarda.org
E-mail: aarda@aarda.org

American Diabetes Association (ADA)
2451 Crystal Dr., Ste. 900
Arlington, VA 22202
Toll-Free: 800-DIABETES
(800-342-2383)
Website: www.diabetes.org
E-mail: askada@diabetes.org

American Gastroenterological Association (AGA)
4930 Del Ray Ave.
Bethesda, MD 20814
Phone: 301-654-2055
Fax: 301-654-5920
Website: www.gastro.org
E-mail: member@gastro.org

American Liver Foundation (ALF)
National Office
39 Broadway
Ste. 2700
New York, NY 10006
Toll-Free: 800-465-4837
Phone: 212-668-1000
Website: www.liverfoundation.
org
E-mail: info@liverfoundation.org

American Porphyria Foundation (APF)
4915 St. Elmo Ave.
Ste. 200
Bethesda, MD 20814
Toll-Free: 866-APF-3635
(866-273-3635)
Phone: 301-347-7166
Fax: 301-312-8719
Website: www.
porphyriafoundation.org
E-mail: porphyrus@
porphyriafoundation.org

American Society for Bone and Mineral Research (ASBMR)
2025 M St., N.W.
Ste. 800
Washington, DC 20036-3309
Phone: 202-367-1161
Fax: 202-367-2161
Website: www.asbmr.org
E-mail: asbmr@asbmr.org

American Society for Reproductive Medicine (ASRM)
1209 Montgomery Hwy
Birmingham, AL 35216-2809
Phone: 205-978-5000
Fax: 205-978-5005
Website: www.reproductivefacts.
org
E-mail: asrm@asrm.org

American Society of Human Genetics (ASHG)
6120 Executive Blvd.
Ste. 500
Rockville, MD 20852
Phone: 301-634-7300
Website: www.ashg.org
E-mail: society@ashg.org

American Thyroid Association (ATA)
6066 Leesburg Pike
Ste. 550
Falls Church, VA 22041
Phone: 703 998-8890
Fax: 703 998-8893
Website: www.thyroid.org
E-mail: thyroid@thyroid.org

Association for Glycogen Storage Disease (AGSD)
P.O. Box 896
Durant, IA 52747
Phone: 563-514-4022
Website: www.agsdus.org
E-mail: info@agsdus.org

Association of Occupational and Environmental Clinics (AOEC)
1010 Vermont Ave., N.W.
Ste. 513
Washington, DC 20005
Toll-Free: 888-347-AOEC
(888-347-2632)
Phone: 202-347-4976
Fax: 202-347-4950
Website: www.aoec.org
E-mail: aoec@aoec.org

CARES Foundation
2414 Morris Ave.
Ste. 110
Union, NJ 07083
Toll-Free: 866-CARES-37
(866-227-3737)
Phone: 908-364-0272
Fax: 908-686-2019
Website: www.caresfoundation.org
E-mail: contact@caresfoundation.org

The Children's Fund for Glycogen Storage Disease Research
20 Sherwood Ln.
Cheshire, CT 06410
Phone: 203-272-CURE
(203-272-2873)
Website: www.curegsd.org
E-mail: info@curegsd.org

Children's Gaucher Research Fund (CGRF)
8110 Warren Ct.
Granite Bay, CA 95746
Phone: 916-797-3700
Fax: 916-797-3707
Website: www.childrensgaucher.org
E-mail: research@childrensgaucher.org

Children's PKU Network (CPN)
3306 Bumann Rd.
Encinitas, CA 92024
Phone: 858-756-0079
Fax: 858-756-1059
Website: www.pkunetwork.org
E-mail: pkunetwork@aol.com

Creutzfeldt-Jakob Disease Foundation Inc. (CJDF)
3634 W. Market St.
Ste. 110
Akron, OH 44333
Toll-Free: 800-659-1991
Fax: 234-466-7077
Website: www.cjdfoundation.org
E-mail: help@cjdfoundation.org

Cystic Fibrosis Foundation (CFF)
4550 Montgomery Ave.
Ste. 1100
Bethesda, MD 20814
Toll-Free: 800-FIGHT-CF
(800-344-4823)
Phone: 301-951-4422
Website: www.cff.org
E-mail: info@cff.org

Endocrine Society
2055 L St., N.W.
Ste. 600
Washington, DC 20036
Toll-Free: 888-363-6274
Phone: 202-971-3636
Fax: 202-736-9705
Website: www.endocrine.org
E-mail: info@endocrine.org

Fatty Oxidation Disorders (FOD) Family Support Group
P.O. Box 54
Okemos, MI 48805-0054
Phone: 517-381-1940
Toll-Free Fax: 866-290-5206
Website: www.fodsupport.org

Genetic Alliance, Inc.
4301 Connecticut Ave., N.W.
Ste. 404
Washington, DC 20008-2369
Phone: 202-966-5557
Fax: 202-966-8553
Website: www.geneticalliance.org
E-mail: info@geneticalliance.org

Graves' Disease & Thyroid Foundation (GDATF)
P.O. Box 2793
Rancho Santa Fe, CA 92067
Toll-Free: 877-643-3123
Toll-Free Fax: 877-643-3123
Website: www.gdatf.org
E-mail: info@gdatf.org

Human Growth Foundation (HGF)
997 Glen Cove Ave., Ste. 5
Glen Head, NY 11545
Toll-Free: 800-451-6434
Fax: 516-671-4055
Website: www.hgfound.org
E-mail: hgf1@hgfound.org

Hypoglycemia Support Foundation, Inc. (HSF)
P.O. Box 451778
Sunrise, FL 33345
Website: www.hypoglycemia.org

International Association for Muscle Glycogen Storage Disease (IAMGSD)
746 Fourth Ave.
San Francisco, CA 94118
Website: www.iamgsd.org
E-mail: info@iamgsd.org

Iron Disorders Institute (IDI)
P.O. Box 4891
Greenville, SC 29608
Website: www.irondisorders.org
E-mail: info@irondisorders.org

Juvenile Diabetes Research
Foundation International
(JDRF)
26 Broadway
14th Fl.
New York, NY 10004
Toll-Free: 800-533-CURE
(800-533-2873)
Fax: 212-785-9595
Website: www.jdrf.org
E-mail: info@jdrf.org

The MAGIC Foundation
4200 Cantera Dr.
Ste. 106
Warrenville, IL 60555
Toll-Free: 800-362-4423
Phone: 630-836-8200
Fax: 630-836-8181
Website: www.magicfoundation.
org
E-mail: contactus@
magicfoundation.org

March of Dimes
National Office
1550 Crystal Dr.
Ste. 1300
Arlington, VA 22202
Toll-Free: 888-MODIMES
(888-663-4637)
Website: www.marchofdimes.org

Muscular Dystrophy
Association (MDA)
National Office
161 N. Clark
Ste. 3550
Chicago, IL 60601
Toll-Free: 800-572-1717
Website: www.mda.org
E-mail: resourcecenter@mdausa.
org

National Adrenal Diseases
Foundation (NADF)
P.O. Box 566
Lake Zurich, IL 60047
Phone: 847-726-9010
Website: www.nadf.us
E-mail: nadfmail@nadf.us

National Gaucher
Foundation (NGF)
5410 Edson Ln.
Ste. 220
Rockville, MD 20852
Toll-Free: 800-504-3189
Website: www.gaucherdisease.
org

National MPS Society
P.O. Box 14686
Durham, NC 27709-4686
Toll-Free: 877-MPS-1001
(877-677-1001)
Phone: 919-806-0101
Website: www.mpssociety.org
E-mail: info@mpssociety.org

National Organization for Rare Disorders (NORD)
55 Kenosia Ave.
Danbury, CT 06810
Toll-Free: 800-999-6673
Phone: 203-744-0100
Fax: 203-263-9938
Website: www.rarediseases.org

National Osteoporosis Foundation (NOF)
251 18th St., S.
Ste. 630
Arlington, VA 22202
Toll-Free: 800-231-4222
Website: www.nof.org
E-mail: info@nof.org

National Urea Cycle Disorders Foundation (NUCDF)
75 S. Grand Ave.
Pasadena, CA 91105
Toll-Free: 800-38-NUCDF
(800-386-8233)
Phone: 626-578-0833
Fax: 626-578-0823
Website: www.nucdf.org
E-mail: info@nucdf.org

The Nemours Foundation / KidsHealth®
Website: www.kidshealth.org

Organic Acidemia Association (OAA)
c/o Kathy Stagni, Executive Director
9040 Duluth St.
Golden Valley, MN 55427
Phone: 763-559-1797
Toll-Free Fax: 866-539-4060
Website: www.oaanews.org
E-mail: mkstagni@gmail.com

Oxalosis and Hyperoxaluria Foundation (OHF)
579 Albany Post Rd.
New Paltz, NY 12561
Toll-Free: 800-OHF-8699
(800-643-8699)
Phone: 212-777-0470
Website: www.ohf.org
E-mail: info@ohf.org

Pediatric Endocrine Society (PES)
6728 Old McLean Village Dr.
McLean, VA 22101
Phone: 703-556-9222
Fax: 703-556-8729
Website: www.pedsendo.org
E-mail: info@pedsendo.org

Pituitary Network Association (PNA)
P.O. Box 1958
Thousand Oaks, CA 91358
Phone: 805-499-9973
Fax: 805-480-0633
Website: www.pituitary.org
E-mail: info@pituitary.org

The Pituitary Society
8700 Beverly Blvd.
Rm. 2051
Los Angeles, CA 90048
Phone: 310-988-9486
Website: www.pituitarysociety.
org

**Society for Inherited
Metabolic Disorders (SIMD)**
c/o Leslie Lublink, SIMD
Administrator
18265 Lower Midhill Dr.
West Linn, OR 97068
Phone: 503-636-9228
Fax: 503-210-1511
Website: www.simd.org
E-mail: leslie.lublink@gmail.com

**United Leukodystrophy
Foundation (ULF)**
224 N. Second St.
Ste. 2
DeKalb, IL 60115
Toll-Free: 800-728-5483
Phone: 815-748-3211
Fax: 815-748-0844
Website: www.ulf.org
E-mail: office@ulf.org

**Wilson Disease Association
(WDA)**
1732 First Ave.
Ste. 20043
New York, NY 10128
Toll-Free: 866-961-0533
Phone: 414-961-0533
Website: www.wilsonsdisease.
org
E-mail: info@wilsonsdisease.org

Index

Index

519